Second Edition

The KEY TOPICS Series

Advisors:

T.M. Craft *Department of Anaesthesia and Intensive Care, Royal United Hospital, Bath, UK*
C.S. Garrard *Intensive Therapy Unit, John Radcliffe Hospital, Oxford, UK*
P.M. Upton *Department of Anaesthetics, Treliske Hospital, Truro, UK*

Anaesthesia, Second Edition

Obstetrics and Gynaecology, Second Edition

Accident and Emergency Medicine

Paediatrics, Second Edition

Orthopaedic Surgery

Otolaryngology and Head and Neck Surgery

Ophthalmology

Psychiatry

General Surgery

Renal Medicine

Trauma

Chronic Pain

Oral and Maxillofacial Surgery

Oncology

Cardiovascular Medicine

Forthcoming titles include:

Neonatology

Thoracic Surgery

Orthopaedic Trauma Surgery

Respiratory Medicine

Neurology

Critical Care

KEY TOPICS IN
PAEDIATRICS

A.L. BILLSON
BA MBBS MRCP (UK) MRCPCH
Senior Registrar in Paediatrics, Royal United Hospital, Bath, UK

A.V. PEARCE
BM MRCP (UK) MRCPCH
Specialist Registrar Community Child Health, Frenchay Health Care Trust, Bristol, UK

C. TUFFREY
BMedSci BM BS MRCP (UK) MRCPCH
Senior House Officer in Neonatology, Southmead Hospital, Bristol, UK

BIOS SCIENTIFIC PUBLISHERS
Oxford • Washington DC

First published 1994 (ISBN 1 872748 58 9)
Reprinted 1996
Second Edition 1998 (ISBN 1 859960 32 4)

A CIP catalogue record for this book is available from the British Library.

ISBN 1 859960 32 4

BIOS Scientific Publishers Ltd
9 Newtec Place, Magdalen Road, Oxford OX4 1RE, UK
Tel. +44 (0)1865 726286. Fax. +44 (0)1865 246823
World Wide Web home page: http://www.bios.co.uk/

DISTRIBUTORS

Australia and New Zealand
Blackwell Science Asia
54 University Street
Carlton, South Victoria 3053

India
Viva Books Private Limited
4325/3 Ansari Road, Daryaganj
New Delhi 110002

Singapore and South East Asia
Toppan Company (S) PTE Ltd
38 Liu Fang Road, Jurong
Singapore 2262

USA and Canada
BIOS Scientific Publishers
PO Box 605, Herndon
VA 20172-0605

Important Note from the Publisher
The information contained within this book was obtained by BIOS Scientific Publishers Ltd from sources believed by us to be reliable. However, while every effort has been made to ensure its accuracy, no responsibility for loss or injury whatsoever occasioned to any person acting or refraining from action as a result of information contained herein can be accepted by the authors or publishers.

The reader should remember that medicine is a constantly evolving science and while the authors and publishers have ensured that all dosages, applications and practices are based on current indications, there may be specific practices which differ between communities. You should always follow the guidelines laid down by the manufacturers of specific products and the relevant authorities in the country in which you are practising.

Production Editor: Priscilla Goldby.
Typeset by Chandos Electronic Publishing, Stanton Harcourt, UK.
Printed by Redwood Books, Trowbridge, UK.

CONTENTS

ABBREVIATIONS

ACTH	adrenocorticotrophic hormone
AD	autosomal dominant
ADH	antidiuretic hormone
ADHD	attention deficit hyperactivity disorder
AFP	α-fetoprotein
AIDS	acquired immunodeficiency syndrome
ALEC	artificial lung expanding compound
ALL	acute lymphoblastic leukaemia
ALT	alanine aminotransferase
AML	acute myeloid leukaemia
ANA	antinuclear antibody
APLS	advanced paediatric life support
AR	autosomal recessive
AS	aortic stenosis
ASD	atrial septal defect
ASO	anti-streptolysin O
AST	aspartate aminotransferase
AV	atrioventricular
AVSD	atrioventricular septal defect
BCG	Bacillus Calmette–Guérin
CAH	congenital adrenal hyperplasia
CAPD	continuous ambulatory peritoneal dialysis
CDH	congenital dislocation of the hip
CESDI	Confidential Enquiry into Stillbirths and Deaths
CF	cystic fibrosis
CFTR	cystic fibrosis transmembrane conductance regulator
CHD	congenital heart disease
CML	chronic myeloid leukaemia
CMV	cytomegalovirus
CNS	central nervous system
CONI	care of the next infant
CP	cerebral palsy
CPK	creatine phosphokinase
CPR	cardiopulmonary resuscitation
CRP	C-reactive protein
CSF	cerebrospinal fluid
CT	computerized tomography
CXR	chest X-ray
DCT	direct Coombs' test
DDAVP	1-deamino-8-D-arginine vasopressin
DI	diabetes insipidus
DIC	disseminated intravascular coagulopathy
DKA	diabetic ketoacidosis

DMSA	dimercaptosuccinic acid
DTP	diphtheria, tetanus, pertussis
EBM	expressed breast milk
ECG	electrocardiogram
EEG	electroencephalogram
ERCP	endoscopic retrograde cholangiopancreatography
ESR	erythrocyte sedimentation rate
ETT	endotracheal tube
FBC	full blood count
FDP	fibrin degradation product
FSH	follicle-stimulating hormone
Gal-1-put	galactose-1-phosphate uridyl transferase
G6PD	glucose-6-phosphate dehydrogenase deficiency
GFR	glomerular filtration rate
GH	growth hormone
GHRH	growth hormone-releasing hormone
GI	gastrointestinal
GMN	glomerulonephritis
GnRH	gonadotrophin-releasing hormone
GOR	gastro-oesophageal reflux
HDN	haemorrhagic disease of the newborn
HIE	hypoxic–ischaemic encephalopathy
HIV	human immunodeficiency virus
HLA	human lymphocyte antigens
HSP	Henoch–Schönlein purpura
HSV	herpes simplex virus
HUS	haemolytic uraemic syndrome
HVA	homovanillic acid
ICP	intracranial pressure
IDDM	insulin-dependent diabetes mellitus
IF	intrinsic factor
IGF-1	insulin-like growth factor 1
IPPV	intermittent positive-pressure ventilation
IRT	immunoreactive trypsin
ITP	idiopathic thrombocytopenic purpura
ITU	intensive therapy unit
IUGR	intrauterine growth retardation
IVH	intraventricular haemorrhage
IVU	intravenous urography
JCA	juvenile chronic arthritis
JVP	jugular venous pressure
LBW	low birth weight
LH	luteinizing hormone
LP	lumbar puncture
LVH	left ventricular hypertrophy

MC&S	microscopy, culture and sensitivity
MCAD	medium-chain acyl CoA dehydrogenase
MCNS	minimal change nephrotic syndrome
MCUG	micturating cystourethrogram
MEN	multiple endocrine neoplasia
MIBG	meta-iodobenzylguanidine
MLD	mild learning difficulty
MMR	measles, mumps, rubella
MRC	Medical Research Council
MRI	magnetic resonance imaging
MSU	mid-stream urine
NAI	non-accidental injury
NEC	necrotizing enterocolitis
NHL	non-Hodgkin's lymphoma
NSAID	non-steroidal anti-inflammatory drug
OFC	occipito-frontal circumference
OPCS	Office of Population Censuses and Surveys
PA	pulmonary atresia
PCP	*Pneumocystis carinii* pneumonia
PCR	polymerase chain reaction
PCV	packed cell volume
PDA	patent ductus arteriosus
PET	pre-eclamptic toxaemia
PFC	persistent fetal circulation
PKU	phenylketonuria
PS	pulmonary stenosis
PT	prothrombin time
PTH	parathyroid hormone
PTT	partial thromboplastin time
PUJ	pelvi-ureteric junction
PUO	pyrexia of unknown origin
RAH	right atrial hypertrophy
RAST	radioallergosorbent test
RDS	respiratory distress syndrome
RhF	rheumatoid factor
ROP	retinopathy of prematurity
RSV	respiratory syncytial virus
RVH	right ventricular hypertrophy
SBE	subacute bacterial endocarditis
SCID	severe combined immunodeficiency
SEA	seronegative enthesopathy and arthropathy
SEN	special educational needs
SIDS	sudden infant death syndrome
SLD	severe learning disability
SLE	systemic lupus erythematosus

SPA	suprapubic aspirate
SSPE	subacute sclerosing panencephalitis
SUDI	sudden unexpected death in infancy
SVT	supraventricular tachycardia
T_4	thyroxine
T_3	tri-iodothyronine
TA	tricuspid atresia
TAR	thrombocytopenia and absent radius syndrome
TBG	thyroid-binding globulin
TFT	thyroid function test
TGA	transposition of the great arteries
TIBC	total iron-binding capacity
TOF	tracheo-oesophageal fistula
TPN	total parenteral nutrition
TSH	thyroid-stimulating hormone
TT	thromboplastin time
UC	ulcerative colitis
UDPGT	uridine diphosphate glucuronyl transferase
U&E	urea and electrolytes
UKCCR	UK Co-ordinating Committee on Cancer Research
UKCCSG	UK Children's Cancer Study Group
US	ultrasound
UTI	urinary tract infection
VATER	**V**ertebral abnormalities, **A**nal atresia, **T**racheo-**E**sophageal fistula, **R**adial and **R**enal abnormalities
VF	ventricular fibrillation
VIII RAG	factor VIII-related antigen
VLBW	very low birth weight
VMA	vanillylmandelic acid
VSD	ventricular septal defect
VTEC	verotoxin-producing *E. coli*
VUR	vesico-ureteric reflux
WBC	white blood cell count

PREFACE TO THE SECOND EDITION

Many of the topics in this second edition have been re-written, revised and updated. In line with current trends in teaching and learning, we have adopted a more problem-orientated approach, which is reflected in revised topic titles (e.g. Heart murmurs replaces Acyanotic congenital heart disease; Cough and wheeze replaces Lower respiratory tract infections).

The contribution of the two new authors (AP and CT) has enabled us to review the key areas of knowledge which we felt should be included in this book. We have also reviewed the list of topics in the light of the syllabus for general professional and higher specialist training which has been produced recently by the Royal College of Paediatrics and Child Health (RCPCH). As a result, some new topics have been added (e.g. Adolescent health, Orthopaedic problems in childhood, Inflammatory bowel disease) and there are more community-orientated topic titles (e.g. Disability, Learning disability, Accidents). We have combined topics from the first edition which more logically go together; for example, blistering conditions and childhood exanthemata are now included in one topic entitled Rashes and blisters; birth injuries, congenital dislocation of the hip, talipes and naevi are included in the Newborn examination topic.

We are grateful to the readers of the first edition, and the doctors and medical students within our departments who have made comments and suggestions for the second edition. We hope that the book continues to be a useful revision aid for those preparing for both undergraduate and postgraduate paediatric examinations (including the Diploma in Child Health, the Part I and Part II MRCP in Paediatrics exams). We anticipate that the information provided will also be the core knowledge required for the new RCPCH exams which will be introduced over the next few years. We are grateful to Jonathan Ray and Lisa Mansell at BIOS for their continued help and encouragement.

Amanda Billson
Alison Pearce
Catherine Tuffrey

PREFACE TO THE FIRST EDITION

This book contains 100 chapters, each providing a concise account of a topic considered to be central to a general paediatric curriculum. The text is aimed primarily at candidates approaching Part II MRCP in Paediatrics, but will also be of great value to those undertaking Part I MRCP in Paediatrics (recently introduced) and the Diploma of Child Health. Medical students and nurses may also find it a useful source of information.

It is assumed that the reader will already have acquired a basic knowledge of paediatrics. The book is therefore intended to act as a revision text, although references to more detailed texts and articles are included for many topics.

We would like to thank our many teachers, past and present, our publishers, BIOS, and the series editors for their help and encouragement.

Anne E.M. Davies
Amanda L. Billson

ABDOMINAL PAIN – ACUTE

Acute abdominal pain may be difficult to assess, particularly in the young infant. Both medical and surgical causes should be considered. The diagnosis of appendicitis is often not considered in pre-school children as they localize pain poorly and the presenting features may not be typical. The risk of perforation and subsequent complications is, therefore, higher in this group.

Causes

- Gastroenteritis.
- Urinary tract infection, pyelonephritis.
- Constipation.
- Urinary retention.
- Lower lobe pneumonia.
- Diabetic ketoacidosis.
- Non-specific abdominal pain (including mesenteric adenitis).
- Acute appendicitis.
- Intussusception.
- Volvulus.
- Testicular torsion.
- Strangulated inguinal hernia.
- Rare causes (e.g. duodenal ulcer, ovarian cyst, pancreatitis).

Acute abdominal pain may also be a feature of some systemic conditions e.g. Henoch–Schönlein purpura, nephrotic syndrome (hypovolaemia, peritonitis), sickle cell disease (peritonitis, sickle cell crisis).

Clinical assessment

A detailed history should be taken, noting the features of the pain (time of onset, site, nature) and any associated symptoms (e.g. fever, urinary symptoms etc). Examination should include assessment of the state of hydration, careful examination of the abdomen, including the external genitalia, and examination of the chest. Repeated or unnecessary digital rectal examinations should be avoided. Subsequent investigations and management depend on the likely cause, but should at least include a urine for protein, glucose, microscopy and culture.

Intussusception

Invagination of one segment of bowel into another, commonly the terminal ileum into the caecum, typically occurs in infants between the ages of 6 and 12 months. Boys are more frequently affected than girls. The cause is unknown but it may be due to lymphoid hyperplasia resulting in an enlarged Peyer's patch during an intercurrent infection. There is usually a short history of episodic screaming, irritability and pallor, during which the child draws up his/her legs in pain. Vomiting, sometimes bile-stained, may occur. The passage of blood and mucous per rectum is a relatively late sign ('redcurrant jelly' stool). A sausage-shaped mass may be palpable in the right hypochondrium and plain abdominal X-rays typically show evidence of small bowel obstruction. There may be a paucity of gas or a soft tissue shadow in the region of the intussusception. Ultrasound may be helpful if the diagnosis is uncertain. An air or barium enema confirms the diagnosis and hydrostatic or air reduction may be attempted if the history is less than 24 hours and there are no signs of peritonism. If this is unsuccessful, the history is long (> 24 hours – risk of perforation), or there are signs of shock or peritonism, surgical reduction is indicated. The child may be severely ill at presentation with shock or peritonitis and should be resuscitated with i.v. fluids and antibiotics prior to surgical reduction. There is a small risk of recurrence of the intussusception after both non-surgical and surgical reduction. Intussusception occasionally occurs in older children when the lead point may be a Meckel's diverticulum, polyp, duplication cyst or lymphoma.

Acute appendicitis

Abdominal pain typically starts centrally and over a few hours becomes localized to the right iliac fossa. The child is anorexic, irritable, looks flushed and may vomit. A low-grade fever is usual and there may be tenderness, guarding and rebound in the right iliac fossa. In patients with a pelvic appendix, diarrhoea may occur and tenderness or a mass may be detected by gentle rectal examination. The pre-school child is very difficult to assess and the diagnosis is often not considered in these children or is made only once the appendix has perforated. Antibiotic administration prior to admission for presumed ear and throat infections may modify the course, leading to the development of an appendix abscess. Psoas spasm may cause the child to present with a limp diverting the attention away from the abdomen to the hip joint. To avoid late diagnosis it important to consider appendicitis even in young infants. The white cell count is usually raised, but this will not distinguish appendicitis from other causes of abdominal pain. Abdominal X-rays are rarely helpful and the decision to operate must be based on repeated careful clinical assessment. Post-operative complications are more common if there is diffuse peritonitis at diagnosis (wound infection, paralytic ileus, localized intraperitoneal abscess formation, adhesions).

Non-specific abdominal pain

This term has been used in recent years to include the group of children with acute abdominal pain which may be similar in presentation to acute appendicitis, but is more diffuse and variable on examination. Diagnosis is made by repeated clinical assessment together with relevant investigations to exclude more definite pathology (e.g. UTI, appendicitis, intestinal obstruction). The pain usually settles spontaneously over 24–48 hours. This group includes children with mesenteric adenitis which is often diagnosed at laparotomy for presumed appendicitis – enlarged mesenteric lymph nodes with free peritoneal fluid are found in the presence of a normal appendix.

Further reading

Stringer MD, Drake DP. Diagnosis and management of acute abdominal pain in childhood. *Current Paediatrics,* 1991; **1:** 2–7.

Williams N. Acute appendicitis in the pre-school child. *Archives of Disease in Childhood,* 1991; **66:** 1270–2.

Related topics of interest

Abdominal pain – recurrent (p. 4)
Constipation (p. 97)
Urinary tract infection (p. 370)
Vomiting (p. 377)

ABDOMINAL PAIN – RECURRENT

Recurrent abdominal pain is a common paediatric problem affecting between 10 and 20% of school-children. The term is usually used to describe recurrent, moderately severe attacks of pain occurring over a period of at least 3 months. These episodes may lead to repeated absence from school. An organic cause to explain the pain is found in <10% of cases and clinical examination between episodes is usually normal. Siblings may have had similar symptoms, and there may be a family history of irritable bowel syndrome in the parents.

Causes

- Non-organic (functional) abdominal pain accounts for > 90% of cases.
- Constipation.
- Urinary tract infection.
- Abdominal migraine.
- Oesophagitis, gastritis.
- Dysmenorrhoea.
- Other rare causes:
  - Food intolerance.
  - Renal tract, e.g. PUJ obstruction, calculi.
  - GI tract – peptic ulceration, inflammatory bowel disease, coeliac disease, intermittent volvulus, gall stones (particularly if underlying haemolytic disorder), Meckel's diverticulum.
  - Ovarian cysts – recurrent pain is not uncommon in the months preceding the menarche due to follicular enlargement.
  - Lead poisoning.
  - Porphyria.
  - Pancreatitis.
  - Referred pain, e.g. from spine, pelvis, pleura.

History

A detailed history is essential asking about the following features of the pain:

- Timing, including relation to meals, does the pain wake the child at night?
- Frequency, e.g. only on school days suggests non-organic pain.
- Duration.
- Site and radiation. Ask the child to point to the site of the pain with one finger. Non-organic pain is typically described using a flat hand in the periumbilical region.
- Nature, e.g. burning epigastric pain suggests possible gastritis/oesophagitis.
- Precipitating and relieving factors.

Enquiry should be made about associated symptoms including vomiting, headache, urinary symptoms (dysuria, frequency, haematuria), bowel habit (stool frequency, colour, consistency), and relationship to periods. A detailed family and social history may reveal some psychological upset or life-event which has precipitated the abdominal pain, e.g. moving to a new school, parental separation.

Examination

Examination should include an assessment of growth (height, weight, nutritional status) and pubertal staging. General physical examination may reveal features to suggest an organic cause, e.g. palpable faecal loading, anaemia, epigastric or renal angle tenderness. However, examination is usually entirely normal. The child is rarely seen during an episode, but it may be helpful to arrange this.

Investigations

If non-organic pain is suspected from the history and examination, investigations may be limited to urine analysis and culture. More detailed investigations may be indicated if there are any features to suggest an underlying organic cause (e.g. full blood count, ESR, renal function and liver function tests, abdominal US, barium contrast studies, oesophageal pH studies). Radiological investigations may be normal between episodes in some conditions (e.g. abdominal X-ray in intermittent volvulus, intravenous pyelogram in a child with renal calculi) and are best used to show evidence of obstruction during an episode of pain.

Management

In non-organic pain, the first consultation should provide the reassurance that the physical examination is normal, and that serious disease is unlikely. The gentle suggestion that the problem may be functional is sometimes appropriate at this stage. At subsequent interviews symptoms can be reviewed – asking the child to keep a diary of episodes for a short period of time is sometimes useful in establishing a pattern to the symptoms. Reassurance that abdominal pain occurs commonly in normal children, combined with suggestions to avoid reinforcing the child's response to pain are usually all that is required. Formal psychological assessment and advice on pain management is occasionally indicated.

Abdominal migraine is a term used to describe recurrent attacks of abdominal pain usually associated with headache and vomiting. Typically there is a family history of migraine. Management includes avoidance of precipitating factors (e.g. certain foods) and the prompt use of analgesics, with or without antiemetics, during attacks. Prophylaxis with pizotifen or beta-blockers may be helpful. Management of other organic conditions, such as constipation, is dealt with elsewhere.

Further reading

Murphy MS. Management of recurrent abdominal pain. *Archives of Disease in Childhood,* 1993; **69:** 409–411.

Related topics of interest

Abdominal pain – acute (p. 1)
Constipation (p. 97)
Gastrointestinal haemorrhage (p. 156)
Headache (p. 182)
Inflammatory bowel disease (p. 221)
Urinary tract infection (p. 370)

ACCIDENTS

Accidents remain the single major cause of death in children, aged 1 to 15 years, in England and Wales, causing more deaths than the two next commonest causes combined. On average two children die every day in accidents and each year an estimated 10 000 children are left with a permanent disability. Accidents contribute substantially to childhood morbidity, leading to one in five Accident and Emergency attendances and 20% of paediatric admissions.

Major causes of severe injury and death are:

- Road traffic accidents (RTAs), as passenger or pedestrian.
- Burns.
- Drowning or near drowning.

Other injuries, especially in the pre-school age group, can occur through lack of safety in the home, e.g. falls or poisonings from chemicals or medicines not locked safely away from children.

Road traffic accidents (RTAs)

Half of accidental deaths and 16% of total deaths in the age group 1 to 15 years are the result of road traffic accidents. RTAs are an important cause of long-term morbidity, being the most common cause of severe head injury in children over the age of one year.

The majority of children involved in RTAs are pedestrians. A child injured as a pedestrian is more likely to be killed or seriously injured than a child cyclist or passenger.

Young children have very poor traffic awareness. Many injuries occur when children are playing unsupervised in the street close to their home and a significant number of accidents occur when children are travelling home from school. Provision of safe play areas, particularly in areas of high density housing, and traffic calming measures to slow vehicles speed, have become important community and public health issues.

Increasing numbers of child passenger injuries are being seen as a direct result of increasing use of private transport in the population. It is essential to emphasize the need for adequate seating with restraints.

Bicycle accidents are relatively infrequent but remain an important cause of morbidity because of the high risk of head injury. Children continue to be taught cycle proficiency in schools nationally. There is clear evidence that cycle helmets help prevent injury, particularly for falls from cycles; however most fatal accidents involve collision with a vehicle.

Emergency management

A structured approach is required when assessing the seriously injured child. The principles of basic life support apply with assessment and management of **A**irway, **B**reathing and **C**irculation. A thorough neurological examination should be undertaken, followed by examination for bony and internal injury; emergency treatment should be undertaken as each problem is identified. Cervical spine injury should be assumed until it is excluded by clinical and radiological examination.

Burns and scalds

Each year approximately 50 000 burnt or scalded children attend emergency departments in the UK, of whom 10% require hospital admission. Burns are the second most common cause of accidental death in children after RTA. The majority of fatal burns occur in home fires, smoke inhalation causing death. Most commonly children are less than 5 years old. Non-fatal burns often involve flammable clothing. Scalds are often caused by hot drinks, kettles or hot bath water. Some burns may be the result of non-accidental injury.

Emergency management of major burns

- Rapid initial assessment must be made as fluid replacement and analgesia should not be delayed.
- Take a clear history of the nature of the injury documenting the time it occurred.

Assessment

1. *Distribution.* Burns to head and neck or genital area need special attention.

2. *Depth.*

- Superficial: injury to epidermis cause redness and no blistering.
- Partial thickness: some injury to the dermis. Skin appears pink and mottled with some blistering seen.
- Full thickness: injury to epidermis, dermis and possibly deeper structures. Skin appears charred and white and is painless.

3. *Surface area* is calculated as a percentage. A useful rule is that the child's palm and adducted fingers is approximately 1% of body surface. The 'rule of 9's' can only be used for children over 14 years of age. A 'burns chart' should be available in the emergency department.

Management

1. *Resuscitation.* Basic life support should be the priority in any emergency: **A**irway, **B**reathing, **C**irculation. Airway and breathing problems occur after burns to the face and mouth or after smoke inhalation in house fires.

2. *Fluid loss.* Burns greater than 10% surface area will need intravenous fluid replacement. For the shocked patient 20 ml/kg bolus of human albumin solution 4.5% or crystalloid is given. Maintenance and replacement fluid for the next 24 hours should be calculated using the following equation:

Replacement fluid in ml = % burn × weight (kg) × 4

Half of the total calculated amount should be given over 8 hours since the burn. Fluid given is usually 4.5% human albumin solution.

3. Analgesia. Intravenous morphine 0.1 mg/kg should be given for anything other than a minor burn. Intramuscular morphine is poorly absorbed particularly at the burn site.

Transfer to a regional burns unit is advisable if child has greater than 10% burns, if greater than 5% full thickness burn or for burns to specific areas, e.g. face or genital area.

Long-term considerations include scarring, contractures and psychosocial consequences.

Prevention

Home safety devices, e.g. smoke alarms; cooker guards; coiled kettle flexes; fire resistant clothing and household items; thermostat control of tap water temperature.

Drowning and near drowning

Drowning is defined as death from asphyxia associated with submersion in a fluid. *Near drowning* is said to have occurred if there is any recovery, however transient, following a submersion incident.

Epidemiology

Drowning is the third most common cause of accidental death in children in the UK, after RTA and burns. The true annual incidence of near drowning accidents in children is uncertain as not all seek medical advice. In England and Wales the annual incidence of submersion accidents in children is approximately 1.5 per 100 000 and mortality is 0.7 per 100 000. The majority of children are less than 5 years old. Events most commonly occur in private swimming pools, garden ponds and inland and open water ways.

Assessment and management

Basic life support should be commenced as soon as the child is taken out of the water after assessment of **A**irway, **B**reathing and **C**irculation. Cardiopulmonary resuscitation should continue during transfer to hospital.

Problems

1. Hypoxia may occur due to alveolar mismatch or secondary pulmonary oedema. Artificial ventilation may be required until spontaneous respiration is established.

2. Hypothermia. Many children will be hypothermic as a result of immersion; rewarming should be undertaken slowly. Full resuscitation must continue until the core temperature is at least 32°C.

3. Electrolyte abnormalities and disorder of acid–base balance may follow fresh or salt water immersion and can contribute to arrhythmias.

4. Convulsions may occur as a result of hypoxia, cerebral oedema and electrolyte imbalance and should be treated appropriately.

5. Infection. Once cultures have been taken, broad spectrum antibiotics should be commenced to cover the risk from contaminated water.

6. Associated injury. Once basic life support has been established you should progress to a secondary assessment for any injuries, e.g. diving injury to head or neck.

A total of 70% of children survive near drowning when basic life support is performed at the water-side. This reduces to 40% when it is not started until arrival in the emergency department. Prognostic indicators include immersion time, time to first gasp, conscious level and temperature on arrival in casualty.

Prevention

Supervision of public and private swimming areas. Fencing or netting around pools and ponds. Encourage children to learn to swim.

Accident prevention

Statistics for accidents in children are alarming. What is more, little change has been seen in the last 20 years. Accident prevention has been identified in the Health of the Nation document as a priority area, with a target set to reduce childhood accident fatality by one third by the year 2005. Research is being directed at identifying the most effective forms of accident prevention. Education for parents and carers on safety awareness has an important role; however, this has had limited impact to date. There is a higher incidence of all childhood accidents amongst children from households in disadvantaged socio-economic groups. This does not reflect that these families do not care but instead identifies issues of poor housing, overcrowding and lack of finance. Some community programmes have been effective which identify high risk households, make home visits, provide education on safety issues and provide free safety devises.

In order to fully develop effective interventions for injury prevention, further data collection is required from national injury surveillance systems.

Non-accidental injury and accidental poisoning are discussed in further chapters.

Further reading

Advanced Paediatric Life Support Handbook, 2nd edn. London: BMJ Publications, 1997.
Parkhouse N. Burns and scalds. *Current Paediatrics*, 1993; **3:** 67–71.
Sibert J. Accidents and Emergencies in Childhood. London: RCP Publications, 1992.

Related topics of interest

Cardiac arrest (p. 61)
Child protection (p. 65)
Poisoning (p. 315)
Shock (p. 344)

ACUTE HEMIPLEGIA

An acute onset of hemiplegia is a serious event, and may arise from a wide variety of underlying causes. Detailed investigations must be undertaken to establish aetiology, although in a proportion of cases no cause will be found.

Aetiology

1. Haemorrhage. Bleeding may arise from an arteriovenous malformation or aneurysm (congenital, traumatic or mycotic). Generalized bleeding disorders (thrombocytopenia, haemophilia, disseminated intravascular coagulation) or administration of anticoagulants may be responsible. Bleeding into a cerebral tumour may cause hemiplegia in a previously asymptomatic patient.

2. Arterial occlusion. This usually occurs as a result of occlusion of a major cerebral artery, e.g. internal carotid or middle cerebral artery. Thrombus may form as a result of infection (cervical adenitis, tonsillar infection), cyanotic congenital heart disease (polycythaemia), sickle cell disease or hypertension. Progressive arterial occlusion occurs in moya-moya disease, in which recurrent episodes of hemiplegia, transient dysphasia and seizures may occur. Emboli may form from mural thrombus in cyanotic congenital heart disease with arryhthmia, acute endocarditis and, rarely, cardiac myxoma. Smaller arteries may be involved in collagen vascular disease, e.g. polyarteritis nodosa, systemic lupus erythematosus.

3. Trauma. Head injury may cause hemiplegia as a result of epidural or subdural haemorrhage. A blunt injury to the paratonsillar area may cause thrombosis of the internal carotid artery. Stretching of the internal carotid artery against the upper cervical vertebrae may occur when there is overextension of the neck with head rotation, and both thrombi and emboli may form. Air embolus after surgical intervention and fat embolus after long bone fractures are rare events.

4. Venous occlusion. Sterile venous thrombosis may occur in dehydration, cyanotic congenital heart disease, diabetic coma and protein S or C deficiency. Infected thrombus may be responsible if there is focal intracranial infection, e.g. purulent meningitis, mastoiditis.

5. Infection. Acute hemiplegia may occur in bacterial meningitis as a result of thrombosis in cortical veins or arteries. The direct focal cerebral invasion of herpes simplex virus may be responsible for an acute hemiplegia, but a post-infectious encephalitis, e.g. measles or varicella, may also be involved.

6. Migraine. Neurological deficits may occur in complicated forms of migraine, and a hemiplegia may be accompanied by sensory changes, dysarthria or aphasia. Although spontaneous recovery is the rule, persistent weakness may rarely occur.

7. Epilepsy and post-ictal states. Acute hemiplegia may follow convulsions (including complicated febrile convulsions) and status epilepticus.

Clinical assessment

The history must establish the presence of any relevant chronic illness, e.g. congenital heart disease or sickle cell disease. There may be a recent history of trauma, infectious disease or vaccination. A family or past medical history of migraine or epilepsy may be important. The mode of onset of the deficit and the presence of associated symptoms is also important, e.g. the sudden onset of headache with rapidly evolving hemiplegia may suggest an intracranial haemorrhage. Physical examination may reveal signs of a generalized bleeding disorder, trauma or local or systemic infection. Cardiological assessment, including blood pressure measurement, is mandatory (there may be extracardiac manifestations of infective endocarditis). Detailed neurological examination may establish the likely vessel of occlusion, e.g. a contralateral hemiparesis with legs affected more than arms in occlusion of the anterior cerebral artery. Cranial auscultation may reveal a bruit associated with an AV malformation.

Investigation

- FBC, ESR, coagulation studies, haemoglobin electrophoresis. Protein C, S and antithrombin III estimation.
- Autoantibodies.
- Microbiology: blood culture, mid-stream urine (MSU), throat swab. Consider lumbar puncture (LP) only if raised intracranial pressure has been excluded. Viral studies.
- U&E, creatinine.
- Radiography of skull and cervical spine.
- EEG.

- ECG.
- Computerized tomography (CT) or magnetic resonance imaging (MRI) of head and cervical spine.
- Angiography or digital subtraction angiography to delineate vessels accurately.
- Lipid studies, if no cause is found and there is a family history of stroke.

Management

The initial management of acute hemiplegia depends on the underlying aetiology, aiming to arrest the disease process while limiting intracranial damage, e.g. in a patient with herpes simplex encephalitis, intravenous acyclovir is accompanied by close attention to fluid balance, management of raised intracranial pressure and treatment of seizures. If there is residual neurological impairment, physiotherapy should be instituted.

Further reading

Brett EM. Vascular disorders of the nervous system in childhood. In: Brett EM, ed. *Paediatric Neurology*, 3rd edn. Edinburgh: Churchill Livingstone, 1991; 571–88.

Related topics of interest

Fits, faints and funny turns (p. 144)
Headache (p. 182)
Meningitis and encephalitis (p. 265)

ACUTE RENAL FAILURE

Acute renal failure occurs when a sudden decrease in renal function leads to loss of biochemical homeostasis. Oliguria or anuria leads to accumulation of nitrogenous waste products and disturbance of water and electrolyte balance. It may occur as a result of renal hypoperfusion (prerenal), parenchymal damage (renal) or obstruction of the renal tract (post-renal). If not corrected, renal hypoperfusion will lead to acute tubular necrosis and, if the insult is severe, cortical necrosis will follow. Acute on chronic renal failure may be precipitated by dehydration or an intercurrent infection.

Problems

- Fluid overload (cardiac failure, oedema, hypertension).
- Hyperkalaemia.
- Acidosis.
- Risk of infections.

Aetiology

1. Prerenal (renal hypoperfusion)

- Hypovolaemia, e.g. severe gastroenteritis, nephrotic syndrome, burns.
- Septicaemic shock.
- Cardiac failure.
- Renal vein thrombosis.

2. Renal

- Acute glomerulonephritis.
- Severe pyelonephritis.
- Cortical ischaemia, e.g. shock, haemorrhage, trauma.
- Nephrotoxins, e.g. gentamicin, gold, methotrexate.
- Haemolytic uraemic syndrome.

3. Post-renal (obstructive uropathy)

- Posterior urethral valves.
- Uric acid crystals, e.g. tumour lysis syndrome in the treatment of leukaemia.
- Ureteric obstruction, e.g. stones, ureteroceles.

Clinical features

The history and examination may suggest the aetiology. Features of acute renal failure include oliguria (urine output less than 200 $ml/m^2/day$), oedema and fluid overload, acidotic breathing and drowsiness. Acute hypertensive encephalopathy may occur.

Investigation

- Urine. Haematuria and/or proteinuria suggest underlying renal disease. Microscopy will confirm the presence of red cells and may identify casts. Pyuria suggests infection, which should be confirmed on urine culture.
- Blood and urine U&E, creatinine and osmolality. Urea and creatinine will be raised in line with the severity of

renal failure. There may be dilutional hyponatraemia, and hyperkalaemia will be exacerbated by acidosis. In prerenal failure the urinary sodium concentration will be low (< 30 mmol/l), whereas in renal failure the kidneys tend to leak sodium and the concentration will be higher (> 30 mmol/l). In prerenal failure the urine is appropriately concentrated (urine to plasma osmolality ratio > 1.15, urine to plasma urea ratio > 10), but in renal failure the ratios will be lower.

- FBC and clotting studies. The haematocrit may be a useful guide to hypovolaemia. There will be thrombocytopenia and deranged clotting if there is associated disseminated intravascular coagulopathy (DIC).
- Acid–base status. Metabolic acidosis.
- Liver function tests, calcium, phosphate, albumin.
- Blood culture.
- Radiology. Renal tract US may detect dilatation of the renal tract in obstructive uropathy. Renal size and cortical thickness may reveal intrinsic renal disease (dysplasia, polycystic disease, acute on chronic renal failure). Renal isotope scans are useful to detect underlying chronic renal disease and to follow recovery from the acute episode. Cystoscopy and micturating cystourethrography are indicated for the diagnosis and treatment of posterior urethral valves. Chest radiographs may show pulmonary oedema and cardiomegaly if fluid overload precipitates heart failure.

Management

1. Fluids. Hypovolaemia should be corrected immediately with plasma expansion 10–20 ml/kg. If the patient is hypoalbuminaemic (e.g. nephrotic syndrome) use 20% albumin. Central venous pressure monitoring enables more accurate assessment of intravascular volume. When fluid replacement is adequate and oliguria persists, diuretics such as frusemide may improve urine output. Accurate fluid balance is essential and weight should be monitored to avoid fluid overload. Urinary catheterization allows accurate measurement of urine output. Maintenance fluids should replace insensible losses (300 ml/m^2/day) plus urine output.

2. Hyperkalaemia. This can lead to arrhythmias and cardiac arrest and so should be carefully monitored. ECG changes (peaked T waves, depressed R waves, prolonged QRS and PR intervals) or a serum potassium > 7 mmol/l are indications for emergency treatment while dialysis is arranged:

- Intravenous calcium gluconate 0.5 ml/kg over 2–4 minutes (reduces the cardiotoxic effect of hyperkalaemia) followed by dextrose and insulin, which reduces the serum potassium by promoting uptake into cells. The blood glucose level should be monitored carefully to avoid hypo/hyperglycaemia.
- Nebulized salbutamol given 2-hourly will reduce the serum potassium and can be used in conjunction with dextrose and insulin.
- Calcium resonium orally or rectally increases the elimination of potassium from the body.

3. Acidosis will correct with the reduction of uraemia. If severe, correct with sodium bicarbonate.

4. Hypertension occurs as a result of salt and fluid overload. If strict fluid balance and diuretics are inadequate antihypertensive drugs such as beta-blockers or vasodilators can be used. If hypertension remains severe and uncontrolled with drug treatment, dialysis is indicated.

5. Risk of infections. Treat suspected infections promptly with broad-spectrum antibiotics to prevent catabolism. Use aminoglycosides with caution.

6. Nutrition. Intake should be adequate to minimize catabolism. Uraemia causes anorexia and vomiting so intravenous feeding may be necessary.

7. Dialysis. Peritoneal dialysis is the method of choice in children. Indications for dialysis include uncontrolled hyperkalaemia, acidosis or fluid overload.

Outcome

The outcome depends on the underlying cause. A child with acute tubular necrosis secondary to hypovolaemia will recover renal function in 7–14 days. Polyuria occurs during the recovery phase and careful monitoring of fluid balance and electrolytes is necessary. Acute renal failure secondary to rapidly progressive glomerulonephritis or renal cortical necrosis has a worse prognosis.

Further reading

Robson AM, Cameron JS. Acute renal failure in the neonate and older child. In: Cameron S, Davison AM, Grunfeld JP, Kerr D, Ritz E, eds. *Oxford Textbook of Clinical Nephrology*. Oxford: Oxford University Press, 1992: 1110–23.

Related topics of interest

Chronic renal failure (p. 82)
Hypertension (p. 199)
Shock (p. 344)

ADOLESCENT HEALTH

Adolescence is the term employed by the World Health Organization (WHO) to refer to young people between the ages of 10 and 19 years. This is perceived as a vulnerable time, packed with challenges and decisions to make. The majority of teenagers consider themselves in excellent health, psychologically well-balanced and educationally well-informed. It is important to take this into consideration when discussing issues of consent. Many of the 'Health of the Nation' targets specifically focus on areas of health needs in this age group, including reducing smoking; reducing death rates from accidents; reducing the overall suicide rate and reducing pregnancy rates.

Risk-taking is a normal part of adolescence but may damage health. Knowledge about risk does not necessarily alter behaviour.

Smoking

Ninety per cent of adult smokers started before the age of 19 years. Studies have shown that the incidence in teenagers increases with age from 10% in 13-year-olds to 22% in 16-year-olds. More girls smoke than boys in all age groups. Reasons for smoking include improving self image, releasing stress and peer pressure. Even in this age group, lung function in regular smokers has been shown in one study to be worse than non-smokers. Teenagers who smoke regularly are also more likely to abuse alcohol and cannabis.

Alcohol

Most children have their first taste of alcohol at home supervised by their parents in their early teens. Although the prevalence of under age drinking remains stable, the quantity consumed on each occasion has increased. Adolescent intoxication is associated with poor school performance and increased risk-taking behaviours leading to injury, crime and sexual encounters.

Drug misuse

Teenage drug use is on the increase due to increased availability and fashion influences. Recent studies show that between 40–50 % of school children say they have taken drugs at some stage and even greater numbers have been offered them. Drug misuse leads to a whole spectrum of associated problems including poor school performance, addiction, financial problems, crime, accidental poisoning and infection including Hepatitis B and HIV.

Sexual health

1. Contraception. Teenagers are having their first sexual experience at ever younger ages, emphasizing the importance of making advice on contraception easily accessible. Despite this, 25% do not use contraception; for those who do, the oral contraceptive pill is most frequently used. Girls under the age of 16 who request the oral contraceptive pill but do not wish their parents to be informed must be assessed by the prescriber to be 'Gillick competent'. Thus the prescriber must feel sure that the girl fully understands the implications of taking and not taking this medication. In all cases it is strongly advised that the girl should discuss her decision with her parents.

2. *Teenage pregnancy*. The UK has one of the highest teenage pregnancy rates in Europe and a reduction in the incidence was one of the targets in the Health of the Nation government White Paper. Countries with lower rates are those with more open sex education programmes for young people. Compared to 20 years ago, there are increasing numbers of conceptions in this age group, and also an increasing number of terminations of pregnancy. There is an increased incidence in areas of high unemployment, in teenagers from lower socio-economic groups and where the teenager was herself the result of a teenage pregnancy. The evidence for an increased risk of adverse outcome for both the health of mother and baby is contradictory, but some studies have suggested that there is an increased risk of antepartum haemorrhage, pre-eclampsia, premature birth, and post-natal depression. There is also an increased risk of sudden infant death syndrome, child abuse and the child is more likely to be admitted to hospital, often with multiple admissions.

Prevention involves not only increasing knowledge and access to family planning services, but also more opportunities for young people in employment and other life options.

Mental health

It is estimated that in any one year 10–20% of adolescents have a specific mental health problem. Within this group, 2–8% have major depression; 1.9% have obsessive–compulsive disorders; 0.5–1.0% anorexia and 1% bulimia. It is estimated that 2–4% of adolescents have attempted suicide at some time and 7.6 per 100 000 in the 15 to 19 age group, mainly boys, do commit suicide. These increasing suicide rates in young men are noted throughout Europe.

Chronic disease

The experience of adolescence for children who suffer from chronic diseases will be similar to that of healthy children but there may be additional hurdles to be overcome.

Problems

- Specific issues related to the condition (e.g. driving and epilepsy).

- Independence in managing medication or equipment.
- Transfer of care from paediatric to adult services.
- Careers and employment.
- Fertility (e.g. cystic fibrosis, previous treatment for cancer).

Anorexia nervosa

Definition

Anorexia nervosa is a disorder characterized by deliberate weight loss, induced and/or sustained by the patient.

Epidemiology

Most frequent in adolescent females and young women but also recognized in adolescent/young males.

Aetiology

Complex biological, socio-cultural and psychological factors need to be taken into consideration.

Clinical assessment

A characteristic presentation is with:

- Restricted diet.
- Excessive exercise.
- Induced vomiting and/or abuse of laxatives.
- Distortion of body image.
- Body weight less than 15% expected.

The condition is associated with undernutrition resulting in endocrine and metabolic changes:

- Secondary amenorrhoea.
- Poor skin.
- Poor hair.
- Parotid enlargement.
- Hypotension.
- Fluid and electrolyte abnormalities.

Severe emaciation can be life threatening, leading to renal or cardiac failure.

Management

The aim of treatment is to improve the patient's physical and emotional state. Therefore a multidisciplinary approach is adopted involving child psychiatrist, paediatrician, dietician, general practitioner, community psychiatric and paediatric nurses. The majority of cases are very resistant to treatment. Residential care or hospital admission may be required intermittently to ensure adequate food intake and weight gain, at the same time restricting exercise.

Outcome

Anorexia nervosa is very unpredictable and in its chronic state often persists in adult life.

Further reading

Birch DML. Adolescent behaviour and health. *Current Paediatrics*, 1996, **6:** 80–83.
Jones R, Finlay F, Simpson N, Kreitman T. How can adolescents' health needs and concerns best be met? *British Journal of General Practice*, 1997, **47:** 631–4.
MacFarlane A. *Adolescent Medicine*. London: RCP Publications, 1996.
Rutter M, Taylor E, Hersov L. Anorexia and bulimia nervosa. In: *Child and Adolescent Psychiatry: Modern Approaches*. Oxford: Blackwell Science, 1994; 425–37.

Related topics of interest

Accidents (p. 7)
Children and the law (p. 69)
Chronic fatigue syndrome (p. 80)
Poisoning (p. 315)

ADRENAL DISORDERS

The adrenal cortex produces mineralocorticoid, glucocorticoid, and sex hormones (androgens). Clinical disease results from relative excess or lack of these hormones.

- Aldosterone, the principal mineralocorticoid, is produced by the outer zone of the adrenal cortex (zona glomerulosa). It causes increased sodium reabsorption, and potassium and hydrogen ion loss from the distal renal tubule. Aldosterone is released in response to angiotensin II, which is produced following renal renin release and subsequent pulmonary angiotensin I conversion.
- Cortisol, the principal glucocorticoid, is secreted by the zona fasciculata. It modulates stress and inflammatory responses. It is a potent stimulator of gluconeogenesis and antagonizes insulin. Cortisol production is under diurnal control by the hypothalamo-pituitary axis [hypothalamic corticotrophin releasing hormone (CRH), and pituitary adrenocorticotrophic hormone (ACTH)].
- The adrenal androgens (dehydroepiandrosterone sulphate (DHEAS) and androstenedione) are secreted by the innermost zone of the cortex (zona reticularis). These are converted by the liver to testosterone in boys and oestrogen in girls, and production increases markedly at puberty. Androgen production is controlled by ACTH.

Congenital adrenal hyperplasia (CAH)

This is a group of autosomal recessive disorders of adrenal corticosteroid biosynthesis, due to deficiency of one of five enzymes in the cholesterol to cortisol pathway. By far the commonest is 21-hydroxylase deficiency (incidence of 1 in 12 000 live births). This enzyme is also involved in the cholesterol to aldosterone pathway and a deficiency in the zona glomerulosa will lead to aldosterone deficiency and a salt-losing tendency. A less common cause of CAH is 11β-hydroxylase deficiency which does not usually cause a salt-losing tendency but hypertension may be a prominent feature.

Presentation

- Ambiguous genitalia at birth (virilized female).
- Vomiting, dehydration and salt loss (salt-losing crisis) in the first few weeks of life.
- Collapse during stress, e.g. intercurrent illness, surgery.
- Virilization in early childhood. Males may present with false precocious puberty. Females may develop signs of androgen excess (acne, hirsutism, delayed menarche, irregular periods).
- Hypertension.

Investigations

- Cortisol low or normal. Unstressed levels may be normal.
- Raised plasma steroid precursors. Accumulation of metabolites proximal to the enzyme block (particularly 17 OH-progesterone in 21-hydroxylase deficiency).
- ACTH raised due to reduced feedback inhibition of

ACTH by cortisol. ACTH stimulates the metabolism of 17 OH-progesterone by alternative pathways leading to the overproduction of androgens and virilization in 21-hydroxylase deficiency.

- Urinary steroid metabolites. The pattern of metabolites will help identify the precise enzyme defect. Pregnanetriol is the main metabolite of 17 OH-progesterone.
- Aldosterone low, renin raised, if salt-losing.
- Genetics. The gene encoding the 21-hydroxylase enzyme system and a pseudogene have been located on the short arm of chromosome 6. Recombinations between these two genes result in deletions and mutations which can now be identified, making antenatal diagnosis possible.

Management

1. Ambiguous genitalia. CAH is the commonest cause of ambiguous genitalia. Sex assignment with chromosomes and pelvic ultrasound is extremely important. Parents are often devastated by the problem, but should be encouraged not to register the birth or name the child (particularly with an ambiguous name, such as Leslie) until the sex has been decided. Surgery (clitoral reduction, labial separation) may be necessary to achieve functionally and cosmetically normal external genitalia.

Other causes of ambiguous genitalia are rare, e.g. exogenous androgens, maternal or fetal androgen-secreting tumours, testosterone synthesis defects, true hermaphrodite. The karyotype is not always the most important factor in sex assignment in these conditions. The decision is based on the possibility of achieving the most normal external genitalia, and reproductive capacity where possible, with surgery and hormonal therapy.

2. Emergency treatment of salt-losing crisis. All babies with ambiguous genitalia should be considered to be at risk of a salt-losing crisis. The first sign of an impending crisis is a rising potassium. Mineralocorticoid (fludrocortisone) treatment and salt replacement before the serum sodium falls will avert a hypotensive crisis. As boys do not exhibit ambiguous genitalia, the diagnosis is often not made until they present with a salt-losing crisis. Dehydration and hypotension require plasma volume expansion with dextrose and saline. Hydrocortisone should be given intravenously.

3. Maintenance hormone therapy. Oral hydrocortisone is given to replace cortisol secretion and to suppress excessive ACTH production. The dose must be increased during periods of stress, e.g. intercurrent infection, general anaesthesia. 17 OH-progesterone levels are monitored in some centres, to ensure adequate suppression of ACTH, but growth and pubertal development are probably better indicators. Inadequate suppression results in rapid growth, advancement of skeletal maturity, and early puberty. If salt-losing, mineralocorticoid replacement (oral fludrocortisone) is necessary and renin levels are monitored to ensure adequate replacement. Oral sodium supplements are commonly needed in the first year of life.

4. Antenatal diagnosis. The main aim of antenatal diagnosis is to prevent virilization of a female infant. In a family with a child with CAH due to 21-hydroxylase deficiency, the genetic mutation should be identified. As soon as a further pregnancy is confirmed the mother should be commenced on oral dexamethasone. Chorionic villus sampling is performed at about 12 weeks to identify the presence of the mutation and the sex of the child. If the fetus is not affected the dexamethasone can be stopped. If the fetus is female and affected, the dexamethasone is continued to term and this will prevent virilization. If the fetus is male and affected, the treatment can be stopped but hormone replacement therapy will need to be commenced in the early neonatal period to prevent a salt-losing crisis.

Cushing's syndrome

This is uncommon in children. Clinical features are due to excessive glucocorticoid leading to protein catabolism, increased carbohydrate production, fat accumulation, and potassium loss (moon face, thin skin, easy bruising, hypertension (60%), hirsutism, obesity, poor growth velocity, buffalo hump, muscle weakness, diabetes, osteoporosis, aseptic necrosis of the hip, pancreatitis). The commonest cause is corticosteroid treatment (e.g. for frequently relapsing nephrotic syndrome). Rare causes of endogenous glucocorticoid excess include adrenal hyperplasia, adrenal cortex tumours, and pituitary ACTH hypersecretion (Cushing's *disease* implies an ACTH-secreting pituitary tumour). Investigations may include midnight and 08.00 plasma cortisol and ACTH levels, 24-hour urinary free cortisol, and a dexamethasone suppression test. Management depends on removing the cause either medically or surgically.

Adrenocortical failure

Failure of the adrenal cortex may be due to a primary adrenal disorder (Addison's disease (autoimmune), CAH, adrenal haemorrhage), or it may be secondary to hypothalamo-pituitary disorders leading to ACTH insufficiency (e.g. tumours of the hypothalamo-pituitary axis, congenital hypopituitarism, surgery or radiotherapy, and corticosteroid treatment). There may be complete failure of the adrenal cortex or selective failure of glucocorticoid, mineralocorticoid, or androgen synthesis. Onset may be insidious with fatigue, weight loss, nausea, and hyperpigmentation, or acute with an Addisonian crisis (hypotension, hypoglycaemia, hyperkalaemia) during a period of stress such as an infection. Management of acute adrenocortical insufficiency consists of resuscitation with fluids, hormone replacement, and correction of hypoglycaemia and electrolyte disturbances.

Primary hyperaldosteronism (Conn's syndrome)

This is very rare in children and is usually due to a zona glomerulosa adenoma. Features include sodium and water retention, hypertension, hypokalaemia, muscle weakness, polyuria, and impaired growth. Hyperaldosteronism results in a hypochloraemic, hypokalaemic alkalosis. The main differential diagnosis is Bartter's syndrome in which hyperaldosteronism is secondary to juxtaglomerular apparatus hypertrophy with raised renin levels and, in contrast to Conn's syndrome, the blood pressure is normal.

Further reading

Brook CGD. The adrenal gland. In: *A Guide to the Practice of Paediatric Endocrinology*. Cambridge University Press, 1993; 97–118.

Appan S, Hindmarsh, PC, Brook CGD. Monitoring treatment in congenital adrenal hyperplasia. *Archives of Disease in Childhood,* 1988; **64:** 1235–9.

Brook CGD. Intersex. In: *A Guide to the Practice of Paediatric Endocrinology*. Cambridge University Press, 1993; 1–17.

Related topics of interest

Shock (p. 344)
Vomiting (p. 377)

ALLERGY AND ANAPHYLAXIS

Allergy may be defined as a state of altered reactivity to a particular substance which is mediated by an immunological response to that specific allergen or antigen. The reaction is usually reproducible. The substance causing the reaction may have been ingested, inhaled or come into contact with skin or mucous membranes.

Problems

- Asthma.
- Eczema.
- Allergic rhinitis and conjunctivitis.
- Food allergy and intolerance.
- Drug allergy.
- Anaphylaxis.
- Psychosocial effects.

Types of allergic reaction

There are four types defined by the different immunological mechanisms involved. Type I is produced when allergens react with IgE on the surface of mast cells and basophils, causing immediate release of vasoactive substances. Examples are some food allergies and allergic rhinitis. Anaphylaxis is the most extreme result. Type II, which includes autoimmune haemolytic anaemia and post-streptococcal glomerulonephritis, occurs when circulating antibody reacts with antigen which is bound to a cell surface. Type III reaction is immune complex mediated and includes the vasculitis of autoimmune diseases. Type IV is delayed or cell mediated hypersensitivity and involves sensitized T lymphocytes. Typical examples are tuberculin hypersensitivity and organ transplantation rejection.

1. Allergic rhinitis. Intense irritation in the nose and congested conjunctivae, sneezing and post-nasal drip are typical features. The latter stimulates the cough reflex. The allergen is commonly grass or tree pollen. Treatment includes oral antihistamines and topical steroids or sodium cromoglycate.

2. Urticaria. Also known as hives or nettle rash, urticaria is an itchy, erythematous rash with weals. There may be associated angioedema in severe cases. There may be a history of atopy. Precipitants include physical agents (sunlight, mechanical pressure – dermographism, cold), drugs (e.g. aspirin), foods, insect bites and plants. Treatment is by avoidance of the allergen and oral antihistamines.

3. Anaphylaxis. Anaphylaxis is the extreme end of the allergy spectrum and is potentially fatal. The number of children in the UK who suffer from severe reactions is increasing and it has been estimated that as many as 1 in 300 is susceptible. The commonest allergens involved are nuts, eggs and wasp and bee stings. Exposure to even a trace amount of the allergen may be life-threatening in the susceptible child. Initial clinical features are irritation and itching of the mouth, malaise, weakness and vomiting, followed by bronchospasm, upper airway oedema, hypotension and shock. Emergency treatment is to secure the airway, ensure oxygenation and to administer intramuscular or subcutaneous adrenaline at a dose of 0.1 ml/kg of 1:10 000 solution. Repeated doses may be needed. Intravenous fluids are needed to support the circulation and hydrocortisone, antihistamines and nebulized salbutamol are often also given. After recovery the child should be observed for at least a further 4 hours as anaphylaxis may recur within that time.

Specific allergens

1. Food allergy. A small but increasing number of children, particularly those who are atopic, have true food allergy. Foods such as citrus fruit, shell fish or monosodium glutamate may cause just a rash or vomiting. Some children have more severe reactions particularly to eggs and to nuts which can result in anaphylaxis. Peanut allergy is an increasing concern and atopic families are being advised to avoid exposing infants to peanuts for as long as possible and nursing mothers should avoid peanut containing foods. Although some children grow out of these allergies, most are life long. Parents can be taught to administer i.m. adrenaline via a pen device and a susceptible child's school teachers should also be trained in its use. Since both eggs and nuts and their derivatives are used in a huge range of foods, parents must be vigilant to prevent exposure.

2. Food intolerance. This is a reproducible response to a specific food which is not psychologically based. It is not a true allergy as there are no immunological changes. Cow's milk protein intolerance is the commonest in childhood. Symptoms such as loose stools, vomiting, rash and poor weight gain may occur after the introduction of cow's milk into the diet. Iron deficiency anaemia may occur. Treatment is by total exclusion of cow's milk and use of a soy-based or casein hydrolysate formula. The latter may be preferable as some children are also intolerant of soya protein. The diet should be administered under the supervision of a dietician to ensure adequate intake of calcium and vitamins. Most children are able to tolerate cow's milk again by the age of 3 years.

3. Drug allergy. Reactions most often involve the skin and range from a non-specific maculopapular rash to a Stevens–Johnson syndrome. Anaphylactic reactions may also occur. When assessing whether a child is allergic to a drug, it is important to distinguish between a true allergic reaction and side effects of the drug. For example, antibiotics often cause nausea and loose stools which parents may interpret as an allergy. Many people have also been incorrectly labelled as allergic to penicillins having had a rash which was due to a viral infection. Amoxycillin typically causes a maculopapular rash with Epstein–Barr virus infection. All people with a true drug allergy should have this clearly written on the front of all medical notes.

4. House dust mite allergy. Atopic children are often allergic to the antigen on the faeces of the house dust mite which is ubiquitous in the home. Large quantities are found in bedding and carpets and in the dust particularly in bedrooms. Symptoms include cough, wheeze and rhinitis. The amount of allergen present can be reduced by frequent hoovering, damp dusting, using plastic mattress covers and ensuring rooms are well ventilated.

Investigation of allergic conditions

The history is usually sufficient for diagnosis but further confirmatory tests may be indicated.

- Skin tests. The weal and flare response to allergen extracts is tested. Specificity and sensitivity are poor.
- Radioallergosorbent test (RAST). This is a semiquantative assay for allergen specific IgE. It has many of the same problems as skin tests.
- Provocation tests. These are useful particularly in assessing whether a child is still allergic to a particular substance after abstention for a period of time. The allergen is applied directly to the skin or the mucosa of the nose or mouth. The child is monitored for symptoms.

Full resuscitation equipment must be available in case of anaphylaxis.

Further reading

David TJ. *Food and Food Additive Intolerance in Childhood.* Oxford: Blackwell Scientific Publications, 1993.

Parikh A, Scadding GK. Seasonal allergic rhinitis. *British Medical Journal,* 1997; **314:** 1392–5.

Sampson H. Editorial: Managing peanut allergy. *British Medical Journal*, 1996; **312:** 1050–1.

Related topics of interest

Asthma (p. 38)
Cardiac arrest (p. 61)
Eczema (p. 132)
Shock (p. 344)

ANAEMIA

The haemoglobin level is high at birth (15–19 g/dl) and falls to a nadir at about 2–3 months of age, but it seldom falls to below 10 g/dl in healthy infants. Anaemia may result from failure of red cell production, increased red cell breakdown or haemorrhage. It is often asymptomatic, but clinical features include tiredness, lethargy and pallor. Breathlessness and cardiac failure are more common if the onset of anaemia is acute (e.g. acute haemolysis). The commonest cause of anaemia in childhood is iron deficiency.

Aetiology

1. Failure of production

- Aplastic anaemia (congenital, acquired, e.g. drugs, parvovirus infection in spherocytosis).
- Iron deficiency (dietary lack, chronic blood loss).
- B_{12} deficiency (Crohn's disease).
- Folate deficiency (coeliac disease, anticonvulsants, haemolysis).
- Bone marrow invasion (leukaemia, neuroblastoma, tuberculosis).
- Erythropoietin deficiency (renal disease).
- Chronic infection.

2. Increased breakdown (haemolysis)

(a) Hereditary

- Membrane defects (spherocytosis).
- Haemoglobinopathies (sickle cell anaemia, thalassaemia).
- Enzyme deficiencies (glucose-6-phosphate dehydrogenase (G6PD) deficiency, pyruvate kinase deficiency).

(b) Acquired

- Immune (rhesus, ABO, blood transfusion incompatibility).
- Autoimmune (drugs, e.g. methyldopa; infections, e.g. mycoplasma).

(c) Other

- Burns.
- Artificial heart valves.
- Haemolytic uraemic syndrome.
- Snake venom.

3. Blood loss

- Perinatal (feto-maternal, twin to twin, placental/cord accidents, haemorrhagic disease of the newborn).
- Epistaxis.
- Trauma.
- Gastrointestinal (acute/chronic).
- Haematuria.
- Bleeding disorders (haemophilia, thrombocytopenia).

Iron deficiency anaemia

Seventy-five per cent of the total body iron at birth is found in the circulating haemoglobin, with the remainder stored as ferritin and haemosiderin. This is sufficient to meet requirements for the first 4–6 months of life, and infants should be weaned at this time. Most cases of iron deficiency anaemia are due to poor dietary intake and present in late infancy and early childhood. Prolonged breast-feeding without the introduction of adequate solids will lead to iron deficiency, but infant formula milks are fortified with iron. Doorstep cow's milk is not recommended for infants under 12 months of age as it is low in iron and may cause microscopic gastrointestinal bleeding. Also children who drink a lot of milk tend to have a poor intake of solids and are frequently iron deficient.

Iron absorption occurs in the duodenum and jejunum and is enhanced by gastric acid, protein and ascorbates. Only 5–10% of the dietary iron is normally absorbed, and a high intake of phytates (e.g. chapattis) or phosphates in the diet will reduce absorption further. Premature and low birth weight infants have reduced iron stores and should routinely receive supplements in the first year of life. Less common causes of iron deficiency are chronic blood loss (including hookworm infestation) and malabsorption.

Iron deficiency anaemia is treated with oral iron supplements, which should be given for at least 3 months to correct anaemia and replace iron stores. Blood transfusion is rarely necessary. There is some evidence to suggest that iron deficiency anaemia is associated with mild to moderate developmental delay.

Investigation

- FBC. Microcytic, hypochromic anaemia. It is important to exclude β-thalassaemia trait (the microcytosis and hypochromia are more marked for the degree of anaemia) and anaemia of chronic disease.
- Stools for occult blood, faecal fat, ova, cysts and parasites, e.g. hookworms.
- Serum iron low, total iron-binding capacity (TIBC) high, ferritin low. Iron and TIBC are both normal in thalassaemia trait and low in chronic disease.
- Free erythrocyte protoporphyrin is increased.

Folate and B_{12} deficiency

Megaloblastic anaemia is uncommon but is usually due to folate deficiency. Poor dietary intake may be exacerbated by rapid growth, fever, infection, diarrhoea and haemolysis, all of which increase folate requirements. Folate absorption occurs in the small intestine and is impaired in malabsorption states, e.g. coeliac disease, Crohn's disease, blind loop syndrome. Several drugs are associated with folate deficiency, e.g. phenytoin, methotrexate, co-trimoxazole.

B_{12} is combined with intrinsic factor (IF) from gastric parietal cells and is absorbed in the terminal ileum. Deficiency is uncommon as stores are sufficient for 2–3 years, but may result from inadequate intake (vegans) or failure of absorption (IF deficiency, blind loop syndrome, Crohn's disease). IF deficiency (pernicious anaemia) is rare in childhood.

Investigation

- FBC. Macrocytosis.
- Red cell folate.
- Serum B_{12} and folate.
- Deoxyuridine suppression test for folate deficiency.
- Schilling test for IF deficiency.

Haemolytic anaemia

The bone marrow can compensate for excessive red cell destruction by increasing erythropoiesis six- to eightfold before anaemia develops. The cause of haemolysis may be hereditary or acquired (see p. 31). The commonest hereditary haemolytic anaemia in the UK is hereditary spherocytosis. This is an autosomal dominant membrane defect which can present at any age. Anaemia is variable, splenomegaly is common and jaundice is usually mild. Exacerbations of haemolysis are associated with intercurrent infections. Pigment gallstones are common. Aplastic crises may occur, usually precipitated by parvovirus infection or folate deficiency. Folate supplements are routinely given. Splenectomy extends the life of the red cells and may be necessary if the haemolysis is severe, but should be delayed for as long as possible because of the risks (particularly pneumococcal infection).

G6PD is a red cell enzyme which protects the cell membrane from oxidant stress. G6PD deficiency is due to X-linked mutations, which are most common in African, Mediterranean and Oriental races. It may present with neonatal jaundice or with acute haemolysis on exposure to certain drugs (e.g. antimalarials, salicylates, sulphonamides), following ingestion of fava beans or during intercurrent infections.

Investigation

- FBC, film and reticulocyte count. Raised reticulocytes, fragmented red cells, spherocytes.
- Serum bilirubin. Raised unconjugated bilirubin, raised urinary urobilinogen.
- Blood group and direct Coombs' test (DCT). Blood group incompatibility produces haemolysis in the first days of life (see Neonatal jaundice, p. 276).
- Osmotic fragility test for membrane defects.
- Red cell enzyme assays.
- Haemoglobinuria. Occurs when intravascular haemolysis leads to saturation of the haemoglobin carrier protein, haptoglobin.
- Cold agglutinins. May be detected following mycoplasma infection.

Further reading

Booth IW, Aukett MA. Iron deficiency anaemia in infancy and early childhood. *Archives of Disease in Childhood,* 1997; **7**: 549–54.

Related topics of interest

Bleeding disorders (p. 53)
Neonatal jaundice (p. 276)
Purpura and bruising (p. 330)
Sickle cell anaemia and thalassaemia syndromes (p. 348)

ARRHYTHMIAS

Sinus tachycardia

The usual heart rates per minute are:

Newborn	100–150
Toddler	85–125
3–5 years	75–115
Over 5 years	60–100

A sinus tachycardia is a sinus rhythm that is faster than normal and is the normal physiological response to a requirement for increased cardiac output, e.g. exertion. The commonest cause is fever, and others include anaemia and hypovolaemia.

Sinus bradycardia

A persistently slow heart rate is uncommon in infants, but it may fall transiently, particularly during sleep, to as low as 60 beats/min. Important pathological causes include raised intracranial pressure and hypothermia.

Supraventricular tachycardia (SVT)

This is the most common abnormal tachycardia of childhood. Thirty to forty per cent of cases present within the first few weeks of life, and underlying structural heart disease is uncommon. It may present *in utero* as hydrops fetalis, or with cardiogenic shock in the neonatal period. More commonly it presents with increasing tachypnoea, poor feeding and pallor in early infancy. The older child usually presents with pallor and palpitations. The tachycardia may result from enhanced automaticity of the atrium (atrial tachycardia) or be sustained by a re-entry circuit involving an accessory atrioventricular (AV) connection (junctional tachycardia). The QRS complexes are narrow in contrast to those in ventricular tachycardias.

Junctional tachycardias

The commonest cause of SVT in childhood is an accessory connection between the ventricle and the atrium leading to an AV re-entry tachycardia. Rates of between 220 and 300 beats/min are seen during episodes of SVT. The QRS complexes are regular and narrow, with a one-to-one relationship with P waves. The accessory connection may occur anywhere around the AV ring. If it is capable of supporting both antegrade and retrograde conduction between the atrium and ventricle, the ECG during sinus rhythm will show a short PR interval and a delta wave (Wolff–Parkinson–White syndrome). If conduction is restricted to the retrograde direction, this ventricular pre-excitation will not be seen. Occasionally there is an underlying structural abnormality, most commonly Ebstein's anomaly of the tricuspid valve.

Atrial tachycardias

Atrial tachycardia, flutter and fibrillation are uncommon in the first year of life. Predisposing factors include cardiac surgery, structural lesions in which the atria are distorted or distended and myocarditis. There is variable conduction to the ventricles resulting in irregular QRS complexes with loss of the one-to-one relationship with P waves.

Management of SVT

1. Document the tachycardia with a 12-lead ECG. Exclude ventricular tachycardia (widened QRS complexes, abnormal QRS axis for age, AV dissociation).

2. Vagal manoeuvres. Elicit the diving reflex (bag of ice on face, immerse face in cold water) or use carotid sinus massage. If unsuccessful, proceed to drug treatment.

3. Adenosine. This acts by slowing conduction through the AV node, thus disrupting the re-entry circuit. It has a rapid onset of action and a very short half-life so side-effects are transient (flushing, tachypnoea, bradycardia, complete AV block). The tachycardia may reinitiate and the dose should be increased at 2-minute intervals until a sustained response is achieved.

4. Other drugs. Verapamil is effective but it is negatively inotropic and suppresses both sinus and AV node function, leading to a risk of profound bradycardia and hypotension. It is no longer recommended in infancy and is contraindicated in the presence of beta-blockers. Digoxin has been used to treat SVT for many years. It is usually effective and is a positive inotrope but its onset of action is slow (up to 12 hours), and if given inappropriately in ventricular tachycardia it can precipitate ventricular fibrillation. If the child is not compromised by the SVT and the diagnosis is certain, intravenous digitalization is indicated if adenosine fails. If the child is compromised or if the diagnosis is uncertain proceed to DC shock or pacing. Digoxin should not be used in Wolff–Parkinson–White syndrome. Flecainide has been recommended in the past but is not currently licensed for children.

5. DC cardioversion (1–2 J/kg). Atrial arrhythmias seldom respond to vagal manoeuvres, and adenosine and digoxin merely slow the ventricular rate. DC cardioversion may be effective in restoring sinus rhythm.

6. *Oesophageal pacing* is effective but usually only available in cardiac centres.

Prevention of further episodes

Recurrent attacks may be prevented by treatment with digoxin or propranolol. Surgical ablation of the accessory connection is sometimes possible.

Heart block

Impaired conduction within the AV node and bundle of His may take three forms.

First-degree heart block

The PR interval is prolonged for age and heart rate (usually > 0.20 seconds). It occurs in up to 10% of normal children, but may be secondary to rheumatic heart disease, congenital heart disease (e.g. Ebstein's anomaly) or digitalis toxicity.

Second-degree heart block (Wenckebach phenomenon)

There is progressive prolongation of the PR interval until one P wave is not succeeded by a QRS complex.

Third-degree (complete) heart block

Complete AV dissociation may be congenital, or acquired following surgery or myocarditis. It is associated with maternal systemic lupus erythematosus and appears to be due to the transfer of maternal anti-Ro or anti-DNA antibodies.

Further reading

Archer N. Management of supraventricular tachycardia. *Current Paediatrics,* 1995; **5** (1): 59–63.

Cardiac emergencies. In: Advanced Life Support Group. *Advanced Paediatric Life Support,* 2nd edn. London: BMJ Publications, 1997; 99–106.

Till JA, Shinebourne EA. Supraventricular tachycardia: diagnosis and current acute management. *Archives of Disease in Childhood,* 1991; **66:** 647–52.

Related topics of interest

Cardiac arrest (p. 61)
Cyanotic congenital heart disease (p. 104)
Heart failure (p. 190)
Heart murmurs (p. 194)

ASTHMA

Asthma is a chronic disease characterized by episodic reversible airway obstruction. The aetiology remains uncertain, but it is likely to be a combination of genetic and environmental factors. Airway narrowing can be precipitated by many factors which provoke bronchoconstriction, mucosal oedema and mucous plugging. Asthma is a major cause of paediatric morbidity, affecting at least 10–20% of children in the UK. Acute asthma is one of the most common paediatric emergencies.

Problems

- Episodic wheezing.
- Acute severe asthma.
- Poor growth.

History

Asthma is primarily a clinical diagnosis based on a history of recurrent wheeze, cough (often at night) and dyspnoea. There may be clear precipitating factors such as viral infections, cigarette smoke, exercise, excitement and allergens e.g. pollen, animal hair. There may have been significant respiratory illness in the neonatal period, or viral bronchiolitis during the first year of life. The child may also suffer from eczema, hay fever or urticaria, or there may be atopic symptoms in family members. Frequency of symptoms and the degree of interference with normal activity should be established. Systemic enquiry is important to exclude symptoms suggestive of other causes of wheeze, e.g. cystic fibrosis, immunodeficiency.

Examination

During an acute episode, tachypnoea, tachycardia, intercostal and subcostal recession with use of accessory muscles of respiration are frequent findings. Auscultation reveals widespread wheezing. In acute severe episodes, cyanosis, poor air entry (silent chest) and inability to talk are signs of life-threatening asthma. Examination between episodes is often normal. Growth should be documented, and a check made for signs of undertreated asthma (Harrison's sulcus, pectus carinatum) or signs of an alternative diagnosis, e.g. clubbing in cystic fibrosis.

Investigation

In most patients with a clear history no investigation is needed.

- Chest radiographs are not routinely requested in acute asthma but can be helpful in cases of severe asthma or persistent symptoms to exclude a complication, e.g. pneumothorax or foreign body.

- Peak flow. Expected mean values are related to height. Bronchodilators may demonstrate reversible airway narrowing, and a home diary card is of value to monitor progress.
- Skin prick tests may help to identify allergic triggers.
- Pulse oximetry is valuable as a non-invasive assessment of oxygenation.
- Arterial blood gases. Needed in severe episodes, usually if considering mechanical ventilation.

Management

National guidelines for the management of childhood asthma were first produced in 1993 and were reviewed in 1995 (see Further reading). The key issues are:

- The importance of correct diagnosis.
- A stepwise approach to treatment.
- Primary prevention of asthma, e.g. discouragement of parental smoking, allergen avoidance including house dust mite.
- The use of self-management plans.

1. The stepwise approach to the treatment of chronic asthma. The emphasis should be on gaining control of symptoms quickly – this may mean starting treatment at higher doses and then stepping down.

Children under 5 years:

- Step 1: Occasional use of β2 agonists (e.g. salbutamol, terbutaline) as relief bronchodilator.
- Step 2: Prophylaxis with regular inhaled anti-inflammatory agents. Sodium cromoglycate may be tried initially for a period of 6 weeks but if no improvement is seen change to an inhaled steroid, e.g. beclomethasone or budesonide. β2 agonists as relief bronchodilators as needed.
- Step 3: Increase the dose of inhaled steroid (fluticasone may be used as an alternative) or consider adding a long-acting inhaled beta-agonist (e.g. salmeterol). A short course of oral prednisolone may be considered at this stage to gain control of symptoms. Relief bronchodilators as needed.
- Step 4: Inhaled steroids in high dose together with regular inhaled bronchodilators. Consider addition of slow-release xanthines or nebulized β2 agonists.

- Stepping down: Regularly review symptom control and consider stepping down treatment every 3–6 months if the child is symptom-free.

Children over 5 years: The recommended steps are basically the same as for younger children. In step 2, when starting prophylaxis, inhaled steroids are usually preferred to sodium cromoglycate. Inhaled ipratropium bromide and oral long-acting β2 agonists are other alternatives to consider at step 4. An additional step 5 recommends regular oral steroids.

2. *General advice.* The method of drug delivery should be carefully considered depending on the child's age. Metered dose inhalers are very difficult for children to use correctly and should not be prescribed without a spacer device. The use of spacer devices is particularly important when using high-dose inhaled steroids. Newer spacer devices can be used even in very young infants with the addition of a soft face mask. Syrups are much less effective and have greater systemic effects. If symptoms are not controlled, check inhaler technique and compliance before increasing doses.

An integral part of asthma management is education of families with an asthmatic child. The importance of compliance with regular medication should be emphasized. Parents should be advised on the action they should take in the event of an acute asthma attack (e.g. how and when to increase treatment, when to request medical help). Written asthma plans can be very helpful. Parents should also be able to recognize the signs of a severe attack (e.g. difficulty in speaking, cyanosis, exhaustion).

Advice should be given on avoidance of provoking factors, including regular vacuuming, using mattress covers, and encouraging the parents to give up smoking. Growth should be carefully monitored. Concerns are often expressed about the effects of steroids on growth but it is important to remember that poorly controlled asthma will also impair growth.

Most children are managed in primary care in GP asthma clinics. Referral to a paediatrician is appropriate for some children, e.g. if the diagnosis is in doubt (especially if the child is < 6 months old), the asthma is unstable or interferes with normal life, high doses of inhaled steroids or frequent oral steroids (> 4 courses per year) are required, or there are any other concerns.

3. Management of acute asthma. Most children with a mild attack respond to a nebulized bronchodilator ± a short course of oral steroids. If hospital admission is indicated high-flow oxygen, with regular nebulized bronchodilators and oral steroids, is the first line of treatment. If there are features of a severe attack or the child does not respond to the first line of treatment intravenous steroids, and infusions of aminophylline or salbutamol should be considered. Transfer to an intensive care unit is indicated for a child with status asthmaticus who is at risk of impending respiratory failure (persistent hypoxia, exhaustion, hypercapnia). Intubation and ventilation are occasionally necessary.

Further reading

Hodges I. The aetiology of childhood asthma. *Current Paediatrics,* 1996; **6:** 247–51.

Rees J, Price J. Asthma in children: treatment. *British Medical Journal,* 1995; **310:** 1522–7.

The British Guidelines on Asthma Management 1995 Review and Position Statement. Published by committee members representing: the British Thoracic Society, the National Asthma Campaign, the Royal College of Physicians of London in association with the General Practitioners in Asthma Group, the British Paediatric Respiratory Society and the Royal College of Paediatrics and Child Health. *Thorax,* 1997; **52:** S1–21.

Related topics of interest

Allergy and anaphylaxis (p. 27)
Cough and wheeze (p. 100)
Cystic fibrosis (p. 107)
Upper respiratory tract infection (p. 367)

ATAXIA

Ataxia is the incoordination which results from sensory loss or cerebellar dysfunction. The presentation in childhood may be acute or chronic, congenital or acquired, intermittent or progressive. Clinical findings may include a wide-based gait, nystagmus, dysarthria and generalized hypotonia. There is difficulty in performing fine motor tasks (handwriting, finger-nose test) and rapidly alternating movements (dysdiadochokinesia). A thorough history and neurodevelopmental assessment will indicate a likely aetiology in many cases.

Acute ataxia

Causes of acute ataxia

1. *Drugs,* e.g. anti-epileptics, piperazine, alcohol and solvent abuse.

2. *Infection.* Cerebellar abscess, meningitis or encephalitis (especially varicella) may cause ataxia in addition to other signs such as fever, meningism and altered consciousness.

3. *Acute cerebellar ataxia of childhood.* A dramatic onset of severe bilateral truncal ataxia occurs 1–3 weeks after a viral infection (echo, Coxsackie and influenza A and B have been implicated). It is usually seen in a young child aged 1–2 years who is systemically well. CSF may show a mild pleocytosis with a later rise in protein. Investigation must exclude other causes. Most recover within 2 months.

4. *Hydrocephalus* may present with ataxia.

5. *Neoplasm.* Tumours in the posterior fossa, e.g. medulloblastoma, may present with ataxia and signs of raised intracranial pressure.

6. *Head injury.* Ataxia may persist for some months.

7. *Basilar artery migraine.* Features of brain stem dysfunction may dominate the clinical picture and ataxia, dysarthria, tinnitus and vertigo may occur. Attacks are typically related to menstruation in adolescent girls who often have a strong family history of migraine.

8. *Epilepsy.* Post-ictal state or minor epileptic status may cause ataxia.

9. Hysteria. Signs are often bizarre and are not consistent.

10. Dancing eye syndrome (myoclonic encephalopathy of infancy). This may follow a viral infection or may occur with neuroblastoma (often occult). Chaotic, rapid jerking of extraocular muscles and limbs is seen while the child is awake or asleep. Recurrent ataxia with neurodevelopmental problems may result.

11. Metabolic disease, e.g. Maple syrup urine disease, urea cycle defects, Hartnup disease. Ataxia may be intermittent.

12. Sensory ataxias, e.g. Guillain Barré.

Investigations

- CT or MRI brain.
- Lumber puncture, if the brain scan is normal.
- Toxicology screen.
- Viral serology.
- Metabolic screen (see below).
- Urinary VMA, in Dancing eye syndrome.

Chronic ataxia

Causes

1. Ataxic cerebral palsy accounts for 10% of cerebral palsy and underlying causes are diverse. There are three main groups: ataxic, ataxic diplegic and dysequilibrium syndrome. The latter is associated with autosomal recessive inheritance, cerebellar hypoplasia, spasticity and learning disability.

2. Congenital cerebellar abnormalities, e.g. Joubert's syndrome (autosomal recessive agenesis of the cerebellum associated with learning disability and episodic tachypnoea), Dandy Walker malformation.

3. Metabolic disease, e.g. leucodystrophies, Batten's disease, abetalipoproteinaemia, Refsum's disease, Wilson's disease. Ataxia may occur with other signs and symptoms depending on the condition.

4. Demyelinating disease. Multiple sclerosis is rare in children but may present with intermittent ataxia in adolescents.

5. *Friedrich's ataxia*. A progressive ataxia of the limbs and trunk is associated with dysarthria, weakness, and wasting and pyramidal tract dysfunction of the legs. There is a loss of joint and position sense, absent tendon reflexes and extensor plantar responses. Associated features include scoliosis, pes cavus, diabetes mellitus and cardiomyopathy which may lead to arrhythmias. Symptoms usually commence before the age of 15 and gradual deterioration of neurological and cardiovasular function renders most patients chairbound by 20–30 years of age. Inheritance is autosomal recessive and the gene has been localized to chromosome 9q13-21.

6. *Ataxia telangectasia*. Progressive cerebellar ataxia appears in early childhood, and may be associated with oculomotor apraxia, mental retardation and later, loss of joint position sense and dementia. Telangectasia appear at the age of 3–5 years, notably on the face, flexures of knees and elbows, and the pinnae. There is poor humoral and cellular immunity and one third of patients develop malignancy, e.g. lymphoma. Investigations show depressed levels of IgA and IgM with a raised level of α-fetoprotein. Death before adulthood is common. Inheritance is autosomal and the gene has been localized to chromosome 11q22-23.

Investigations

Selected investigations may include:

- MRI brain scan.
- α-fetoprotein and immunoglobulins which will be abnormal in ataxia telangectasia.
- Metabolic screen: Blood for lactate, ammonia, amino acids, lysosomal enzymes, phytanic acid; urine for amino and organic acids; CSF lactate.
- Copper and caeruloplasmin if Wilson's disease is being considered.
- Blood film for acanthocytes if abetalipoproteinaemia is suspected.

Further reading

de Sousa C. The ataxic child. *Current Paediatrics*, 1995; **5** (3): 160–4.

Related topics of interest

Big heads, small heads (p. 49)
Disability (p. 124)
Malignancy in childhood (p. 254)

BEHAVIOUR

Many behavioural problems are variations of an expected pattern of development, especially during the toddler years. Parents may have unrealistic expectations of the child's performance. Recognized behaviour problems in school age children include school refusal, bullying, conduct and attention deficit disorders. Behaviour difficulties may occur as a result of low self-esteem, learning difficulties, poor supervision or difficulties at home.

The following are common behaviour problems in young children:

- Sleep problems.
- Eating problems.
- Temper tantrums.
- Toileting issues.

History

Providing an opportunity for parents to talk about their child's behaviour difficulties and acknowledging how they feel is very important. Taking a medical and developmental history is useful to exclude an underlying cause. Special consideration should be given to social factors, e.g. marital breakdown, family bereavement or birth of a new sibling. Reports from teachers and carers, other than parents, may reveal that a certain behaviour is displayed only for the parents.

Assessment

Discuss current behaviour management strategies with parents and help to find a way forward. Build on their existing skills and strengths. Parents need reassurance that problems can improve with behaviour modification and that their contribution is vital to success. The basis for most programmes is to have a consistent approach, rewarding good behaviour, e.g. praise, attention or stars on a chart and avoid rewards or attention for unwanted behaviour.

Sleep problems

1. Settling and waking problems. It may be difficult to settle young children off to sleep in the evening. They may wake frequently during the night demanding attention and drinks. A regular bedtime routine with a bath, calming down and reading a story is most likely to be successful. If the child then wakes regularly, rewarding with drinks or play should be avoided.

2. Night-time attacks. Night terrors and sleep-walking occur during deep non-rapid eye movement sleep, during the first hours of going to sleep. The child remains asleep during the episode and has no recollection of events the next morning.

Nightmares occur during rapid eye movement sleep, the child wakes fully with vivid recollection of the dream and reassurance of the child's safety is important. Parents should be assured that night terrors, sleep walking and nightmares usually remit spontaneously.

Eating problems

Toddlers frequently refuse to eat or eat a limited range of food, causing great anxiety for their parents. Most children will be thriving, and parents should be encouraged to offer meals regularly, ideally as part of family meal-time, without coaxing, scolding or forcing. General review of health and dietary advice is needed if there is failure to thrive.

Temper tantrums

These are common from 1 to 5 years of age during moments of intense frustration. Reinforcement of the behaviour occurs if the parents give in to the child's desires, and this should be avoided. Removing the child from the centre point of attention into a separate room may help this behaviour.

Toileting problems

1. Enuresis. Nocturnal enuresis, involuntary emptying of the bladder at night, is a common problem. It is estimated to affect 10% of 5-year-old children, 5% of 10-year-olds and 1% of 15-year-olds. Bedwetting is more common in boys and there is often a family history. The majority of cases are due to delay in bladder maturation. Approximately 1–2% of cases will have an underlying organic cause, e.g. urinary tract infection, congenital urinary tract anomaly or neurogenic bladder. A thorough history, examination and urinalysis can exclude these. Management may involve general measures such as avoiding a bedtime drink and parents lifting the child and putting them on the toilet late at night when they go to bed. In persistent cases alarm devices or the use of medication, Desmopressin, may prove useful. Nocturnal enuresis can prove distressing for the child, especially not being able to stay overnight with friends or relatives. For the parents there is the inconvenience of changes of bed clothes with additional financial burdens for mattress covers and laundry. Reassurance must be given that enuretic problems will resolve.

2. Encopresis. Encopresis is the term used when formed stools are deposited in abnormal places. It should be distinguished from constipation with overflow. Reassure the child and parents that problems usually resolve using a basic management programme; encourage the child to sit on the toilet at regular intervals, giving a first reward for sitting, and a further reward for passing a stool on the toilet. The use of star charts may prove useful. If symptoms continue despite intervention consider more closely whether the child has emotional difficulties.

Hyperactivity

Many children are incorrectly given the label hyperactive when their behaviour represents part of the normal spectrum of activity of early childhood. However some children are restless and have poor concentration which may lead to learning and behavioural difficulties. The cause of hyperactivity is uncertain and it is likely to be complex, involving genetic, neurochemical and psychosocial factors. A few children improve with dietary manipulation and an increasing number of children are diagnosed as having attention deficit hyperactivity disorder.

Attention deficit hyperactivity disorder (ADHD)

Children with ADHD are overactive, restless and generally disruptive. They have poor concentration and attention skills, they are easily distracted, rarely finish tasks and do not seem to listen to instructions. As a result of this behaviour children may have learning difficulties, sleep problems, conduct disorders and poor relationships with family members and peers.

1. Assessment. Clinical assessment includes neurodevelopmental and mental state assessment as well as physical examination. Children with suspected ADHD may be diagnosed by a paediatrician or child psychiatrist using strict criteria outlined in international psychiatric guidelines (DSM IV and ICD 10). It is helpful to gather information from teachers on the child's behaviour in school. The condition is more common in boys and children with developmental delay. No specific cause has been identified and it is likely to be multifactorial with genetic and environmental influences.

2. Management. Behavioural modification strategies for home and school should be introduced. Parent and family support groups are available. Some children benefit from medication with psychostimulants; methylphenidate (Ritalin™) is most frequently prescribed. Other drugs used include dexamphetamine and pemoline. All children on medication should continue with behavioural strategies and need regular clinic review.

Further reading

Bramble D, Pearce J. Attention deficit hyperactivity disorder: a rational guide to paediatric assessment and treatment. *Current Paediatrics*, 1997; **7:** 36–41.
Green C. *Toddler Taming*, 1st edn. London: Vermillion, Ebury Press, 1995.
Polnay L, Hull D. *Emotional and Behavioural Difficulties in Community Paediatrics*, 2nd edn. London: Churchill Livingstone, 1993; 388–417.

Related topics of interest

Developmental assessment (p. 111)
Developmental delay (p. 115)

BIG HEADS, SMALL HEADS

All babies and young children should have their head circumference measured as part of child health surveillance and when medically examined. Head growth is rapid in the first year of life after which it plateaus. Serial measurements of head circumference should be recorded along with height and weight, on the appropriate centile chart and any deviation from the expected head size and shape should prompt a thorough assessment to determine the cause. In the newborn, the skull sutures are not fused to allow moulding of the head during delivery. They remain open to allow the brain to grow in the first few years. The anterior fontanelle is of variable size but is easily felt in the newborn and average time of closure is 18 months. The posterior fontanelle is much smaller and is usually closed by 6–8 weeks. Hydrocephalus and hypothyroidism may cause persistence beyond this age.

Small heads

A child may be born with an abnormally small head or the head may not grow at the expected rate. Microcephaly may be congenital or acquired. History should include pregnancy, birth and neonatal history, family history and any past illnesses. As well as careful measurement of head circumference and examination of shape, suture lines and fontanelles, the child should be examined for dysmorphic features and other congenital anomalies which might point to a syndromic diagnosis. The height and weight should also be measured to ascertain whether head growth is in proportion to that of the body.

Causes

- Familial. Autosomal dominant and recessive forms of microcephaly.
- Genetic abnormalities, e.g. Trisomy 18, Smith–Lemli–Opitz syndrome.
- Congenital infection, e.g. rubella, CMV.
- Teratogens, e.g. maternal phenylketonuria, fetal alcohol syndrome.
- Perinatal insult, e.g. hypoxic ischaemic encephalopathy.
- Postnatal infection, e.g. meningitis.
- Craniosynostosis if involving multiple sutures.

Investigation

- Serology for congenital infection screen.
- Chromosomes.
- MRI of the brain.
- Skull X-rays may show fusion of sutures in craniosynostosis.

Large heads

A child may be born with a large head, which is most often familial, or they may have accelerated head growth. Examination should focus initially on signs of acute hydrocephalus (dilated scalp veins, 'sun-setting' eyes, tense fontanelle). If they are not present signs of rarer causes such as neurocutaneous syndromes should be looked for.

Causes

- Familial (measure the parents' heads).
- Hydrocephalus.
- Hydrancephaly may be confused clinically with hydrocephalus but is a condition where the brain tissue is replaced by fluid.
- Neurocutaneous syndromes, e.g. neurofibromatosis.
- Storage disorders, e.g. Alexander's disease, Canavan's disease.

Hydrocephalus

Hydrocephalus is an increase in CSF volume with enlargement of the ventricular system. CSF is produced by the choroid plexuses and passes from the lateral ventricles through the foramina of Monro into the 3rd ventricle. It exits via the aqueduct of Sylvius and flows into the 4th ventricle and then to the subarachnoid space and basal cisterns. Absorption is through the arachnoid villi into the cerebral sinuses. Hydrocephalus can therefore occur from CSF overproduction, failure of absorption (communicating hydrocephalus) or obstruction to flow (non-communicating hydrocephalus).

Aetiology

1. *Congenital*

- Aqueduct stenosis is due to thickening of the tissue causing compression and distortion of the canal.
- Arnold Chiari malformation of the cerebellum causes outflow obstruction of the 4th ventricle due to elongation of the medulla and downwards displacement of the cerebellar tonsils.
- Dandy Walker syndrome consists of cerebellar hypoplasia and a cystic 4th ventricle with outflow obstruction.
- Others. Aneurysm of the vein of Galen, arachnoid cysts, and bone deformities of the base of the skull (e.g. in achondroplasia).

2. *Acquired*

- Neoplasia. Tumours may obstruct CSF flow. Papilloma of the choroid plexus is a rare cause of excess CSF production.
- Infection. Adhesions may obstruct CSF pathways after bacterial or TB meningitis or following intrauterine infection, e.g. toxoplasma.
- Intraventricular haemorrhage causes hydrocephalus when the blood clot blocks CSF flow and prevents reabsorption by blocking the arachnoid villi.

Clinical features

The child presents with an enlarging head circumference with open, large, tense fontanelles. They may be vomiting, drowsy, irritable and have delayed motor milestones.

Investigations

- Ultrasound scan if the fontanelle is open, will confirm hydrocephalus.
- CT or MRI scan will show any underlying cerebral abnormalities. MRI is particularly useful for showing aqueduct stenosis and lesions around the 3rd ventricle.

Management

The underlying cause of hydrocephalus should be treated where possible, but most cases also require a shunt to divert the CSF. The usual type of shunt is ventriculo-peritoneal with flow of CSF controlled by one way valves in the tubing which control the pressure at which CSF is released. Ventriculoatrial shunts are rarely used now. Drug therapy (e.g. acetazolamide) only has a short term effect on reducing CSF production. It is sometimes used to treat neonates with acute hydrocephalus secondary to IVH where the majority will eventually have arrest or regression of the hydrocephalus.

Complications of CSF shunts

Epilepsy occurs in 20–35% of patients with shunts. Eighty per cent of children require at least one shunt revision in the first 10 years. Other complications are:

1. Blockage. The shunt may become blocked at either end, by adhesions, omentum, or brain tissue. There may also be valve malfunction. Symptoms of acute or chronic hydrocephalus occur and urgent neurosurgical assessment is needed.

2. Infection tends to occur within weeks of shunt insertion and usually results from perioperative shunt contamination. *Staphylococcus epidermidis* or *aureus* is commonly responsible. Symptoms of malaise, vomiting and pyrexia occur, with an associated neutrophil leucocytosis and raised ESR and CRP. Diagnosis involves sampling from the shunt reservoir. Treatment involves removal of the shunt and insertion of an external ventricular drain.

Abnormal head shape

Abnormal head shape is usually caused by external deforming forces and the abnormal shape tends to resolve spontaneously. However, rarer conditions such as craniosynostosis should also be considered.

- *Deforming forces* which may be responsible include intrauterine positioning or infant sleeping position, or more rarely torticollis or hemifacial microsomia. Since the 'Back to Sleep' campaign to reduce the risk of SIDS, there has been an increase in the incidence of plagiocephaly (parallelogram shaped head when viewed from above) with flattening of the occiput.
- *Craniosynostosis* is premature closure of the sutures. The resulting head shape will depend on which sutures are involved, e.g. scaphocephaly with sagittal suture fusion, plagiocephaly with unilateral coronal or lambdoidal suture fusion. Multiple sutures are involved in the craniosynostosis syndromes such as Apert's and Crouzon's.
- *Box shaped skull* is seen in chronic subdural haematomata.

Further reading

Guazzo EP. Recent advances in paediatric neurosurgery. *Archives of Disease in Childhood*, 1993; **69:** 335–8.

Jones BM, Hayward R, Evans R, Britto J. Occipital plagiocephaly: an epidemic of craniosynostosis? *British Medical Journal*, 1997; **315:** 693–4.

Related topics of interest

Congenital infection (p. 93)
Developmental delay (p. 115)
Disability (p. 124)
Malignancy in childhood (p. 254)

BLEEDING DISORDERS

Disorders of coagulation may be hereditary or acquired. The most important hereditary conditions are haemophilia A, Christmas disease and von Willebrand's disease. Acquired coagulation defects may be due to deficiency of the vitamin K-dependent clotting factors (e.g. haemorrhagic disease of the newborn, liver disease), or a consumptive coagulopathy (disseminated intravascular coagulation, DIC).

Haemophilia and Christmas disease

Haemophilia A (factor VIII deficiency) is a sex-linked recessive condition which occurs in 1 in 20 000 males. A family history is obtained in over 50% of cases. Christmas disease (factor IX deficiency = haemophilia B) is also sex-linked recessive but is much less common. These coagulopathies may present in infancy with excessive superficial bruising, or bleeding following circumcision. Once the child is mobile, haemarthroses are common and bleeding post tonsillectomy may be life-threatening. Bleeding from cuts or from mucosal surfaces (e.g. epistaxis) is less common, but haematuria does occur. Female carriers are asymptomatic but can be detected by reduced factor VIII or IX activity.

Problems

- Haemarthroses.
- Muscle haematomas.
- Joint deformity and ankylosis.
- Elective surgery.
- Risk of viral infections from blood products.
- Family and social disruption.

Investigation

- Prolonged partial thromboplastin test (PTT).
- Normal prothrombin time (PT), thromboplastin time (TT) and fibrinogen.
- Bleeding time normal.
- Platelet count normal.
- Liver function tests normal.
- Clotting factor assays. In haemophilia A, levels of factor VIII coagulation activity (VIIIc) produced by the liver are low. Levels of factor VIII-related antigen (VIII RAG) produced by endothelial cells and factor VIII von Willebrand's factor (VIII VWF) which mediates platelet adhesion are normal.

  In Christmas disease, factor IX levels are low and some patients produce an abnormal factor IX (IXCAg). Assays of other vitamin K-dependent factors (II, VII, X) are sometimes necessary to exclude a hepatic disorder.
- Gene analysis is now available, making antenatal diagnosis possible.

Management

Christmas disease tends to have milder clinical manifestations than haemophilia A, but the general management principles are the same. The severity of haemophilia is linked to the degree of clotting factor deficiency: < 1% of normal causes severe problems, 1–5% causes moderate problems and 5–20% only mild symptoms. Factor VIII or factor IX concentrates are now used instead of cryoprecipitate in the treatment of acute bleeds. The amount of concentrate required depends on the desired rise in factor VIII or IX:

$$\text{Units of factor VIII} = \frac{\text{weight (kg) x desired rise in factor VIII (\%)}}{1.5}$$

Following a head injury or severe bleed a level of over 60% is aimed for. Bleeds in the throat are particularly serious as they may cause respiratory embarrassment. Following a haemarthrosis or soft-tissue injury, levels of 30–50% should be achieved. Haemarthroses cause pain and, if severe, the joint should be splinted to maintain a good position and to relieve pain. Opiate analgesia may be needed, but intramuscular injections should be avoided. Passive exercises and later active exercises are a vital part of recovery and prevention of joint deformity and ankylosis. Factor VIII or IX inhibitors can develop, which makes treatment much more difficult.

Tranexamic acid is an antifibrinolytic agent which is useful in controlling mucosal bleeds but is not useful for other bleeds and is contraindicated in haematuria.

Mild to moderate haemophilia may respond to desmopressin (DDAVP) which can be infused to cover minor procedures such as dental extraction.

Haemophilia and HIV infection

The use of multidonor cryoprecipitate and lyophilized factor VIII or IX concentrates, before the recognition of the HIV virus, has led to the infection of a significant number of haemophiliacs. In the UK in 1990, 17% of the 863 haemophiliacs under the age of 14 years and 42% of the 424 haemophiliacs between 15 and 19 years were HIV positive. Twenty of these children and adolescents had developed AIDS and there had been nine AIDS-related deaths. However, no child under 5 years was HIV positive, and as a result of exclusion of high-risk donors, HIV antibody testing and the treatment of clotting factor concentrates to remove viruses, no further cases of infection have been reported since 1986.

Haemophiliacs have also been at risk of chronic liver disease from transfer of hepatitis B and C in blood products.

They should be immunized against hepatitis B, and it is hoped that the treatment methods used to eliminate HIV from clotting factors will also eliminate other viruses such as hepatitis C.

von Willebrand's disease

This is a rare autosomal dominant disorder (approximate incidence 1 in 150 000) which is due to failure of synthesis of normally functioning factor VIII VWF. Levels of factors VIIIc and VIII RAG are also low. Mucocutaneous bleeds, particularly epistaxes, are a recurrent problem. These may be managed with nasal cautery, tranexamic acid, DDAVP or cryoprecipitate.

Investigations

- Prolonged PTT.
- Normal PT, TT, and fibrinogen.
- Prolonged bleeding time.
- Impaired ristocetin-induced platelet aggregation.
- Assays of factors VIIIc, VIII RAG, and VIII VWF.

Haemorrhagic disease of the newborn (HDN)

The vitamin K-dependent coagulation factors (II, VII, IX, X) are low at birth and fall further over the first 3 days of life. Vitamin K levels then rise as a result of synthesis by gut bacteria and absorption from the diet. HDN typically presents with gastrointestinal bleeding between the second and fourth days of life. Occasionally intracranial bleeding can occur. Babies who are breast fed, premature or have been exposed to perinatal asphyxia are at greatest risk. Prophylactic vitamin K is now given to all newborn babies shortly after birth. The recent suggestion of an association between intramuscular vitamin K and an increased risk of leukaemia has not been substantiated.

Investigations

- Prolonged PT.
- Prolonged PTT.

Further reading

Jones P. HIV infection and haemophilia. *Archives of Disease in Childhood,* 1991; **65:** 364–8.

Related topics of interest

Purpura and bruising (p. 330)
Shock (p. 344)

CALCIUM METABOLISM

Ninety-nine per cent of the total body calcium is present in the skeleton. The other 1% in extracellular and intracellular fluids plays a vital role in enzyme reactions, coagulation and neuromuscular functioning. Vitamin D, parathyroid hormone (PTH) and calcitonin act on bone, kidneys and gastrointestinal tract to maintain serum calcium concentrations within narrow limits. Hypocalcaemia and hypercalcaemia may be associated with disorders of vitamin D metabolism, parathyroid disease or non-endocrine disorders such as chronic renal failure. Hypocalcaemia is a more common problem than hypercalcaemia in childhood and, apart from excessive ingestion of vitamin D, causes of hypercalcaemia are rare.

Calcium

Serum calcium is present in three fractions which are in dynamic equilibrium: 50% ionized (active), 40% protein bound (inactive), 10% complexed to phosphate, citrate, etc. Routinely, total serum calcium is measured, but ionized calcium can be measured directly. Acidosis increases ionized calcium (H^+ ions compete for albumin binding sites) and alkalosis decreases ionized calcium. Hypoproteinaemia may lead to a low total serum calcium while ionized calcium levels remain normal. Fasting blood taken with the least amount of venous stasis gives the most accurate level.

Vitamin D (calciferol)

This is the collective term for ergocalciferol (vitamin D_2) and cholecalciferol (vitamin D_3), which occur naturally in foods, e.g. fish, eggs, butter. Absorption via the upper small intestine is impaired by steatorrhoea. Vitamin D_3 is also produced in skin by UV light acting on a precursor. Vitamin D is activated by hydroxylation in the liver to 25-hydroxy D and then in the proximal renal tubules to 1,25-dihydroxy D.

Actions

Increases serum calcium by:

- Increasing intestinal absorption.
- Increasing mobilization from bone (PTH dependent).
- Decreasing renal excretion.

Parathyroid hormone (PTH)

PTH is an 84-amino-acid peptide secreted by the chief cells of the parathyroid glands. It is coded for by a gene close to that for insulin on chromosome 11. PTH is cleaved from larger, biologically inactive precursors and released into the circulation with carboxy-terminal fragments. It is metabolized predominantly by the liver. There is diurnal variation in PTH secretion with higher levels in the early morning. Secretion is increased by hypocalcaemia, catecholamines, vitamin D metabolites and cortisol, and is suppressed by hypercalcaemia.

Actions

(a) Increases serum calcium by:

- Increasing resorption from bone.
- Decreasing renal excretion.
- Stimulating renal 1,25-dihydroxy D synthesis.

(b) Increases renal excretion of phosphate and bicarbonate.

Calcitonin

Calcitonin is a 32-amino-acid peptide synthesized and secreted by the parafollicular (C) cells of the thyroid gland, encoded by a gene on chromosome 11. Secretion is suppressed by hypocalcaemia, and increased by hypercalcaemia, gastrointestinal hormones, oestrogens and β-adrenergic agonists.

Actions

- Inhibits calcium resorption from bone.
- Increases renal excretion of calcium, phosphate, magnesium, sodium, potassium.
- Promotes effect of vitamin D on intestinal absorption of calcium.

The importance of calcitonin in homeostasis remains unclear as neither thyroidectomy nor calcitonin hypersecretion affect serum calcium levels. It may protect against unwanted bone resorption when demands for calcium are high, e.g. pregnancy, lactation.

Hypocalcaemia

Aetiology

- Hypoparathyroidism.
  Decreased secretion = true hypoparathyroidism.
  Decreased peripheral action of PTH = pseudohypoparathyroidism.
- Vitamin D deficiency – lack of sunshine, dietary deficiency, malabsorption.
- Acute or chronic renal failure.
- Renal tubular disorders, e.g. Fanconi syndromes.
- Hypomagnesaemia (e.g. due to i.v. feeding, drugs such as cisplatin) leads to PTH resistance and decreased PTH secretion.
- Long-term anticonvulsant treatment (phenytoin).
- Citrated blood.

Clinical features

Neonatal hypocalcaemia is a relatively common transient problem which may cause irritability, jitteriness and fits, but it is often asymptomatic. In older children, if the onset is rapid, there will be neuromuscular manifestations such as paraesthesia around the mouth, hands and feet, cramps, carpopedal spasms, tetany (Trousseau's and Chvostek's signs), and convulsions.

Hypoparathyroidism may be sporadic or familial, transient or permanent. It may be idiopathic or secondary (e.g. neck surgery or irradiation, hypomagnesaemia). It may be associated with DiGeorge syndrome, mucocutaneous candidiasis, Addison's disease, and other autoimmune diseases. Chronic hypocalcaemia associated with hypoparathyroidism results in ectodermal changes (dry skin, coarse hair, brittle nails, tooth enamel hypoplasia), cataracts, basal ganglia calcification, and mental retardation. Resistance to PTH (pseudo-hypoparathyroidism) produces a similar clinical picture which may be associated with characteristic dysmorphic features (Albright's hereditary osteodystrophy results in short stature, round facies, obesity, shortening of the fourth metacarpals). Some patients have this typical phenotype but have no evidence of PTH resistance or biochemical abnormality (pseudo-pseudo-hypoparathyroidism).

Rickets

Rickets is due to defective growth plate mineralization secondary to decreased calcium or phosphate availability.

(a) Calciopenic rickets:

- Vitamin D deficiency.
- Defective conversion of vitamin D to 1,25-dihydroxy D (e.g. renal failure).

(b) Phosphopenic rickets:

- Increased renal phosphate loss (Fanconi syndrome, vitamin D-resistant rickets = X-linked hypophosphataemic rickets).
- Inadequate phosphate intake (premature infants).

Clinical features of rickets include craniotabes, delayed closure of the anterior fontanelle and swelling of the metaphyses (particularly the wrists). Later features include softening and deformity of long bones, chest deformity and enlargement of the rib ends (rickety rosary).

Investigation

- Ionized calcium.
- Total protein/albumin.
- Phosphate, alkaline phosphatase. Low phosphate with raised alkaline phosphatase suggests rickets. Phosphate will be raised in both hypoparathyroidism and pseudo-hypoparathyroidism.

- Serum U&E, creatinine and urinalysis to exclude a primary renal cause (chronic renal failure, Fanconi syndrome).
- Serum magnesium. Hypocalcaemia will be difficult to correct until hypomagnesaemia is corrected.
- Serum PTH. Low or undetectable in hypoparathyroidism, high in pseudohypoparathyroidism, high in calciopenic rickets (secondary hyperparathyroidism), normal in phosphopenic rickets.
- Urinary cAMP and phosphate increase in response to PTH in hypoparathyroidism but not in pseudohypoparathyroidism.
- Plasma vitamin D metabolites. Low levels found in dietary rickets, liver disease, malabsorption and anticonvulsant treatment.

Management

1. Acute. Intravenous calcium gluconate infusion, correct hypomagnesaemia.

2. Long-term. Depends on cause, e.g. vitamin D analogues (calcitriol) used in calciopenic rickets and renal disease, phosphate supplements given in vitamin D resistant rickets, calcium supplements and vitamin D analogues used to treat hypoparathyroidism.

Hypercalcaemia

Aetiology

- Primary hyperparathyroidism (parathyroid hyperplasia, adenoma).
- Idiopathic infantile hypercalcaemia.
- Familial hypocalciuric hypercalcaemia (due to defective renal excretion of calcium).
- Hypervitaminosis D.
  (a) Increased intake (e.g. overtreatment of hypoparathyroidism, rickets).
  (b) Increased synthesis (increased conversion of 25-hydroxy D to 1,25-dihydroxy D seen in some patients with sarcoidosis, tuberculosis or malignancy).
- Other – congenital hypothyroidism, PTH-related protein produced by some tumours, maternal hypoparathyroidism.

Clinical features

Features include nausea and vomiting, constipation and polyuria. Irritability and failure to thrive are common in infants. Renal stones, bone pain and pathological fractures may occur. Nephrocalcinosis and ectopic calcification will occur if hypercalcaemia is long-standing, with subsequent renal failure. Idiopathic hypercalcaemia of infancy associated with mental retardation, cardiovascular abnormalities and dysmorphic features is known as William's syndrome. Primary hyperparathyroidism may be familial and is associated with the multiple endocrine neoplasia syndromes (MEN 1 and 2).

Investigation

- Phosphate, alkaline phosphatase.
- Total protein/albumin.
- Serum PTH. Low in vitamin D intoxication; inappropriately normal or raised in presence of hypercalcaemia indicates hyperparathyroidism.

Management

1. Acute. i.v. hydration with saline promotes calcium excretion, ± steroids, calcitonin, biphosphonates.

2. Long-term. Remove underlying cause.

Further reading

Bishop N. Bone disease in preterm infants. *Archives of Disease in Childhood,* 1989; **64**: 1403–9.

Kruse K. Disorders of calcium and bone metabolism. In: Brook CGD, ed. *Clinical Paediatric Endocrinology,* 3rd edn. Oxford: Blackwell Scientific Publications, 1995; 735–81.

Related topics of interest

Chronic renal failure (p. 82)

Polyuria and renal tubular disorders (p. 319)

CARDIAC ARREST

Cardiac arrest in childhood is usually secondary to hypoxia and is rarely due to primary cardiac disease. The outcome for respiratory arrest alone is often good, but the outcome for cardiac arrest is generally poor, even in children who are successfully resuscitated, as tissue hypoxia and acidosis prior to arrest frequently lead to subsequent multisystem failure. Following successful cardiopulmonary resuscitation (CPR), management aims to achieve and maintain homeostasis to optimize chances of recovery. Advanced paediatric life support (APLS) courses are run regularly in the UK to help doctors, nurses and paramedics deal with seriously ill and injured children more effectively. Prevention of cardiac arrest by earlier recognition of a seriously ill child will help reduce morbidity and mortality. The current CPR recommendations of the Advanced Life Support Group are given here.

Aetiology

1. Respiratory failure

- Respiratory distress, e.g. asphyxia, epiglottitis, asthma, bronchiolitis.
- Respiratory depression, e.g. raised intracranial pressure, convulsions, poisons.

2. Circulatory failure – shock

- Hypovolaemic.
- Cardiogenic.
- Septicaemic.
- Anaphylactic.

Basic life support

1. Call for assistance, approach the child with care and remove from continuing danger.

2. Airway. If the child is unresponsive to the question "Are you alright?" or gentle shaking, open and maintain the airway using the head tilt/chin lift manoeuvre. The jaw thrust manoeuvre is safer if there may be a cervical spine injury.

3. Breathing. Look, listen and feel for signs of breathing. If opening the airway has not led to resumption of breathing give five long mouth to mouth/nose breaths.

4. Circulation. Feel for a central pulse for 5 seconds (brachial or femoral in infants, carotid in older children). If absent commence cardiac compression at a rate of 100 per minute. A precordial thump is not recommended in children. Cardiac compression in infants is achieved by using two fingers to depress the sternum by 1.5–2.5 cm at a point one finger-breadth below the nipple line. Alternatively, the infant is held with both the rescuer's hands encircling the chest so the thumbs can compress the sternum in the correct position.

In small children the heel of one hand is used to compress the sternum one finger-breadth above the xiphisternum to a depth of 2.5–3.5 cm. In larger children the heels of both hands are used to compress the sternum two finger-breadths above the xiphisternum to a depth of 3–4.5 cm. A ratio of five compressions to one breath should be maintained (20 CPR cycles per minute).

Advanced life support

1. Airway and breathing. Look, listen, and feel for airway obstruction, respiratory arrest, depression or distress. If there is respiratory arrest or depression despite airway opening manoeuvres, commence ventilation with high-concentration oxygen via bag and mask or orotracheal intubation. Uncuffed tubes are preferred up to puberty as they cause less oedema at the cricoid ring. If intubation is impossible or unsuccessful consider needle cricothyroidectomy. Look for evidence of chest or neck trauma, and assess symmetry of chest movement and breath sounds.

2. Circulation. If there are no palpable central pulses, cardiac compression should be continued at a rate of 100 per minute, not stopping while a breath is given. Establish venous access. Commence pulse oximetry and ECG monitoring.

3. Arrhythmias. The child should have a secure airway and be adequately ventilated with high-concentration oxygen before any drugs are given. For children aged 1–10 years the weight (kg) can be estimated as 2 x (age + 4).

Arrhythmias

Asystole

Asystole is the most common arrhythmia in a childhood arrest. Prolonged severe hypoxia and acidosis cause progressive bradycardia leading to asystole.

- Adrenaline 10 mcg/kg i.v. or i.o. (intraosseous) or 100 mcg/kg via ETT. 10 mcg = 0.1 ml of 1:10 000.
- 3 minutes CPR, i.e. 60 cycles, consider sodium bicarbonate 1 mmol/kg i.v. or i.o. if profound acidosis is likely or if indicated by the venous pH (it may not be given via the ETT), and consider i.v. fluids.
- Adrenaline 100 mcg/kg i.v. or i.o.
- Further doses of adrenaline 100 mcg/kg i.v. or i.o. given every 3 minutes (i.e. 60 × 5:1 CPR cycles).
- Atropine is no longer in the asystole protocol.

Ventricular fibrillation (VF)

Ventricular fibrillation (VF) is uncommon in childhood but may occur in those with cardiac disease or recovering from hypothermia, or poisoned with tricyclics.

- Defibrillate 2 J/kg.
- Defibrillate 2 J/kg.
- Defibrillate 4 J/kg.
- Adrenaline 10 µg/kg i.v. or i.o.
- Three further shocks (4 J/kg).
- Adrenaline 100 µg/kg i.v. or i.o.
- Three further shocks (4 J/kg) 1 minute later.

VF due to hypothermia may be resistant until the core temperature is increased. Antiarrhythmic agents (e.g. lignocaine) and sodium bicarbonate should be considered in drug overdose.

Electromechanical dissociation

No output in the presence of QRS complexes on the ECG most commonly occurs in profound shock. It may also occur with tension pneumothorax, cardiac tamponade, drug overdose, hypothermia and electrolyte imbalance.

- Adrenaline 10 µg/kg i.v. or i.o., or 100 µg/kg via an ETT.
- Volume expansion with 20 ml/kg crystalloid i.v. or i.o.
- Look for the underlying cause and treat appropriately.
- Adrenaline 100 µg/kg i.v. or i.o. every 3 minutes (i.e. 60 x 5:1 CPR cycles).

Post-resuscitation management

1. Monitor blood pressure, heart rate and rhythm, oxygen saturation, arterial pH and gases, toe–core temperature and urine output. CVP monitoring is often useful. The role of intracranial pressure (ICP) monitoring is controversial.

2. Investigations. Chest radiograph, FBC (haematocrit and platelets), group and save serum for cross-match, U&Es, clotting screen (DIC, hepatocellular damage), blood glucose, liver function tests, ECG.

3. Maintain oxygenation.

4. Maintain circulation. Normalize acid–base and electrolyte balance and correct hypovolaemia. Inotropic support may be needed.

5. Normalize blood glucose and body temperature.

6. Maintain adequate analgesia and sedation. Detect and treat raised ICP.

Stopping resuscitation

CPR should be discontinued if there is no detectable cardiac output or cerebral activity after 30 minutes. Prolonged resuscitation attempts are indicated in the hypothermic child (continue until core temperature is at least 32°C) or those who have been poisoned with central depressant drugs.

Further reading

Basic life support. In: Advanced Life Support Group. *Advanced Paediatric Life Support – the Practical Approach,* 2nd edn. London: BMJ Publications, 1997; 21–9.

The management of cardiac arrest. In: Advanced Life Support Group, *Advanced Paediatric Life Support – the Practical Approach,* 2nd edn. London: BMJ Publications, 1997; 45–53.

Related topics of interest

Coma (p. 89)
Shock (p. 344)

CHILD PROTECTION

A child is considered to be abused if he or she is treated in a way that is unacceptable in a given culture at a given time.

Both boys and girls can be victims of abuse and young children are most at risk, as they are dependent on adults for their care. Most children are abused by either or both parents. Many abusing parents have a history of being abused themselves as a child. Children from all social levels may be affected, although abuse is more likely in those who are socially deprived.

Each year one child per 1000, under the age of 4 years, suffers severe physical abuse; however the true prevalence of child abuse is difficult to establish as much goes undetected. It is important to recognize child abuse to ensure further protection of that child and other children in the household. All professionals working with children, teachers, youth workers, health and social workers need to be aware of the warning signs of abuse. Recognized types of child abuse include:

- Physical abuse. Actual or likely physical injury to a child or failure to prevent physical injury (or suffering) to a child, including deliberate poisoning, suffocation and Münchausen's syndrome by proxy.
- Sexual abuse. Actual or likely sexual exploitation of a child or adolescent. The child may be dependent and/or developmentally immature.
- Neglect. Failing to provide the love, care, food or physical circumstances that will allow a child to grow and develop normally. This includes failure to protect from accidents.
- Emotional abuse. A child's behaviour and emotional development are severely affected by the parents persistent neglect or rejection. Emotional abuse may lead to failure to thrive or short stature.

Children are often victims of more than one form of child abuse.

Presentation of abuse

1. Bruising. Accidental bruises are common on shins and foreheads; bruising to the face, ears, shoulders, back and buttocks are more suggestive of non-accidental injury. Patterns from fingertips, bites, straps or sticks may be seen. Bruising of the thighs or genitalia should raise suspicion of child sexual abuse. Colour is an unreliable indication of the age of bruising.

2. Fractures. Accidental fractures usually present with the child upset and the injury is appropriate for the age and activity of that child. Non-accidental fractures are amongst the most serious of injuries sustained through physical abuse. They are sometimes difficult to detect and a skeletal survey may prove useful in cases of concern. Multiple fractures of varying ages; spiral, metaphyseal or epiphyseal fractures of long bones; rib fractures and skull fractures, associated with intracranial injury, are all highly suggestive of child abuse. Differential diagnoses include birth trauma, osteogenesis imperfecta, copper deficiency and other bone disease.

3. *Burns and scalds.* Non-accidental burns and scalds may occur by various methods, e.g. cigarette-tip burns, scalding bathwater or holding part of child directly under a heat source. Blistering of the lesion may cause diagnostic confusion with staphylococcal bullous impetigo.

4. *Failure to thrive.* Some children who are victims of child abuse fail to reach their expected growth potential. This process is complex and multifactorial, including inadequate calorie intake, recurrent illness, poverty and psychosocial difficulties.

5. *Child sexual abuse.* Behavioural changes, a disclosure by the child or local symptoms of vulval or anal soreness may lead to suspicion of the diagnosis. Examination must be approached with the utmost sensitivity; frequently there are no specific physical signs. Important signs include genital bruising, abrasion or laceration, hymenal dilatation or scars, reflex anal dilatation or identification of a sexually transmitted disease.

6. *Münchausen's syndrome by proxy.* Various symptoms and signs are fabricated to bring the child to the attention of medical staff on repeated occasions, e.g. seizures, apnoea, vomiting and diarrhoea. These may be brought about through suffocation or poisoning. The perpetrator, usually the mother, gives the impression of being caring and attentive. These people are not mentally ill, but they do have characteristic personalities.

7. *Intracranial injury.* Infants, usually under one year of age, may present with seizures or in a coma as a result of an intracranial bleed. Bleeding may occur as a result of a traumatic skull fracture or from shaking the baby. It is important to examine the eyes for evidence of retinal haemorrhage. Full examination including a skeletal survey is required. Differential diagnoses include birth trauma, congenital anomaly or coagulation disorder.

Clinical assessment

A history and examination should be conducted in the normal way, taking into account the developmental age of the child. Delay in presentation; an inconsistent story or examination findings that do not fit the history of injury, should all arouse the suspicion of non-accidental injury (NAI).

A full social history should be taken, including details of all carers involved with the child. The child's height and weight should be documented as well as their appearance, clothing, hygiene and behaviour.

Any injuries should be carefully recorded on a topographical chart, measuring bruises and indicating their colour. Retinal haemorrhages are easier to view after mydriatic drops in infants. In suspected sexual abuse repeated examinations should be avoided, and examination of the external genitalia should be performed at the end of the examination, taking suitable swabs at the time.

Investigation

- FBC, coagulation screen to exclude underlying blood dyscrasia in children with bruising.
- Skeletal survey to identify unrecognized fractures. Periosteal new bone formation is the earliest sign, at 10–14 days. Radioisotope bone scan may detect recent fractures in the presence of a normal skeletal survey.
- Serum copper and bone biochemistry may prove useful if there are fractures.
- Medical photographs.
- Cranial imaging if intracranial haemorrhage suspected.
- Microbiological and forensic swabs in suspected sexual abuse.

Management

Immediate medical treatment of injuries may be needed. The protection of the child is the next priority following discussion with other agencies, social services and police specialist child protection teams. For some children an 'Emergency Protection Order' is required to ensure a place of safety. In cases where child abuse is suspected, a multidisciplinary case conference is arranged. This allows the sharing of information about the incident and the family from all professional agencies; a risk assessment is made and a child protection plan formulated. This may include placing the child's name on the child protection register. An action plan should be made and all agencies will be allocated work to undertake with the child and family to ensure on-going protection.

Further reading

Hobbs C, Hanks H Wynne J. *Child Abuse and Neglect: A Clinician's Handbook*, 1st edn. London: Churchill Livingstone, 1993.

Meadow R. *ABC of Child Abuse*, 3rd edn. London: BMJ Publishing Group, 1997.

Royal Collage of Physicians. *Physical Signs of Sexual Abuse in Children*, 2nd edn. London: Royal College of Physicians, 1997.

Related topic of interest

Children and the law (p. 69)

CHILDREN AND THE LAW

Laws regarding children are of particular importance in issues of child protection, but they may also concern aspects of education, adoption, child safety and consent. The most significant piece of legislation in recent years has been the Children Act 1989, a wide-reaching reform of many previous acts of parliament regarding children, and of related court procedures.

The Children Act 1989

The Children Act 1989 was implemented in October 1991. Its aims are to restructure the court proceedings regarding child protection, providing a unified and practical approach for all agencies involved.

The general principles of the Children Act 1989 are:

- The children's welfare is of paramount importance.
- The children should be brought up with their families whenever possible. Local authorities should promote this, provided it is consistent with the children's welfare.
- Delay in court proceedings for child protection issues is harmful and should be avoided whenever possible.
- Courts should refer to a checklist of matters regarding children's welfare.
- Court orders should not be made unless they positively contribute to children's welfare.
- The concept of parental responsibility (replacing parental rights) is retained even if children become the subject of a care order.
- Children should give their own consent to medical investigation and treatment, if they have sufficient understanding.

Emergency protection procedures

Voluntary agreements with parents may allow a period of assessment of risk to the child, without the need for a court order, but in some cases access may be denied, or the child may need a temporary place of safety, and specific court actions may be required.

- The Emergency Protection Order (EPO) may be made in cases of immediate physical risk. The order lasts for up to 8 days, but may be challenged after 72 hours. The courts may extend it by a further 7 days, but only once. Applicants may be Social Services officers or the NSPCC. Police also have powers to remove the child into police protection for 72 hours if it is believed that the child may otherwise suffer significant harm.

- A Child Assessment Order (CAO) lasts for 7 days and enables an assessment of the child's health and welfare to take place in cases of suspicion of significant harm, often overriding the objections of the parents. However the CAO may not override the wishes of the child, if he or she is of sufficient understanding to make an informed decision. The local authority or the NSPCC may apply.

Care proceedings (either a Care Order or a Supervision Order) may be required if the child is suffering, or likely to suffer, significant harm.

- A Care Order places the parental responsibility with Social Services (in addition to the parents), and usually removes the child from home to foster homes, or a children's home, at least temporarily. There is usually a contract between Social Services and the parents, following full multidisciplinary review at a case conference.
- A Supervision Order gives Social Services the right to visit a child and impose conditions relevant to the child's management, e.g. nursery or clinic attendance.
- Interim Care Orders may be made, placing the child in local authority care while a full investigation of the child's risk and needs is undertaken.

Private law orders

The court can decide also to make private law orders concerning the child's welfare (the four Section 8 orders).

- A Residence Order determines with whom the child is to live.
- A Contact Order decides what contact the child may have with other people.
- A Specific Issues Order is required for any specific care issue for an individual child, e.g medical care or consent issues.
- A Prohibited Steps Order may forbid any specific step which may be taken by the parents which is not in the interests of the child, e.g. unsupervised visiting.

The law and education

The Education Act 1944

This Act stated that every child over 5 years old must receive full-time education until the end of the spring or summer term following the child's 16th birthday.

The Education Act 1981

This followed the Warnock report of 1978 recommending that "all children should have education appropriate to their needs", aiming to educate children in normal schools whenever possible. If it is known by health authority staff that a child over 2 years old is likely to have special educational needs, staff should inform the Local Education Authority (LEA) after obtaining permission from the parents. The LEA should then obtain written information from all professionals involved with the child before preparing a Statement of Educational Need, which is sent to the parents, and a school most appropriate to those needs is then nominated by the LEA. Parents have 30 days in which to appeal against the statement. Statements should be reviewed annually.

The Education Act 1993

'The Code of Practice'. This brought major changes to the way LEAs in England and Wales identify, assess and make provision for children with special educational needs (SEN). The Code offers practical advice to all those involved in the statementing process: schools, health and social services and parents.

The aim of this act is to enable all concerned to:

- improve the quality and coherence of the education of children with SEN in mainstream school;
- ensure that statutory assessment is focused and relevant;
- make the statement and review process more relevant and efficient.

Consent

Consent for children aged 16 years and younger is a controversial topic. Issues were highlighted in the Gillick Case (1986) which challenged doctors prescribing contraception for girls under 16 years of age, without consulting the parents. As a result the phrase 'Gillick competent' was founded. A child is judged to be competent if they have acquired sufficient maturity, intelligence and understanding to consent. However, for any child this does not happen at a fixed age. The Children Act states that a child with "sufficient understanding to make an informed decision" can refuse to submit to a care order. The degree of understanding and intelligence required will also vary according to the complexity of the issue, e.g. a tooth extraction or a major operation. It remains unclear how and by whom competency should be assessed. Ultimately, the decision rests with the health professional.

Further reading

Hendrick J. *Child Care Law for Health Professionals*, 1st edn. Oxford: Radcliffe Press, 1993.
Leslie SC. Child protection – The Children Act 1989. *Current Paediatrics*, 1993; **3** (3): 168–70.
Working Together Under the Children Act 1989. London: HMSO, 1991.

Related topics of interest

Adolescent health (p. 19)
Child protection (p. 65)
Learning disability (p. 236)

CHROMOSOMAL ABNORMALITIES

A normal human karyotype has a complement of 46 chromosomes (22 autosomal pairs and one pair of sex chromosomes XX or XY). Down's, Turner's and Klinefelter's syndromes were the first chromosome abnormalities identified, in 1959. With the advent of new molecular techniques many more chromosomal abnormalities have now been identified. Chromosomal abnormalities occur in approximately 6 per 1000 live births. The true incidence post conception is higher than this, but many result in spontaneous abortion. A chromosomal abnormality usually gives rise to multiple congenital malformations. Many can now be detected on prenatal testing, by ultrasound and amniocentesis.

Types of chromosome disorder

1. Numerical

- Polyploid
  Triploidy (69 chromosomes)is lethal.
- Aneuploid
  Trisomy 21(Down's syndrome).
  Monosomy of X chromosome(Turner's syndrome).
  47 chromosomes (Klinefelter's syndrome).

2. Structural

- Deletion
  Terminal deletion of 5p in cri-du-chat syndrome.
  Interstitial deletion 11p in Wilms' tumour.
- Translocation
  Balanced translocations cause no abnormality.
  Unbalanced may result in abortion or a syndrome.
- Fragile site
  Fragile X, mental retardation syndrome.
- Inversion.
- Duplication.
- Ring chromosome.

Down's syndrome (trisomy 21)

Down's syndrome is the commonest autosomal trisomy, affecting 1 in 650 live births, with the same number of fetuses failing to reach term. Most cases are due to non-dysjunction of chromosome 21 during meiosis. Only 5% of cases are due to translocation, in which chromosome 21 is translocated on to chromosome 14 or occasionally 22. The risk of having an affected child increases with maternal age, but 50% of affected infants are born to mothers under 35 years because of the higher birth rate in this age group. The overall risk is 1 in 650, but at 20 years it is only 1 in 2000. This rises steeply with maternal age to 1 in 450 risk at 35 years, 1 in 100 at 40 years and 1 in 30 at 45 years. The recurrence risk following one child with Down's syndrome is 1% if due to non-dysjunction but 10% if the mother carries a translocation. The recurrence risk if the father is the translocation carrier is 2–3%.

Amniocentesis should be offered to women with increased risk, i.e. age over 35 years, previous affected child, known balanced translocation carrier.

Clinical features

- Characteristic facial features. Epicanthic folds, flat occiput, protruding tongue.
- Eyes. Brushfield spots, nystagmus, myopia, early cataracts.
- Hands and feet. Brachydactyly, clinodactyly (incurved little fingers), abnormal dermatoglyphics, sandal toes (wide gap between first and second toes).
- Hypotonia. Motor delay, feeding difficulties, recurrent chest infections, increased risk of congenital dislocation of the hip and hernias.
- Gastrointestinal abnormalities. Increased risk of atresias (especially duodenal) and Hirschsprung's disease.
- Congenital heart defects (50%). Particularly septal defects, Fallot's tetralogy.
- Learning difficulties. Usually mild or moderate but rarely severe. High incidence of Alzheimer's disease in third and fourth decades.
- Glue ear. High incidence of conductive deafness.
- Leukaemia. Increased risk.

Edward's syndrome (trisomy 18)

This is the second commonest autosomal trisomy but the incidence is only 1.2 per 1000 live births. It is more common in girls than boys. The majority die in the neonatal period but a few have survived several years. It is associated with increased maternal age but the recurrence risk is low.

Clinical features

- Polyhydramnios and intrauterine growth retardation (IUGR).
- Craniofacial abnormalities. Low-set ears, prominent occiput, narrow head, micrognathia, narrow slanting palpebral fissures.
- Limb abnormalities. Clenched hands with overlapping fingers, rocker bottom feet, hypoplastic nails, flexion deformities.
- Congenital heart defects.
- Gastrointestinal abnormalities – especially exomphalos.
- Renal abnormalities.
- Severe learning difficulties.

Patau's syndrome (trisomy 13)

The incidence is 0.07 per 1000 live births and it is mainly due to non-dysjunction. The majority die in the first few days or weeks of life. Maternal age is less of a predisposing factor than for trisomies 18 and 21 and the recurrence risk is low.

Clinical features

- IUGR.
- Holoprosencephaly. Developmental defect of the forebrain resulting in a single cerebral hemisphere. Cyclops in the most severe form.
- Craniofacial abnormalities. Microcephaly, hypotelorism, small nose, cleft lip and palate (80%), microphthalmos.
- Scalp defects.
- Polydactyly.
- Renal and cardiac abnormalities.

Turner's syndrome (XO)

This is the only monosomy that is compatible with life. The incidence is 0.4 per 1000 live births and it is a common finding in first-trimester abortuses. Phenotypic abnormalities vary but are usually mild. The lifespan may be normal but sterility is almost invariable. Fifty-five per cent are 45XO, but the rest are mosaics or have other abnormalities. Pre-natal ultrasound may identify cystic hygroma, chylothorax, ascites or hydrops.

Clinical features

- Cystic hygroma and hydrops in second trimester.
- Lymphoedema at birth, especially hands and feet and back of neck (nuchal) swelling which can be detected on antenatal ultrasound.
- Short stature due in part to skeletal dysplasia. Growth may improve with growth hormone.
- Webbed neck, low posterior hairline, widely spaced nipples, nail changes, cubitus valgus (increased elbow carrying angle), tendency to keloid scarring.
- Congenital heart disease, particularly coarctation of the aorta (hypertension).
- Renal tract abnormalities. Common but not usually clinically significant, e.g. duplex ureters, horseshoe kidney.
- Streak ovaries, primary amenorrhoea and failure of development of secondary sexual characteristics. Puberty is induced with oestrogen replacement but the patient remains infertile. Osteoporosis in adult life occurs in the absence of oestrogen replacement.
- Intelligence. Normal or mild learning difficulties.

Fragile X syndrome

This is an inherited X-linked disorder which was first described in 1969. It is the commonest cause of learning difficulties in males after Down's syndrome, estimated to affect 1 in 2000 individuals, male and female. Analysis of chromosomes with special culture techniques identifies a fragile site on the long arm of the X chromosome (Xq27 folate-sensitive fragile site) in a proportion of cells (5 – 20%). Fragile sites may be seen in female carriers but the absence of sites does not exclude carrier status. The gene for Fragile X, FMR-1, has been isolated and is made up of CGG, trinucleotide repeats. In a premutation state the number of repeats is between 50 and 200. A true mutation will have anything from 200 to several thousand repeats. This process is called 'anticipation'. Premutation is usually sub-clinical, may be found in a carrier, and is likely to become an unstable mutation in offspring.

Clinical features

- Learning difficulties. Moderate to severe in males, mild to moderate in a third of female carriers.
- Craniofacial features. Large head (OFC often above 97th centile), large jaw and ears, prominent forehead.
- Large testes. Particularly after puberty.
- Connective tissue dysfunction. May present like Ehlers–Danlos or Marfan's syndromes. Mitral valve prolapse is not uncommon.

For information on molecular techniques see related topic Gene defects (p. 160).

Further reading

Chu CE, Connor JM. Molecular biology of Turner's syndrome. *Archives of Disease in Childhood,* 1995; **72:** 285–6.

Jones KL. *Smith's Recognisable Patterns of Human Malformation*, 5th edn. Philadelphia: WB Saunders, 1996.

Kingston H. *ABC of Clinical Genetics*, 2nd edn. London: BMJ Publishing Group, 1994; 22–31.

Winter RM. Fragile X mental retardation. *Archives of Disease in Childhood,* 1989; **64:** 1223–4.

Related topics of interest

Dysmorphology and teratogenesis (p. 128)
Fetal medicine (p. 141)
Gene defects (p. 160)
Growth – short and tall stature (p. 171)
Learning disability (p. 236)

CHRONIC DIARRHOEA

Persistent diarrhoea presents to the health professional when the frequency or looseness of the child's stools is perceived by the parent to be excessive. However, there is a wide variation in the 'normal' pattern, depending on the age and diet of the individual child. Constipation with 'overflow', i.e. semiliquid stool seeping past an impacted faecal mass, often with incontinence, may present as chronic diarrhoea, and this diagnosis should be considered at an early stage.

Toddler diarrhoea (chronic non-specific diarrhoea of infancy)

Typically, a pattern of variable diarrhoea occurs in a child of 6–24 months who is otherwise well and thriving. Constipation and diarrhoea may alternate, and both mucus and undigested food matter are often seen in the stool. The diarrhoea is rarely nocturnal. Diagnosis depends on the demonstration of normal growth and a clinical exclusion of other pathology. Sucrose intolerance and infestation with *Giardia* may cause chronic diarrhoea with normal growth, and these conditions may need to be excluded by appropriate investigation (see below). Parents should be reassured that the problem is likely to resolve spontaneously, and a simple explanation of intestinal motility is often helpful. Exclusion of cow's milk and egg under dietetic supervision may help in those children with a history of atopy. Other children may benefit from a diet high in polyunsaturated fat or from avoiding fruit juices with a high fructose:sucrose ratio.

Protracted diarrhoea

This is defined as the passage of four or more loose stools a day for over 2 weeks, with associated failure to thrive. Occasionally at presentation, the child may be severely ill, and resuscitation must then precede thorough investigation. A wide range of conditions must then be considered.

Aetiology of protracted diarrhoea

1. Infection. *Giardia lamblia,* enteropathogenic *Escherichia coli*, hookworm.

2. Protein intolerance. Coeliac disease, cow's milk or soy protein intolerance.

3. Carbohydrate intolerance. Lactase deficiency, secondary lactose intolerance.

4. Drugs. Laxatives, antibiotics, cytotoxics.

5. Inflammation. Ulcerative colitis, Crohn's disease, graft-versus-host disease.

6. Surgical conditions. Hirschsprung's disease, malrotation, blind loop syndrome.

7. Endocrine disorders. Hyperthyroidism, Addison's disease.

8. Immunodeficiency. AIDS, severe combined immunodeficiency.

9. Pancreatic insufficiency. Cystic fibrosis, Schwachman syndrome.

10. Other disorders. Congenital chloridorrhoea, lymphangiectasia, small bowel lymphoma, abetalipoproteinaemia, autoimmune enteropathy, microvillus atrophy, Münchausen by proxy syndrome.

Clinical assessment

The history must establish the exact timing of the onset of diarrhoea, e.g. from birth, after recent acute gastroenteritis or following travel abroad. Introduction of new food substances such as gluten or cow's milk may also be relevant. Systematic enquiry should seek to exclude features of generalized chronic disease such as cystic fibrosis. Family history may be important in coeliac disease (approximately 10% of siblings are at risk), the inborn errors of metabolism and cystic fibrosis. A clear account of the stool frequency, consistency and presence of blood or mucus must be obtained, and any associated features (abdominal pain, allergic manifestations) should be noted. Examination must include assessment of nutritional status (weight, length, head circumference, skinfold thickness and mid-arm circumference) and dehydration. There may be specific signs of disease, e.g. respiratory signs in cystic fibrosis, but often no diagnostic clues are present.

Investigation

Certain selected investigations only may be required, depending on clinical assessment.

- FBC, with film, ESR. Coagulation studies, especially prior to jejunal biopsy.
- U&E, creatinine and acid–base balance.
- Serum calcium, phosphate, alkaline phosphate, ferritin and folate. Trace metals (zinc, copper).
- Antigliadin antibodies, endomysium antibodies.

- Stool specimens for microbiology (MC&S, virology, parasites), electrolytes, reducing substances, chromatography, fat globules.
- Sweat test.
- Radiological investigations: abdominal radiograph, barium meal and follow-through.
- Immunological profile, including functional assessment.
- Jejunal biopsy.
- Pancreatic function tests, e.g. stool chymotrypsin, pancreolauryl test, aspiration of duodenal juice.
- Other tests: colonoscopy and biopsy, breath hydrogen test, thyroid function tests, congenital infection screen, gastrointestinal hormone profile, gut auto-antibody screen.

The management approach will be determined by the degree of illness of the child and the facilities available locally. It may be appropriate in certain cases to refer the child to a centre where specialist diagnostic and supportive services are available.

Further reading

Devane SP, Candy DCA. Investigation of chronic diarrhoea. *Current Paediatrics,* 1992; **2** (4): 189–93.

Puntis JWL. Assessment of pancreatic exocrine function. *Archives of Disease in Childhood,* 1993; **69:** 99–101.

Related topics of interest

Coeliac disease (p. 86)
Constipation (p. 97)
Cystic fibrosis (p. 107)
Failure to thrive (p. 138)
Gastroenteritis (p. 152)

CHRONIC FATIGUE SYNDROME

The symptom complex now known as chronic fatigue syndrome (CFS), has only relatively recently been recognized and recognition of the syndrome in children is more recent than that in adults. It has been given a variety of names including myalgic encephalomyelitis and post-viral fatigue syndrome but these names imply a known pathology or aetiology and in many cases this cannot be demonstrated. Epstein–Barr virus infection can result in a similar clinical picture which has led to the hypothesis that CFS is due to a viral infection. Because many aspects of the condition are still unexplained, theories of causation and ideas on management are controversial. However, children affected by the disease can be considerably disabled for sometimes prolonged periods of time and it is important that health professionals are supportive and provide appropriate information and treatment. For most children, management is best done in primary care, but for children who are severely affected a multidisciplinary approach involving GP, paediatrician, child psychiatrist, school and other health care professionals is required.

Clinical features

CFS is commoner in girls and in childhood, usually presents in the early teenage years. There is a higher incidence in the higher socio-economic groups. For most children, onset is sudden with an acute illness, but the fatigue must have been present for at least 2 months for it to be said to be chronic. Recovery may take several months or sometimes years although symptom severity may fluctuate. The fatigue is out of proportion to the activity precipitating it and lasts for longer than would normally be expected. In addition the child may have other symptoms including:

- Headaches.
- Abdominal pains, nausea.
- Excessive and unrefreshing sleep.
- Sore throat and cervical lymphadenopathy.
- Myalgia, arthralgia.
- Poor concentration, low mood.

Examination should look for evidence of other conditions which present with similar symptoms, e.g. primary muscle disease, hypothyroidism or renal failure. Psychiatric diagnoses such as depression and school phobia should also be excluded and may require assessment by a child psychiatrist.

Investigations

The diagnosis is one of exclusion so that depending on the history certain investigations may be needed to rule out other causes of the symptoms. For example:

- FBC and film.

- Serology for Epstein–Barr virus.
- Plasma viscosity.
- U&E, creatinine, calcium.
- LFTs.
- Thyroid function.
- Creatine kinase.

Management

1. Rest and activity are both important. At the beginning of the illness the child may need to spend a large part of the day resting. Normal activities should then be slowly started. A useful guide for the child is that they should be able to repeat the amount done on one day, the following day. If they are too tired the following day they have done too much. A staged return to normal activities including school should be planned. Sessions of physical or mental activity should be followed by rest. Swimming is a very helpful form of exercise. In severe cases, a physiotherapist is helpful in formulating exercise programmes.

2. Drug treatment. Various drugs have been tried but are not found to be effective. In children where sleep is a particular problem or in those who have low mood, amitriptylline may be helpful.

3. Educational support. Most children will be able to continue at school but some may need to attend part-time for a period at the beginning of their illness. If they are unable to attend school at all it is important to involve the home tutoring service to prevent too great a disruption in their schooling.

Further reading

Vereker MI. Chronic fatigue syndrome: a joint paediatric–pyschiatric approach. *Archives of Disease in Childhood,* 1992, **67:** 550–555.

Related topic of interest

Adolescent health (p. 19)

CHRONIC RENAL FAILURE

Renal insufficiency results from loss of functioning nephrons, but there is remarkable renal reserve. The glomerular filtration rate (GFR) can fall by over 50% before nitrogenous waste products (urea and creatinine) accumulate and is reduced to 25% before symptoms and signs of renal failure occur. The incidence of chronic renal failure in the UK is 2–3 children per million population per year.

Problems

- Anaemia.
- Hypertension.
- Hyperkalaemia.
- Growth failure.
- Renal osteodystrophy.
- Hyperuricaemia.
- Type IV hyperlipidaemia.

Aetiology

- Glomerulonephritis (30–35%).
- Reflux nephropathy / chronic pyelonephritis (~ 20%).
- Renal tract malformations (25–30%) – hypoplastic, dysplastic or cystic kidneys, obstruction, e.g. posterior urethral valves.
- Hereditary renal disorders (~10%), e.g. Alport's syndrome, cystinosis.
- Haemolytic uraemic syndrome (1–2%).
- Cortical or tubular necrosis (1–2%).

Clinical features

The onset of symptoms is usually insidious, but acute deterioration may be precipitated by intercurrent infection or dehydration.

1. GFR 20–25% of normal (chronic renal failure)

- Polyuria, polydipsia, enuresis, failure to thrive, hypertension.

2. GFR 5–20%

- Anorexia, metabolic acidosis, failure to thrive, bone pain (renal osteodystrophy).

3. GFR < 5% (end-stage renal failure)

- Oliguria and oedema, anaemia, lethargy, itching, nausea. Dialysis or transplantation is necessary for survival.

Investigation

- U&E creatinine, bicarbonate. Raised urea and creatinine, hyperkalaemia, metabolic acidosis.
- Glomerular filtration rate. Measured by either creatinine clearance or ^{51}Cr-EDTA clearance (height^2 (m)/40 gives a rough guide to the GFR).

- Serum calcium, phosphate, alkaline phosphatase. Hyperphosphataemia, hypocalcaemia, raised alkaline phosphatase. Hyperphosphataemia results from impaired renal excretion and leads to decreased absorption of calcium. Hyperphosphataemia also causes a secondary increase in parathyroid hormone (PTH) secretion, which promotes calcium resorption (renal osteodystrophy). Bone resorption is increased by acidosis. Relative vitamin D resistance occurs as a result of impaired renal hydroxylation of 25-OH calciferol to 1,25-OH calciferol, resulting in reduced calcium absorption from the gut. Although the total serum calcium is low, symptoms are rare since acidosis increases the proportion of ionized calcium.
- Full blood count. Normochromic normocytic anaemia due to decreased red cell production and shortened red cell lifespan. Iron and folic acid deficiency may result from poor dietary intake. Erythropoietin levels are low.
- Uric acid. Raised and may worsen renal failure by causing a uric acid nephropathy.
- Lipids. Raised triglycerides and cholesterol.
- Radiology. Renal tract ultrasound, intravenous urography (IVU), MCU and isotope scans, may help identify cause. Radiographs of wrists, hands and knees to identify renal osteodystrophy.
- Renal biopsy.

Management

Chronic renal failure is rarely reversible so management is aimed at preserving the remaining renal function and minimizing metabolic disturbances. These children are best managed by an established multidisciplinary team within a specialist renal unit.

1. Hypertension. This is due to the primary renal disease or to salt and water overload. If treated promptly and effectively the rate of progression of renal failure may be slowed and there may even be a modest rise in GFR. Beta-blockers and diuretics are used, with a vasodilator such as hydralazine if severe. Acute hypertensive crises may occur and require urgent intravenous therapy.

2. Renal osteodystrophy. The clinical consequences of renal failure on bone and calcium metabolism are:

- Osteitis fibrosa cystica (due to secondary hyperparathyroidism).

- Rickets (due to vitamin D resistance).
- Ectopic calcification (due to an increased calcium/phosphate product despite hypocalcaemia).

Early recognition is important, and serum calcium, phosphate, and alkaline phosphatase should be monitored in addition to radiology. A rise in PTH may be the best early indicator. Specific treatments include dietary restriction of phosphate, oral phosphate-binding agents (e.g. calcium carbonate) and vitamin D derivatives (1,25 dihydroxy vitamin D (calcitriol) or 1α-OH calciferol (alphacalcidol)).

3. Anaemia. Iron and folic acid supplements are given (serum ferritin should be monitored to prevent iron overload). Erythropoietin can be given intravenously, subcutaneously or intraperitoneally to maintain the haemoglobin. Transfusions may aggravate hypertension and fluid overload.

4. Nutrition. An adequate calorific intake is essential to maintain growth and good nutritional status. Dietary supplements and nasogastric feeding should be considered early. The degree of protein restriction depends on the GFR, and fluid intake depends on the urine output and state of hydration. The calcium intake should be adequate and phosphate intake restricted. Vitamin supplements are given in the form of Ketovite liquid and tablets. Oral bicarbonate supplements may be required if acidosis is marked. Growth hormone may help maintain height velocity.

5. Hyperkalaemia. Severe or worsening hyperkalaemia is an indication for dialysis. Dextrose and insulin, calcium resonium, and nebulized salbutamol can be used to reduce serum potassium levels acutely.

6. Dialysis. At least five children per million population are accepted on to dialysis programmes in Europe each year. Indications for dialysis vary, but it should be considered when fluid overload, electrolyte disturbances, acidosis and symptomatic uraemia remain uncontrolled despite conservative treatment. Continuous ambulatory peritoneal dialysis (CAPD) is the preferred method, and only a small minority receive haemodialysis. Complications of CAPD include peritoneal catheter site infections and peritonitis.

7. *Renal transplantation.* Renal transplantation is now the established treatment for end-stage renal failure in children. In the UK more than 80% of first cadaver donor kidneys are functioning at 1 year and there is an almost 100% success rate with live related donor kidneys.

Further reading

Maxwell H, Rees L. Growth hormone treatment in infants with chronic renal failure. *Archives of Disease in Childhood,* 1996; **74** (1): 40–3.

Mehls O, Fine RN. Chronic renal failure in children. In: Cameron S, Davison AM, Grünfeld JP, Kerr D, Ritz E, eds. *Oxford Textbook of Clinical Nephrology.* Oxford: Oxford University Press, 1992; 1605–21.

Rees L, Rigden SPA, Ward G, Preece MA. Treatment of short stature in renal disease with recombinant growth hormone. *Archives of Disease in Childhood,* 1990; **65:** 856–60.

Trompeter RS. Renal transplantation. *Archives of Disease in Childhood,* 1990; **65:** 143–6.

Related topics of interest

Calcium metabolism (p. 56)
Glomerulonephritis (p. 164)
Urinary tract infection (p. 370)

COELIAC DISEASE

The basic aetiology of coeliac disease is unknown. Malabsorption is accompanied by characteristic morphological abnormalities in the small intestinal mucosa, which revert to normal when gluten is removed from the diet. Relapse occurs when gluten-containing foods are reintroduced into the diet. The prevalence in the UK is fairly constant at 1 in 2000, with a much higher incidence in Ireland and a much lower incidence outside Europe. Ten per cent of patients have an affected first-degree relative, and there is a high prevalence (> 80%) of HLA groups B8, DR3, and DQw2 and also of DR7 and DR2G in affected patients.

Problems

- Malabsorption.
- Abdominal pain and distension.
- Growth failure.
- Dermatitis herpetiformis.
- Malignancy.

Pathology

The proximal small bowel mucosa is predominantly affected, and it is the α-gliadin peptide fraction of the gluten in wheat, rye, barley and oats which causes damage. Histologically there is subtotal villous atrophy, with loss of the villous pattern. There is compensatory crypt hypertrophy, and the surface columnar epithelial cells become cuboidal, with increased intraepithelial lymphocytes. There are increased numbers of plasma cells and lymphocytes in the lamina propria.

Clinical features

At a variable period after introduction of cereals into the diet, failure to thrive may become a feature, accompanied in many cases by abdominal symptoms. Wasting is sometimes marked, e.g. over the buttocks. Stools may be loose, pale, bulky and offensive. Abdominal distension, anorexia, vomiting and abdominal pain are common symptoms. Typically, the child is miserable and irritable. Iron deficiency anaemia with hypochromic indices is a frequent finding and may be the major presenting feature, although folate levels may also be low. Hypoalbuminaemia with oedema, hypoprothrombinaemia and vitamin D deficiency are rarer findings.

Investigation

- FBC, red cell folate, ferritin.
- Coagulation screen – abnormalities should be corrected before jejunal biopsy is performed.
- Serum albumin, calcium, phosphate, alkaline phosphatase.
- Antigliadin, antiendomysium and antireticulin antibodies.
- Jejunal biopsy.

Other screening tests such as the xylose absorption test and barium follow-through studies may also be abnormal, but are not routinely performed.

Diagnostic criteria

The European Society of Paediatric Gastroenterology and Nutrition (ESPGAN) revised and clarified the practical approach to diagnosis of coeliac disease in 1989. The initial step in diagnosis remains the finding of characteristic small bowel mucosal changes on histological examination of a biopsy specimen. This should be followed by an unequivocal clinical remission on a strict gluten-free diet. A gluten challenge is not mandatory in all patients, but is recommended if there was doubt about the initial diagnosis, e.g. no initial biopsy performed, or doubtful histology. Also, in children under 2 years old, there is a high incidence of other causes of enteropathy, e.g. post-infectious and cows' milk-sensitive enteropathy, and a later gluten challenge is advisable. When gluten challenge is performed, a control biopsy taken when the patient is on a gluten-free diet is essential, taking a further specimen 3–6 months after challenge (or earlier if clinical relapse), and again at 2 years after challenge if the patient remains well. Very late relapses (up to 7 years) have been reported, and prolonged clinical monitoring is needed. The presence of circulating antibodies to gliadin, reticulin, endomysium and jejunum is a valuable adjunct to the clinical assessment, and is of value for preliminary screening, in monitoring clinical response and in detecting relapse and non-compliance.

Management

The clinical response to a gluten-free diet is usually seen within a few weeks, with an improvement in temperament, abdominal symptoms and weight gain. Replacement haematinics may be needed initially. Expert dietary advice should be given, and parents should make contact with the Coeliac Society for further practical help. Adolescents may question the need to continue their diet, and this is a further indication to consider a challenge biopsy. Once the diagnosis is firmly established the diet should be life-long as dietary compliance may possibly be protective against coeliac-associated malignancies (T-cell lymphoma and carcinoma of jejunum and oesophagus) in adult life. Dermatitis herpetiformis responds to the diet, but also to dapsone.

Further reading

Challacombe DN. Screening tests for coeliac disease. *Archives of Disease in Childhood,* 1995; **73:** 3–4.
Report of the Working Group of ESPGAN. Revised criteria for diagnosis of coeliac disease. *Archives of Disease in Childhood,* 1990; **65:** 909–11.
Tighe R, Ciclitira PJ. Molecular biology of coeliac disease. *Archives of Disease in Childhood,* 1995; **73:** 189–91.

Related topics of interest

Chronic diarrhoea (p. 77)
Failure to thrive (p. 138)

COMA

The major causes of altered consciousness level in childhood are head injury, CNS infections, hypoxic–ischaemic events and metabolic disturbances. Acute encephalopathy is manifested by a combination of altered consciousness level and seizures, and is a major cause of death and neurological sequelae. Primary management of coma is aimed at cardiopulmonary resuscitation and support. Secondary management aims to determine and treat the cause.

Aetiology

- Infection (35%). Meningitis, encephalitis.
- Cerebral anoxia and ischaemia. Shock, cardiorespiratory arrest, drowning.
- Trauma. Accidental, non-accidental.
- Drugs and poisons. Alcohol, barbiturates, lead, Munchausen by proxy.
- Metabolic
  - Diabetes mellitus (hypoglycaemia, ketoacidosis).
  - Hepatic failure, Reye's syndrome.
  - Uraemia (e.g. haemolytic uraemic syndrome).
  - Hyponatraemia.
  - Inborn errors of metabolism.
  - Post-burns encephalopathy.
- Vascular. Intracranial bleeding (e.g. arteriovenous malformation), thrombosis (e.g. DIC, sagittal sinus).
- Acute hypertension.
- Epilepsy. Post-ictal, status epilepticus.
- Intracranial tumour.
- Haemorrhagic shock encephalopathy.

Primary assessment and management

1. Airway. Clear and maintain.

2. Breathing. Give oxygen. Intubation and ventilation should be considered if the child is not breathing adequately, there are no cough or gag reflexes, the child is unresponsive or there are signs of impending tentorial herniation.

3. Circulation. Insert an i.v. line, take bloods for investigations (including BM Stix). Check blood pressure and pulse rate. If the patient is hypotensive give a 20 ml/kg plasma bolus over 5–10 minutes. If the patient is hypoglycaemic, give an i.v bolus of 10% dextrose and then commence a 10% dextrose infusion.

4. Obtain a brief history of the illness/accident from an accompanying adult (parent, paramedic) while initial assessment and management are proceeding, including any relevant past medical history, drugs and allergies.

5. Assessment of neurological status. Assess consciousness level using the AVPU system (alert, responds to voice, responds to pain, or unresponsive). Assess coma score prior to sedative or paralysing drugs, using the Glasgow coma scale (best motor, verbal and eye-opening responses – a modified scale is available for children under 4 years). Note any decorticate (flexed arms, extended legs) or decerebrate (extended arms and legs) posturing. Note pupillary dilation, inequality or unresponsiveness (third nerve compression) which suggests tentorial herniation of the ipsilateral hippocampal gyrus. Small pupils are seen with narcotic, barbiturate and phenothiazine poisoning. Bilaterally dilated pupils are seen post-ictally, in late barbiturate poisoning and with irreversible brain damage. Tentorial herniation may also cause a sixth nerve palsy. Hypertension, bradycardia and an irregular respiratory pattern are signs of cerebellar tonsil herniation through the foramen magnum ('coning').

6. Clinical examination. Note any evidence of sepsis (rash, neck stiffness) or trauma (including CSF leakage from ears or nose). The breath may smell of alcohol. Hepatomegaly is a feature of Reye's syndrome and some inborn errors of metabolism.

7. Treat any identifiable causes, e.g. DKA, and treat any seizures. If sepsis is suspected or no other cause can be found for the coma treat with broad-spectrum antibiotics and consider i.v. acyclovir.

- FBC and clotting studies.
- U&E, creatinine, calcium.
- Glucose.
- Blood culture.
- Arterial blood gas.
- Group and save serum (cross-match if the patient has sustained major trauma).

Secondary assessment and management

The cause of coma may be apparent from the primary assessment, but if it is not then a thorough history and examination with further investigations should follow. Further neurological assessment should include oculocephalic (doll's eye) reflexes (avoid in children with neck injuries), fundoscopy (papilloedema may not occur if there is an acute rise in ICP, retinal haemorrhages may indicate non-accidental injury) and examination for lateralizing signs. If the cause is thought to be trauma (accidental or non-accidental), a thorough search should be made for other injuries, including intra-abdominal injury. Whatever the cause of coma, it is vital to maintain homeostasis.

- Ensure good oxygenation.
- Maintain blood pressure.
- Normalize acid–base and electrolyte balance.
- Maintain blood glucose.
- Maintain body temperature.
- Detect and treat raised ICP.

Further investigation

- Urine culture.
- Urinalysis. For glucose, protein, blood.
- Blood and urine for toxicology.
- Liver function tests and ammonia.
- Lactate, pyruvate.
- Radiology (CT scan, US, chest radiographs).
- Lumbar puncture. Contraindicated until evidence of raised intracranial pressure is excluded by CT scan. CSF for bacteriology, virology, metabolic investigations.

Raised intracranial pressure (ICP)

Most causes of coma are accompanied by a degree of raised ICP, resulting from either an expanding space-occupying lesion (e.g. haematoma) or cerebral oedema. The aims of treatment are to maintain adequate cerebral blood flow for the brain's metabolic needs and to prevent the ICP rising to a level which will result in brain herniation. Cerebral blood flow is dependent on both cerebral perfusion pressure (CPP = mean arterial blood pressure minus ICP) and cerebrovascular resistance (controlled by vascular autoregulation, which may be impaired by trauma, hypoxia or ischaemia).

The child should be nursed head up with the head in the midline to encourage cerebral venous drainage. A raised arterial $P\text{CO}_2$ will cause cerebral vessels to dilate, leading to a further rise in ICP. The role of hyperventilation to maintain a low $P\text{CO}_2$ is controversial since it may reduce an already critical cerebral blood flow, but a low–normal level is recommended. Mannitol reduces cerebral oedema by raising the plasma osmolality and drawing water into the intravascular space, but dangers include hyperviscosity and prerenal failure. Barbiturates (e.g. thiopentone) reduce the cerebral metabolic rate but may cause systemic hypotension. Hypothermia will reduce metabolic requirements but may be impractical. There is no good evidence that fluid restriction reduces ICP, although it is vital that hypo-osmolar intravenous fluids are avoided. The role of invasive ICP monitoring remains controversial, as the exact level at which brain dysfunction occurs is unclear, but it is useful to monitor the effects of treatments such as mannitol.

Further reading

Coma. In: Advanced Life Support Group. *Advanced Paediatric Life Support – the Practical Approach,* 2nd edn. London: BMJ Publishing, 1997; 119–28.

Sharples PM. Intracranial pressure monitoring in comatose children: concepts and controversies. *Current Paediatrics,* 1991; **1:** 46–8.

Related topics of interest

Hypertension (p. 199)
Inborn errors of metabolism (p. 215)
Meningitis and encephalitis (p. 265)
Shock (p. 344)

CONGENITAL INFECTION

Many organisms can cross the placenta to cause fetal infection, and although severe neonatal symptoms may occur, intrauterine infections are frequently subclinical at birth. The term TORCH includes toxoplasmosis, rubella, cytomegalovirus (CMV) and herpes, but excludes several important pathogens.

Problems

- Spontaneous abortion and stillbirth.
- Congenital malformations.
- Hydrops fetalis.
- Neonatal septicaemia.
- Non-specific neonatal illness, e.g. rash, hepato-splenomegaly.
- Long-term sequelae.

Toxoplasmosis

The protozoon *Toxoplasma gondii* may be transmitted to pregnant women at various stages of its life cycle, including the ingestion of cysts in undercooked meat or oocysts via the faeces of infected kittens. Twenty per cent of pregnant women will already be seropositive following previous, often asymptomatic, infection, but a primary infection during pregnancy may infect the fetus, causing microcephaly, jaundice, hepatosplenomegaly and thrombocytopenia – the classical triad of hydrocephalus, chorioretinitis and intracranial calcification is rare. Diagnosis depends on serological techniques on maternal and neonatal serum, and parasite isolation from blood and tissue. Infection may be treated with spiramycin, alternating with pyrimethamine, sulphadiazine and folinic acid, although efficacy is unproven.

Rubella

Rubella causes a mild viral illness in young children, but maternal rubella infection in the first 16 weeks of pregnancy may lead to fetal damage – up to 90% of pregnancies infected during the first 8–10 weeks are affected. Infants with the congenital rubella syndrome (CRS) are generally small for gestational age, with multiple congenital defects, including cataracts, retinopathy, deafness, microcephaly, congenital heart defects and bony lesions. There may be isolated sensorineural deafness. Diagnosis of congenital rubella may be confirmed by virus isolation from urine or nasopharyngeal secretions, or by the persistence of rubella-specific IgM in the infant during the first 6 months of life. There is no specific treatment. Since the introduction of rubella immunization cases of CRS have fallen in number. Girls between 10 and 14 years should receive rubella vaccine if not previously vaccinated with MMR.

Cytomegalovirus

Cytomegalovirus (CMV) is a herpesvirus that is usually asymptomatic in healthy individuals and, once acquired, may become latent for years. Congenital CMV infection usually results from primary maternal infection at any stage of pregnancy, and affects 3 per 1000 pregnancies in the UK, although only 10% of these will result in long-term sequelae. Clinical features in the neonate may include intrauterine growth retardation, microcephaly, sensorineural hearing loss, hepatosplenomegaly, jaundice, chorioretinitis and thrombocytopenia. Diagnosis is by virus isolation from urine, or the detection of specific IgM in neonatal serum.

Herpes simplex

Neonatal herpes simplex virus (HSV) infection affects 2 per 1000 live births in the UK. The majority of infections are acquired perinatally from the maternal genital tract, although transplacental or post-natal spread may also be responsible. The risk of transmission is greatest if the mother has active, primary genital herpes at delivery, and Caesarean section should be considered in these circumstances. Intrauterine infection may present with skin scars, microcephaly and chorioretinitis at birth. Neonatally acquired HSV infection can cause a severe disseminated infection, which may have a delayed onset of up to 3 weeks. It has a mortality of 50%, even with intravenous acyclovir. Diagnosis is by electron microscopy of fluid from skin vesicles, or virus isolation from nasopharynx or conjunctivae.

Listeriosis

Listeria monocytogenes is a Gram-positive bacterial rod which survives at low temperatures. Outbreaks have been associated with the consumption of paté, soft cheeses and coleslaw. Vertical transmission may occur transplacentally, causing septicaemia in the first 48 hours, or perinatally, usually causing meningitis and/or septicaemia during the second week of life. There may be maternal pyrexia, prolonged rupture of the membranes or meconium staining of liquor. Focal cutaneous granulomas may be seen on the baby's pharynx or skin. Diagnosis is by culture of the organism from tissue, blood, CSF, surface swabs or amniotic fluid. Antibiotic treatment is with intravenous ampicillin and an aminoglycoside.

Parvovirus B19

Human parvovirus B19 is a common virus world-wide, responsible for slapped cheek syndrome (fifth disease), arthralgia and aplastic crises in patients with red cell disorders. Twenty-five per cent of adult infections are asymptomatic. Spread is by respiratory droplet from a patient incubating the virus (before the rash appears), and viral replication then occurs in fetal haemopoietic tissue, occasionally infecting the myocardium. Spontaneous abortion, hydrops fetalis or a neonatal illness with purpura, cardiomegaly and hepatosplenomegaly may result. Diagnosis may be confirmed by antibody measurement (specific IgG and IgM) in maternal, fetal or neonatal serum or by virus identification (B19 DNA or B19 antigen) in blood, tissue or amniotic fluid.

Varicella zoster

Primary maternal varicella zoster virus infection in the first trimester may result in neonatal abnormalities such as cicatricial skin lesions in a dermatomal distribution, microcephaly, cerebellar hypoplasia and skeletal and eye anomalies. Primary infection in the second or third trimester or reactivated latent zoster virus carries less risk. Perinatal chickenpox, however, can cause a devastating neonatal illness with a rash and pneumonitis in babies whose mothers develop a chickenpox rash up to and including 5 days before delivery, or up to 2 days after delivery. These babies should be protected by intramuscular zoster immune globulin as soon as possible after delivery. Early neonatal treatment with acyclovir may not prevent fatalities.

HIV infection – vertical transmission

(see also related topic Immunodeficiency, p. 210)
Transmission of HIV from an infected mother may occur prenatally, perinatally or postnatally. The European Collaborative Study (1992) has reported vertical transmission rates of 13–16% (up to 40% in Africa). Transmission is more likely in the presence of symptomatic disease in the mother, premature delivery, or if HIV is acquired during pregnancy or breast-feeding. Transmission may be reduced by maternal treatment with antiretroviral drugs (e.g. AZT) during pregnancy. Breast-feeding confers an additional risk of transmission of 14% and should be advised against unless the estimated risks associated with bottle-feeding (in the developing world) are felt to be unacceptably high.

Further reading

Hall SM. The diagnosis of congenital infection: three 'old' pathogens with new significance in the 1990s. *Current Paediatrics,* 1993; **3**(3): 171–9.

McIntosh D, Isaacs D. Varicella zoster virus infection in pregnancy. *Archives of Disease in Childhood,* 1993; **68:** 1–2.

Peckham CS, Logan S. Screening for toxoplasmosis during pregnancy. *Archives of Disease in Childhood,* 1993; **68:** 3–5.

Related topics of interest

Immunodeficiency (p. 210)
Neonatal jaundice (p. 276)

CONSTIPATION

Constipation is defined as difficulty or delay in the passage of stool. This may lead to abdominal pain, anal pain or soiling. Soiling is the escape of stool into the underclothing; it is usually liquid stool which seeps around a hard faecal mass (spurious diarrhoea). Encopresis is the passage of normal stool in socially unacceptable places, e.g. behind furniture. In early infancy, constipation may be a sign of an anatomical disorder (e.g. Hirschsprung's disease, anal stenosis) or a systemic disorder (e.g. hypothyroidism). In older infants and children, behavioural factors associated with fear and anxiety about defaecation are by far the most important aetiological factors.

Problems

- Abdominal pain and distension.
- Overflow diarrhoea, soiling – smell, extra washing.
- Poor self-esteem, social exclusion.
- Parental anxiety, frustration and distress.

Pathophysiology

The lower rectum is normally empty. Ingestion of food or fluid stimulates colonic propulsion of stool into the rectum (gastro-colic reflex). Distension of stretch receptors within the rectum leads to rectal contraction and reflex inhibition of the internal sphincter. This is mediated by the nerves of the myenteric plexus. Sensory receptors in the upper rectum produce the sensation of needing to defaecate. The puborectalis muscle, internal and external sphincters are under a degree of voluntary control enabling the individual to maintain continence until it is convenient to pass stool. In chronic constipation the rectum is chronically distended ('megarectum'), the sensory receptors become inactive and the bowel is unable to contract effectively.

Aetiology

1. Behavioural factors. As the final stage of defaecation is under voluntary control, the child may avoid passing stool for a variety of reasons e.g. pain, reluctance to use school toilets, conflict with parents over attempts at toilet training. This 'retaining' behaviour leads to larger, harder stools which are painful to pass leading to further retention.

2. Painful anal lesions. An anal fissure may be the initial factor leading retention of stool. Large, hard stools may then lead to recurrence of the fissure, reinforcing the fear and pain of defaecation. Other causes of anal pain include perianal skin sepsis, penetrative sexual abuse and rectal prolapse.

3. Neurological disorders. Constipation is more common in children with neurological disorders such as generalized hypotonia (e.g. Down's syndrome), cerebral palsy and spina bifida.

4. *Anatomical problems* (e.g. anal stenosis, Hirschsprung's disease). These are uncommon but should be considered if the problem has been present since early infancy particularly if there has been delayed passage of meconium (> 24 hours after birth), failure to thrive, alternating constipation and diarrhoea, or significant abdominal distension. Hirschsprung's disease is due to the incomplete development of ganglion cells in the myenteric plexuses of Meissner (submucosal) and Auerbach (between outer longitudinal and inner circular smooth muscle layers). Failure of relaxation of the bowel to allow defaecation leads to an obstructive picture. With long aganglionic segments of bowel, the condition usually presents in the neonatal period with acute intestinal obstruction, and necrotizing enterocolitis is a major risk. Short and ultra-short segment Hirschsprung's may not present until later in childhood. Hirschsprung's disease has a prevalence of 1 in 5000, and is more common in boys, Down's syndrome, and those with a family history of the condition.

5. *Other.* e.g. hypothyroidism, hypercalcaemia, meconium ileus equivalent in cystic fibrosis.

Clinical assessment

1. *History.* Including onset of symptoms, how often the child has his/her bowels open, size and consistency of stool, any pain or bleeding on defaecation, any soiling, history of attempts at toilet training, current pattern of toileting, general health, diet (adequate fluid, fruit and vegetable intake?).

2. *Examination.* Including neurological examination of lower limbs, abdominal palpation for faecal masses or palpable bladder. Rectal examination should be performed, if the parents and child are willing, including inspection for perianal soreness, fissures etc. The rectum is often loaded with hard stool. In Hirschsprung's disease the rectum is usually empty and there may be a gush of faeces and air on withdrawing the finger.

3. *Investigations.* In most children with constipation investigations are unnecessary as they are rarely helpful. However, an abdominal X-ray may be used to demonstrate the degree of faecal loading. Barium enema or suction rectal

biopsy may be considered if an anatomical lesion is suspected. Histological examination of a rectal biopsy in Hirschsprung's disease reveals excessive acetylcholinesterase activity. Anorectal manometry is rarely used.

Management

Successful management of most children with constipation involves dealing with all the factors that have combined to create the problem (physical and psychological). Regular relaxed toileting, increased fluid intake, stool softeners (e.g. lactulose or docusate) and a local anaesthetic gel to relieve the pain of an anal fissure may be all that is required. If the rectum has been chronically distended, bowel stimulants (e.g. senna in an escalating dose at night) may improve contractility and can be used in combination with stool softeners. If faecal loading is extensive or the stool has become impacted sodium picosulphate (picolax) given orally, glycerine suppositories, microenemas, phosphate enemas, or gentle rectal washouts may be required. Occasionally manual evacuation under general anaesthetic is necessary and anal dilatation with or without rectal biopsy may be considered at the same time. Once the bowel has been cleared, regular bowel habit should be maintained with regular toileting together with stimulant and softening laxatives. Relapses are common and laxatives are often required for at least a year. Dietary advice should be given encouraging increased fibre and a good fluid intake. Star charts or other reward systems may be helpful. Occasionally the help of a child psychiatrist should be sort in the management of more difficult behaviour problems. Treatment of Hirschsprung's disease is surgical resection of the affected segment.

Further reading

Clayden GS. Management of chronic constipation. *Archives of Disease in Childhood,* 1992; **67:** 340–44.

Related topics of interest

Behaviour (p. 45)
Chronic diarrhoea (p. 77)

COUGH AND WHEEZE

Cough is one of the most common symptoms encountered in paediatric clinical practice. A detailed history and examination will aid diagnosis. What does the cough sound like? Is it transient or persistent? Is it worse at night or worse after exertion?

Wheeze is a high-pitched noise characteristically loudest in expiration. It is caused by airway narrowing/obstruction. Asthma is the most common cause of wheeze in childhood; however wheeze is a common symptom of viral repiratory infections in infancy. Wheeze is often but not always associated with cough.

Transient cough

Infection of the upper and/or lower respiratory tract, usually viral, is the most common cause of a transient cough. Infants and young children are particularly vulnerable to both viral and bacterial infections because their immune system is relatively immature.

Pneumonia

Aetiology

- Viral: RSV, influenza, parainfluenza and adenovirus.
- Bacterial: *Streptococcus pneumoniae, Haemophilus influenza, Mycoplasma pneumoniae* and *Staphylococcus aureus.*

Symptoms include fever, cough, wheeze, breathing difficulty, chest or abdominal pain. Signs may be focal or widespread and include reduced air entry, dull percussion note, crepitation or bronchial breathing. A chest X-ray often confirms clinical findings. Positive results from sputum and blood cultures provide help in choosing an appropriate antibiotic. Most bacterial pneumonia can be successfully treated with broad spectrum antibiotics ± supportive treatment with oxygen and intravenous fluids. Penicillin is still recommended for uncomplicated lobar pneumonia; however increasing antibiotic resistance is recognized. Complications of pleural effusion and empyema are uncommon but may require surgical drainage. A single episode of uncomplicated pneumonia should not require radiological follow-up unless symptoms persist.

Bronchiolitis

Respiratory syncytial virus is the usual pathogen responsible for annual epidemics of this lower respiratory tract infection, although adenovirus or parainfluenza may be involved. Young infants are usually affected. Clinical features include fever, coryza, dry cough, poor feeding and apnoea. Tachypnoea, intercostal recession, inspiratory crepitation and expiratory wheeze are typical examination findings.

Recurrent cough and wheeze during the first year after infection occur in up to 80% of infants.

Treatment is supportive, involving correction of hypoxia and maintenance of fluid balance. Assisted ventilation may be required in 1–5%. Specific antiviral treatment with ribavirin may be considered for infants with co-existing cardiorespiratory problems or those who are immunocompromised. However its efficacy is uncertain. Antibiotics are not routinely indicated as secondary bacterial infection is rare.

Persistent cough

A cough which is always present or recurs frequently can cause a great deal of anxiety for child and parents. In some cases identification of the underlying cause may take time.

Aetiology

- Chronic/recurrent infection of respiratory tract including pertussis infection and tuberculosis.
- Asthma/allergy.
- Gastroesophageal reflux with or without aspiration.
- Foreign body.
- Cystic fibrosis or immotile cilia syndrome.
- Immune deficiency.
- Congenital anomalies, e.g. tracheo-oesophageal fistula.
- Psychogenic (habitual).

Investigations

These may include:

- CXR.
- Sputum culture or cough swab/per-nasal swab for pertussis.
- FBC – white cell differential and eosinophilia.
- Sweat test.
- Mantoux test.
- Immunoglobulins (including IgG sub classes and total IgE).
- pH study.
- Lung function tests.

Other investigations may include laryngobronchoscopy, thoracic CT scan or magnetic resonance imaging.

Treatment varies depending on the underlying cause.

Pertussis (whooping cough) Widespread vaccination against *Bordetella pertussis* has led to a notable reduction in the number of notified cases of whooping cough. However sporadic cases still occur in unimmunized infants and children, with a significant morbidity in very young infants. After a two week incubation period, a coryzal phase of 7–10 days is followed by the spasmodic phase, bursts of coughing without inspiratory pauses followed by a 'whoop' as air is drawn into the lungs. Apnoea, cyanosis and seizures as a result of cerebral anoxia may occur. Diagnosis can be confirmed by a positive culture from per-nasal swab and a characteristic absolute lymphocytosis on full blood count. Erythromycin if commenced early may reduce the period of infectivity, otherwise treatment is supportive. Cough may continue for many weeks, pertussis also being known as the 100 day cough.

Tuberculosis

Notification of tuberculosis (TB) in children in the UK remains low. Many schools throughout the UK still have routine Heaf testing and subsequent BCG vaccination. For children born into high-risk categories neonatal vaccination is recommended. High-risk groups include contact with active cases of TB; immigrants from countries with high prevalance; travel, with intended long stay, to country with high prevalance.

Tuberculosis should always be considered for a history of persistent respiratory symptoms with no obvious cause. In these cases a Mantoux test, CXR and sputum cultures can aid diagnosis. Treatment is with rifampicin and isoniazid for 6 months, supplemented with pyrazinamide during the first 2 months of therapy.

Wheeze

Aetiology

- Asthma.
- Lower repiratory tract infection – viral bronchiolitis.
- Foreign body.
- Gastro-oesophageal reflux with aspiration.
- Broncho-pulmonary dysplasia.

Wheeze may also be found in children with cystic fibrosis, immune deficiencies and allergies.

Clinical assessment

A clear history and thorough examination can aid diagnosis.

- Is the wheeze transient or persistent/recurrent?
- Was the child born prematurely?
- Was the wheeze of sudden onset?

- Does the child have a history suggestive of gastro-oesophageal reflux?
- Is there a strong family history of atopy?

Investigation and management

Many children will require no investigation; however in certain circumstances, the following investigations may be considered:

- Response to bronchodilator.
- CXR. Recommended for those children not responding to regular appropriate medication or those with focal clinical signs on examination.
- Naso pharyngeal aspirate (NPA) is used to specifically identify respiratory syncytial virus.
- pH monitoring.
- Bronchoscopy and biopsy.

Treatment varies according to the underlying cause.

Infantile wheeze

Wheezing is common in infancy and may be associated with cough, poor feeding and symptoms of respiratory distress. Wheeze is usually associated with a respiratory infection; however there may be other contributing factors including family history of atopy and parental smoking. Infants with recurrent episodes of wheeze may get labelled as 'happy wheezers'or as having 'wheezy bronchitis'. Supportive management is recommended as the response to bronchodilator therapy is variable. The majority of children who wheeze in early life do not go on to develop childhood asthma.

Further reading

Dinwiddie R. Diagnosis and Management of Paediatric Respiratory Disease. Edinburgh: Churchill-Livingstone, 1990.

Rakshi K., Couriel JM. Management of acute bronchitis. *Archives of Disease in Childhood,* 1994; **71:** 463–9.

Related topics of interest

Asthma (p. 38)
Cystic fibrosis (p. 107)
Immunization (p. 206)

CYANOTIC CONGENITAL HEART DISEASE

Cyanotic lesions account for only about 25% of congenital heart disease (CHD), but many are life-threatening in the first few weeks of life. Even with surgery, 15–20% of infants will die in the first year of life. Cyanosis is clinically detectable when reduced haemoglobin exceeds 5 g/100 ml and is more easily recognized in the newborn with a high haemoglobin than in an anaemic child. Cyanosis may occur because the lungs are underperfused owing to a right-to-left shunt bypassing the lungs (e.g. Fallot's tetralogy) or because there is mixing of the systemic and pulmonary circulations (e.g. transposition of the great arteries with ventricular septal defect, VSD. In the latter case, lung perfusion is normal or excessive. Cyanosis may be apparent in the neonatal period or become increasingly obvious over the first few months of life, particularly when the baby feeds or cries. In the older child, cyanosis is usually obvious at rest, exercise tolerance is reduced and clubbing occurs.

Problems

- Hypoxia.
- Acidosis.
- Heart failure.
- Failure to thrive.
- Polycythaemia.
- Thromboembolic events.
- Hypercyanotic spells.

The blue baby

Cyanosis in the first week of life may be due to respiratory disease, neurological depression (asphyxia, drugs), persistent fetal circulation or cyanotic CHD. The baby with CHD usually has no respiratory difficulty unless there is marked metabolic acidosis or heart failure. There may be a murmur and the second heart sound is usually single. If the atrioventricular septum is intact, the baby will become acutely cyanosed and collapse as the ductus arteriosus begins to close. The most important lesions in descending order of frequency are transposition of the great arteries (TGA), pulmonary atresia (PA) and tricuspid atresia (TA).

Investigation

- Arterial blood gases. Low $P\text{O}_2$ and a normal $P\text{CO}_2$, with or without metabolic acidosis.
- CXR
  - TGA: plethoric lung fields, egg shaped heart + narrow vascular pedicle.
  - PA/TA: oligaemic lung fields.
- ECG
  - TGA: right axis deviation, right ventricular hypertrophy (RVH).
  - PA: normal/left axis, left ventricular hypertrophy (LVH) since pulmonary circulation maintained by left ventricle via patent ductus.

TA: marked left axis deviation leading to a superior axis, LVH, RAH.

- Hyperoxia (nitrogen washout) test. To differentiate between heart and lung disease as the cause of cyanosis. Po_2 > 14 kPa (100 mmHg) in 80–100% oxygen excludes a major right-to-left shunt.
- Echocardiography and cardiac catheterization.

Management

If there is no mixing of oxygenated and deoxygenated blood other than via the ductus arteriosus, prostaglandin E_2 is used to keep the ductus open until a septostomy or surgery can be performed. A balloon atrial septostomy (Rashkind's procedure) can be performed during cardiac catheterization. Initial surgery aims either to increase pulmonary blood flow by a systemic to pulmonary shunt (e.g. Blalock–Taussig shunt) or to correct the defect anatomically (e.g. arterial switch for TGA). Later surgery anatomically corrects the defect or redirects blood through the correct circulations (e.g. Mustard procedure for TGA, Fontan procedure for PA).

Fallot's tetralogy

This is the commonest cyanotic heart defect. The four features of the tetralogy are due to deviation of the infundibular septum (area of interventricular septum between the aortic and pulmonary roots) in an anterocephalad direction:

- Pulmonary stenosis (infundibular septum obstructs the right ventricular outflow tract). Pulmonary atresia represents the severest form.
- VSD.
- Aorta overrides the VSD (receives blood from both right and left ventricles)
- RVH (due to outflow tract obstruction).

Fallot's tetralogy presents with a murmur, increasing cyanosis or hypercyanotic spells. There is a pulmonary systolic murmur and the second heart sound is single. Hypercyanotic spells occur due to infundibular spasm, which results in almost total obstruction of the right ventricular outflow tract. They may be precipitated by exertion and can be life-threatening. An affected baby becomes pale, extremely cyanosed, screams with pain and may lose consciousness. Older children characteristically squat after exertion to relieve symptoms. Squatting increases systemic vascular resistance (thus increasing pulmonary blood flow) and decreases return of unsaturated venous blood from the legs.

Investigation

- CXR. Oligaemic lung fields, boot-shaped heart.
- ECG. Right axis deviation, right atrial hypertrophy, RVH.

Management

Emergency treatment of hypercyanotic spells includes drawing the knees up to the chest, oxygen, i.v. pain relief (e.g. morphine) and i.v. propranolol, which relieves the infundibular spasm. Oral propanolol is used as prophylaxis.

A systemic-to-pulmonary shunt is inserted to improve pulmonary blood flow in infants with marked cyanosis or uncontrolled spells. Total repair of the defect is usually carried out before school age (some centres now do a total repair as a primary procedure in the neonatal period).

Persistent fetal circulation (PFC)

PFC occurs when the pulmonary arterial pressure fails to fall following birth. This leads to persistent right-to-left shunting through the ductus arteriosus and foramen ovale. Predisposing factors include severe lung disease, birth asphyxia, polycythaemia and hypoglycaemia. Cyanosis may be progressive over the first few hours of life, with increasing respiratory distress, acidosis and hypotension. The second heart sound is loud and single. There may be differential cyanosis with a lower Po_2 in the lower body (postductal) than the upper body (preductal). Management includes hyperventilation and pulmonary vasodilators, e.g. tolazoline, nitric oxide, prostacyclin.

Further reading

Cardiac emergencies. In: Advanced Life Support Group. *Advanced Paediatric Life Support,* 2nd edn. London: BMJ Publications, 1997; 111–2.

Mupanemunda RH, Edwards AD. Treatment of newborn infants with inhaled nitric oxide. *Archives of Disease in Childhood,* 1995; **72:** F131–4.

Silove ED. Assessment and management of congenital heart disease in the newborn by the district paediatrician. *Archives of Disease in Childhood,* 1994; **70:** F71–4.

Thorne S, Deanfield J. Long term outlook in treated congenital heart disease. *Archives of Disease in Childhood,* 1996; **75:** 6–8.

Related topics of interest

Heart failure (p. 190)

Heart murmurs (p. 194)

Neonatal respiratory distress (p. 281)

CYSTIC FIBROSIS

Cystic fibrosis (CF) is an autosomal recessive disease, affecting 1 infant in 2500 in the UK. In 1989 the CF gene was identified on the long arm of chromosome 7, and the gene product is a chloride channel – the cystic fibrosis transmembrane conductance regulator (CFTR). The commonest mutation in CF is a deletion of a phenylalanine residue at position 508 (delta F508) and this accounts for 70% of CF mutations in northern Europe and North America.

Problems

- Respiratory.
- Gastrointestinal.
- Hepatobiliary.
- Nutritional.
- Metabolic.
- Arthropathy.
- Reproductive.
- Psychosocial.

Clinical features

Abnormalities affect the exocrine glandular system, mainly the respiratory and gastrointestinal tracts. Neonatal presentation may be with meconium ileus (10–15% of CF cases), prolonged jaundice or as the result of prenatal diagnosis. Later in infancy presentation may be with failure to thrive, steatorrhoea, rectal prolapse, nasal polyps or recurrent respiratory tract infections. Rarely infants present with hyponatraemia and hypokalaemia from excessive electrolyte loss (pseudo-Bartter's syndrome), or with anaemia and hypoproteinaemia secondary to pancreatic insufficiency. In later childhood complications such as chronic sinusitis, biliary cirrhosis, delayed puberty and diabetes mellitus may arise.

Diagnosis

1. Sweat test. Pilocarpine iontophoresis is used to stimulate sweat secretion. Levels of sodium or chloride above 70 mmol/l on a sweat sample weighing 100 mg or more are diagnostic. Values above 50 mmol/l are suspicious, and the test should be repeated. In normal samples the sodium is usually higher than the chloride, but in CF this ratio is often reversed. Tests should be performed by skilled personnel only.

2. Antenatal diagnosis. Chorionic villus sampling at 8–10 weeks gestation or amniocentesis at 16–18 weeks allows direct gene analysis. Population screening for CF carriers has been carried out in pilot studies, and subsequent antenatal diagnosis can then be offered to couples both known to be carriers.

3. Neonatal screening. Elevated levels of immunoreactive trypsin (IRT) in the neonatal period are the result of fetal pancreatic damage *in utero*. Raised IRT levels in affected babies may be found in dried blood spots taken at the time of the Guthrie test. IRT is two to five times higher in neonates with cystic fibrosis. Levels reduce after 1–2 months and become unreliable.

4. Genotyping for CFTR mutation (ΔF508) should be requested for children with a family history of CF and those with a positive sweat test or raised IRT.

Complications

1. Respiratory. Repeated lung infection with *Staphylococcus aureus*, *Pseudomonas aeruginosa* and *Haemophilus influenzae* leads to progressive lung disease with bronchiectasis, clubbing, abscess formation, haemoptysis and eventually cor pulmonale. Chest radiographs may show bronchial wall thickening, mottled shadows, ring shadows and consolidation. Changes over time may be assessed by the use of the Chrispin–Norman score. *Pseudomonas cepacia* may account for a rapid deterioration, while *Aspergillus fumigatus* may cause wheezing from allergic bronchopulmonary aspergillosis.

2. Gastrointestinal and hepatobiliary. Malabsorption with marked steatorrhoea is the main complication, resulting from pancreatic enzyme deficiency. There is malabsorption of fat-soluble vitamins. Rectal prolapse, meconium ileus, biliary cirrhosis, gall stones and portal hypertension may also complicate the disease. Meconium ileus equivalent is a partial obstruction of the terminal ileum and caecum by a faecal mass; its presentation may mimick acute appendicitis.

3. Nutrition. Nutritional support is associated with improved growth and stabilization of lung function. Poor nutritional status results from malabsorption, a high total energy requirement (infection and respiratory effort) and the anorexia and vomiting of advancing lung disease. Energy intakes of 120–150% of estimated daily allowances are recommended to maintain adequate nutrition.

4. Arthropathy. Reduced joint mobility with pain occurs in 1–2% of children with CF, as a result of specific CF arthropathy, hypertrophic pulmonary osteoarthropathy or incidental juvenile rheumatoid arthritis.

5. *Metabolic.* Frank diabetes mellitus requiring insulin occurs in 2–3% of children with CF. Salt depletion may occur at presentation, or as a result of hot climates.

6. *Reproductive.* Ninety-seven per cent of males are infertile and women are subfertile – a primary factor is the production of viscid secretions.

7. *Psychosocial.* The social and psychological implications of the diagnosis are enormous, with far-reaching effects on family life and expectations of the child.

Management

1. *Respiratory.* Physiotherapy with postural drainage and forced expiration techniques is a vital part of treatment. Inhaled bronchodilators and mucolytics may be of value. Oral antistaphylococcal drugs may be given continuously or intermittently. *Pseudomonas aeruginosa* may be treated with oral or intravenous antipseudomonal agents, depending on the clinical condition. Nebulized antibiotics, e.g. tobramycin, may achieve long-term control of *Pseudomonas aeruginosa*. Oral steroids may be needed for severe asthmatic symptoms, and for allergic bronchopulmonary aspergillosis. Regular lung function tests are recommended to monitor progress. Selected patients may benefit from treatment with recombinant human DNAse, a mucolytic agent. Safety and efficacy in improving lung function has been proven in clinical trials; however, it is very expensive.

2. *Nutrition.* A high-energy (normal or high-fat), high-protein diet should be given, accompanied by enteric-coated pancreatic enzymes, e.g. Creon or Pancrease. Vitamin supplements of vitamins A, B, C, D and E should also be given, with additional vitamin K if there is liver disease. If nutrition is still inadequate, high-calorie drinks or nocturnal nasogastric or gastrostomy feeds may be added.

Other specific therapies may be needed, depending on individual circumstances, e.g sclerosant injection of oesophageal varices.

Prognosis

Effective conventional therapies now mean that the median survival for a child with CF is 40 years.

1. *Transitional care.* The increasing numbers of children surviving into adult life highlight the importance of

transitional care. Special CF clinics for young people are recommended as they provide an opportunity to discuss issues such as fertility, employment and continuing care.

2. *Heart lung transplant* is an option for those with end-stage lung disease. Success rates are improving; however progress is limited by eligibility of patients and donor availability.

3. *Gene therapy*. Introducing a normal *CFTR* gene, using a viral or non-viral (liposome) vector, in theory holds the cure for cystic fibrosis. This technique is not without complications and studies are still in their preliminary stages.

4. *Other therapies*. Clinical trials continue to assess the efficacy of other new treatments, e.g. anti-proteases (α_1 anti-trypsin), anti-inflammatory agents (e.g. ibuprofen), and amiloride (to reduce sodium absorption).

Further reading

Graham A, Geddes D. New developments in cystic fibrosis and their potential effects on its management. *Current Paediatrics,* 1993; **3:** 96–101.

MacDonald A. Nutritional management of cystic fibrosis. *Archives of Disease in Childhood,* 1996; **74:** 81–7.

Southern KW. ΔF508 in cystic fibrosis: willing but not able. *Archives of Disease in Childhood,* 1997; **76:** 278–82.

Tanner MS, Taylor CJ. Liver disease in cystic fibrosis. *Archives of Disease in Childhood,* 1995; **72:** 281–4.

Wallis C. Diagnosing cystic fibrosis: blood, sweat and tears. *Archives of Disease in Childhood,* 1997: **76:** 85–91.

Related topics of interest

Adolescent health (p. 19)
Asthma (p. 38)
Chronic diarrhoea (p. 77)
Cough and wheeze (p. 100)
Nutrition (p. 303)

DEVELOPMENTAL ASSESSMENT

Developmental examination involves a system of procedures (history, observations, examination and tests) which are designed to establish the stage of the child's development and identify any deviations from the normal pattern. Developmental assessment involves detailed, expert multidisciplinary investigation of a suspected developmental disorder. A knowledge of the range of normality for each developmental milestone is essential for developmental screening. Briefly, essential milestones are:

6 weeks

- Holds head transiently up to the plane of the trunk in ventral suspension.
- Lies prone with a flat pelvis.
- Smiles back in response to mother.
- Follows object from side to midline.

3 months

- Head held for prolonged period above the plane of the body.
- If pulled to sitting position, minimal head lag only.
- Holds object if it is placed in the hand.
- Turns to sound.
- Hand regard (3-5 months).

6–7 months

- Sits without support by 7 months.
- Rolls prone to supine (6 months), supine to prone (7 months).
- Supports weight when held in standing position.
- Transfers objects from hand to hand.
- Feeds self with biscuit and holds own bottle.
- Babbles of two syllables.

9 months

- Sits steadily unsupported.
- Pulls up to stand, holding on to furniture.
- Compares two cubes, bringing them together.
- Pincer grasp, e.g. picks up currant between index finger and thumb.

1 year

- Walks with one hand held, or creeps 'like a bear' on hands and feet.
- Releases toys into mother's hand.

- Says 2–3 words with meaning, but understands many more.

18 months
- Walks upstairs if hand is held.
- Domestic mimicry.
- Builds tower of 3–4 bricks.
- Obeys two simple commands.
- May be dry by day.

2 years
- Walks up and down stairs alone.
- Draws circular and vertical strokes with a pencil.
- Builds tower of 6–7 bricks.
- Requests food and toilet needs.
- Forms two spontaneous three-word sentences.
- Watches other children at play.

3 years
- Rides a tricycle.
- Undoes buttons, mainly dressing self.
- Copies circles on paper, imitating crosses; may draw a man.
- Builds tower of nine bricks.
- Asks numerous questions. Joins sociable play.

4 years
- Skips. Goes up and downstairs with one foot per step.
- Does up buttons.
- Copies cross on paper.
- Self-caring for toilet needs.
- Plays 'make-believe' games.

History

A developmental history must explore parental concerns about the child's development to date. Milestones which have been achieved should be noted. A full family history must be taken, and should include details of vision, hearing and special educational needs. Maternal age and well-being during the pregnancy may be relevant, and full details of the birth and early neonatal period should be obtained. Significant illnesses or accidents may have occurred since birth. A thorough social history will provide information about the level of stimulation and learning opportunity in the child's home environment. It is important to consider that difficulties with one area of development may affect progress in other areas, e.g. a motor disorder will affect progress in motor skills but also social skills, i.e. feeding and dressing.

Examination

Physical examination should be included in the neurodevelopmental assessment. Initial observation may detect abnormalities of gait and movement, characteristic facies, or eye abnormalities. Examination should include measurements of growth, including head circumference, palpation of the anterior fontanelle and examination of the heart, chest, abdomen, testes and hips.

Neurodevelopmental examination

Formal neurological assessment is best combined with developmental examination in children of most ages. Testing for the persistence of primitive reflexes should be included, where relevant. Cranial nerve function and muscle tone should be tested.

Other tests will depend on the age of the child. Usually only limited equipment is necessary, but should include such items as a set of 1-inch cubed bricks, small pellets of paper, a ring dangling on a thread, and a small handbell. Much information can be obtained by observation of the quality of performance of the various tasks, and the associated vocalization.

The Working Party on child health surveillance (Hall Report) found no clear justifications for routine formal developmental assessment for all children, recommending the evaluation of history, parental concerns and simple milestones only. Referral for expert opinion should be made if there are doubts about normal progress. However, specific tests are in general use for developmental assessment.

- The Denver developmental screening test is widely used for screening normal children.
- Schedule of Growing Skills is a quick and easy popular method for developmental screening.
- Bayley scales of infant development give separate scores for mental and motor development and include an observation of behaviour.
- Griffith's test is widely used for those children in whom an abnormality is found during developmental screening. It gives separate scores for locomotor, personal/social, hearing and speech, hand–eye coordination and performance skills, and a sixth subtest, practical reasoning, is included for 3- to 8-year-olds. Each subtest gives a developmental quotient (DQ) which is averaged into a general quotient (GQ).

- The Mary Sheridan 'from birth to 5 years' scheme is based on the detailed concepts and tests of Gesell and is widely used in the UK.

Children identified as having delay in one or more aspects of development will need repeated clinical developmental assessment of progress.

Further reading

Hall DMB, ed. *Health for all Children. A Programme for Child Health Surveillance,* 3rd edn. Oxford: Oxford University Press, 1996.

Illingworth RS. *The Development of the Infant and Young Child,* 9th edn. Edinburgh: Churchill Livingstone, 1987.

Sheridan M. *From Birth to Five Years. Children's Developmental Progress,* revised 3rd edn. London: Routledge, 1997.

Related topics of interest

Developmental delay (p. 115)
Disability (p. 124)
Hearing and speech (p. 185)
Vision (p. 374)

DEVELOPMENTAL DELAY

Developmental examination may detect a pattern of development which varies from the expected. The progression of milestones may be normal in sequence, but delayed in time when compared with an average child of the same age, or the sequence may be distorted and abnormal. Regression, with loss of previously acquired skills, is a particularly worrying pattern.

Categories of developmental delay

- Isolated motor delay.
- Speech and language delay.
- Global developmental delay.

A detailed developmental history and neurodevelopmental examination are required as outlined in related topic Developmental assessment, p. 111.

Causes of delayed motor development

- Normal or familial variation.
- Previous chronic illness.
- Cerebral palsy.
- Neuromuscular disorders, e.g. Duchenne muscular dystrophy.
- Orthopaedic problems, e.g. congenital dislocation of the hip.
- Emotional.

Speech and language delay

Disorders of speech and language are discussed in related topic Hearing and speech (p. 185). Hearing defects should always be excluded, and the overall pattern of development assessed, to exclude global developmental delay.

Causes of global developmental delay

Global delay involves all aspects of development: fine motor, gross motor, speech and social skills. Many globally delayed children will have learning difficulties of varying degrees. In many cases a specific aetiology will not be found, but it is important to look hard for a specific cause, for reasons of prognosis and genetic counselling. A cause is more often found in those with severe learning difficulties (IQ below 55) than those with mild to moderate learning difficulties (IQ 55–75).

1. Chromosomal abnormalities. Down's syndrome is the commonest chromosomal abnormality to cause developmental delay, followed by the fragile X syndrome. Many less common chromosomal abnormalities associated with specific syndromes are now being recognized.

2. Structural brain abnormalities. Microcephaly, hydranencephaly, agenesis of the corpus callosum and abnormalities of the cortical gyri may be responsible for global developmental delay.

3. Specific syndromes. Numerous specific syndromes associated with global delay have been recognized, e.g. Cornelia de Lange syndrome, Smith–Lemli–Opitz syndrome. The neurocutaneous syndromes (tuberous sclerosis, Sturge–Weber, neurofibromatosis) may also be responsible.

4. Congenital infection. Congenital rubella, toxoplasmosis, cytomegalovirus and herpes simplex infection may cause developmental delay in association with other defects, e.g. cataracts, intracranial calcification.

5. Inborn errors of metabolism. Phenylketonuria and congenital hypothyroidism should now be excluded by the routine neonatal screening programme. Other individual inborn errors are rarer, e.g. the mucopolysaccharidoses, maple syrup urine disease, etc.

6. Cerebral palsy. Some children with cerebral palsy will have global delay.

7. Postnatal causes. Postnatal brain insults such as severe head injury, intracranial haemorrhage, meningitis or encephalitis may cause global developmental delay in a child with previously normal milestones. Milestones may be delayed, but later catch up, e.g. in a child with a previous chronic disease or an emotionally deprived child who subsequently has a secure and loving foster home.

Investigation of global delay

Selected investigations may be considered:

- Chromosomal analysis – for fragile X syndrome.
- Imaging of CNS – by CT or MRI scan – to exclude structural abnormalities.
- Urine for virus excretion (rubella, cytomegalovirus), mucopolysaccharides, amino acids.
- Thyroid function tests.
- Serological tests for congenital infections.
- Creatine phosphokinase in boys – exclude Duchenne muscular dystrophy.

Management

Very few causes of global developmental delay are amenable to specific treatment. Parents and carers need support with coming to terms with this diagnosis. The identification of a specific pathology may provide a prognostic guide, and allow genetic counselling. Practical help may be needed with feeding, sleeping and behavioural difficulties, and the provision of respite care. Financial support may be needed, e.g. the Disability Living Allowance, the Joseph Rowntree Memorial Trust. Special educational provision must be considered at an early stage, based on a Statement of Educational Need.

Developmental regression

The loss of previously acquired skills is an ominous symptom and may occur at any age. The term dementia is often used when it occurs in an older child. A full history including family history and race (e.g. Tay–Sachs disease occurs in Ashkenazi Jews) must be taken. Neurological signs and symptoms such as seizures, ataxia and tremor should be looked for, as should specific problems where appropriate, such as jaundice and Kayser–Fleischer rings if Wilson's disease is a possibility.

Causes

1. Early causes (onset before 2 years of age)

- Infection, e.g. perinatally acquired AIDS.
- Mucopolysaccharidoses, e.g. Sanfillipo's syndrome.
- Inborn errors of metabolism, e.g. galactosaemia, organic and aminoacidurias, congenital hypothyroidism.
- Lipid storage disorders, e.g. Tay–Sachs disease, infantile Gaucher's disease.
- Rett's syndrome.
- Epilepsy, e.g. infantile spasms, Lennox–Gastaut syndrome.
- Leucodystrophies, e.g. late infantile metachromatic leucodystrophy.

2. Later causes (onset after 2 years of age)

- Infection, e.g. SSPE.
- Leucodystrophies, e.g. juvenile metachromatic leucodystrophy, Batten's disease, adrenoleukodystrophy.
- Wilson's disease.
- Huntington's chorea.
- Ataxia telangectasia.

3. Any age

- Structural lesion in brain, e.g. hydrocephalus, cerebral tumour, tuberous sclerosis.

- Toxins, e.g. drugs, lead poisoning.

Investigations

These will depend on the clinical picture but may include:

- CT or MRI of the brain.
- White cell enzymes.
- CSF for protein and measles antibody titre.
- Serum and urine for amino and organic acids.
- EEG.

Rett's syndrome

This is a condition of unknown aetiology which occurs only in girls. There are no biochemical abnormalities and there is no diagnostic test. Because it occurs only in girls, it has been suggested that it may be an X-linked dominant condition, lethal in males. The child is usually normal until the age of 6 months to 1 year when she regresses. Head circumference is also normal at birth with deceleration in growth from about 6 months. The child loses hand skills and develops stereotyped hand-wringing movements. Other features include ataxia, idiosyncratic breathing patterns, epilepsy and, later, scoliosis.

Further reading

Newton R, Wraith J. Investigation of developmental delay. *Archives of Disease in Childhood,* 1995; **72:** 460–5.

Pollak M. *Textbook of Developmental Paediatrics.* Edinburgh: Churchill Livingstone, 1993.

Related topics of interest

Developmental assessment (p. 111)
Disability (p. 124)
Hearing and speech (p. 185)
Learning disability (p. 236)

DIABETES MELLITUS

Childhood diabetes mellitus is almost invariably insulin dependent (type I, IDDM). Insulin deficiency results from irreversible damage to the β-cells of the pancreatic islets of Langerhans. The incidence increases with distance from the equator, is higher in whites than in non-whites and peaks at adolescence (1 in 1200 school-children). The aetiology remains unclear but is likely to involve both genetic predisposition and environmental factors.

Problems

- Hypoglycaemia.
- Ketoacidosis.
- Cerebral oedema.
- Family and social disruption.
- Long-term complications (retinopathy, nephropathy, accelerated atherosclerosis, peripheral neuropathy).

Aetiology

1. Primary

(a) Genetic factors

- Increased incidence in siblings (15–50 times normal) and parents. However, only 10% of affected children have a diabetic first-degree relative.
- Five times more common in monozygotic twins than in dizygotic twins.
- Association with HLA-DR3 and -DR4.

(b) Environmental factors

- Seasonal variation in incidence (autumn/winter peaks).
- Case clustering (geographical variation).
- Association with viral infections, e.g. mumps, coxsackie B4. Destruction of the β-cells may take place over several years with acute decompensation precipitated by a virus or other toxin.

(c) Autoimmune factors

- Associated with autoimmune diseases of thyroid, adrenal and parathyroid glands.
- Cytotoxic islet cell antibodies often found at diagnosis.

2. Secondary

- Cystic fibrosis.
- Genetic syndromes, e.g. Prader–Willi.
- Cushing's syndrome.

Clinical features

The majority of children are diagnosed before the onset of severe ketoacidosis. Characteristic features include thirst, polyuria, weight loss, poor appetite and malaise, developing over days or weeks. Enuresis may recur in a previously dry child. Occasionally a child presents more acutely with rapid onset of ketoacidosis progressing from vomiting, dehydration and hyperventilation to shock, drowsiness and coma over a few hours. Abdominal pain may be a prominent feature, resulting in admission to a surgical ward with an 'acute abdomen'.

Examination should assess:

- Degree of dehydration.
- Level of consciousness.
- Pulse, blood pressure.
- Respiratory rate – Kussmaul respiration (deep sighing respiration due to metabolic acidosis). The breath may smell sweet (acetones).
- Sites of possible infection which may have precipitated acute decompensation.

Investigation

- Urinalysis. Glycosuria strongly suggests the diagnosis. Ketones may be present. Other causes of glycosuria include renal tubular disorders (normal blood glucose).
- Random blood glucose > 11 mmol/l confirms the diagnosis. Glucose tolerance tests are rarely indicated in children.
- U&E. Hyperglycaemia results in polyuria and dehydration. Hyponatraemia results from osmotic diuresis and shift of water from within cells to the extracellular fluid. Despite a total body deficit, the serum potassium is usually normal at presentation because of acidosis.
- Acid–base status. Metabolic acidosis is due to excess lipolysis and production of ketones.
- FBC. White count may be raised even in the absence of infection.
- Blood cultures, urine culture, throat swab ± chest radiography.

Initial management (not ketoacidotic)

In most centres children are admitted to hospital for a few days to allow education of the family and child about diabetes, and to commence insulin injections. Simple practical information should be given about insulin, diet, injection techniques and the symptoms of hypoglycaemia. Diabetic liaison nurses and dietitians are invaluable members of the team. This education continues at home and in outpatients. Initial insulin requirements are ~ 0.5 units/kg/day subcutaneously given as a twice-daily regimen of short- and medium-acting insulins, two-thirds being given before breakfast and one-third before the evening meal. Requirements may be increased by ketoacidosis at presentation, or intercurrent illness, and may be reduced if the diagnosis is made early, with only mild metabolic decompensation. Insulin requirements may be low for the first few months as the pancreas still produces a little insulin ('honeymoon period'). Requirements will then increase as the pancreas finally fails completely.

Ketoacidosis

Diabetic ketoacidosis (DKA) is an emergency which requires prompt recognition and treatment. It may be the presenting feature of IDDM or occur in a known diabetic during an intercurrent illness, or when insulin is not given (in error or deliberately). A common mistake is to stop or reduce the insulin in children who are not eating because they are unwell or vomiting. In this situation they often need more insulin than usual.

- Treat shock with 10–20 ml/kg of plasma or saline.
- Fluids. Intravenous 0.9% saline initially (change to 0.45% saline/2.5% dextrose when blood sugar <11 mmol/l). Calculate fluid deficit (usually 10–15% dehydrated) and normal requirements and replace at a constant rate over 24 hours. Insulin promotes the uptake of potassium into cells so monitor carefully when treatment is commenced and add potassium to fluids. The metabolic acidosis will resolve with correction of dehydration and hyperglycaemia so bicarbonate is rarely needed.
- Insulin. Intravenous infusion commencing at 0.1 units/kg/h.
- Nil by mouth for first 12 hours at least. A nasogastric tube should be passed if vomiting is profuse or gastric dilatation is present.
- Urinary catheterization is unnecessary unless the patient is comatose, a distended bladder is palpable or no urine has been passed within 4–6 hours of commencing treatment.
- Antibiotics if a focus for infection is identified.

Cerebral oedema

There are 6–11 deaths per year from DKA in children under the age of 19 years in the UK. Cerebral oedema is the most important cause of mortality and morbidity. It develops a few hours after commencing treatment in the context of apparent biochemical improvement. It is difficult to predict those at greatest risk, and it may occur in seemingly mild DKA. Rapid fluid replacement and free water overload may contribute, but the antecedents to the development of cerebral oedema are still unclear.

Hypoglycaemia

Hypoglycaemia is a major hazard of insulin treatment in diabetes mellitus and becomes commoner with the quest for better glucose control. It is caused by delayed or missed food, increased exercise, or errors of insulin dosage. Children and parents should be aware of the causes, symptoms and treatment. They should have regular meals, take extra carbohydrate before vigorous exercise, and be given Hypostop, oral glucose or dextrose at the first sign of hypoglycaemia. Recent reports have suggested that the use of human insulins may be associated with loss of awareness of hypoglycaemic symptoms but this has yet to be proven. Hypoglycaemia seldom causes long-term problems although prolonged and severe hypoglycaemia (usually associated with deliberate, massive insulin overdose) will result in cerebral oedema and may cause death.

Long-term follow-up

1. Maintenance of good control. Monitoring is best done by finger-prick blood tests. Urine tests may be used but these are crude, with individual variation in the level at which glucose spills into the urine. Glycosylated haemoglobin (HbA1C) levels give an index of control over a longer period. There is now evidence that improved control reduces the risk of long-term complications (see Further reading, DCCT report). Optimal control should be promoted but this must be balanced against avoidance of recurrent hypoglycaemia and maintenance of an acceptable lifestyle.

2. Growth and development. Physiological and behavioural adjustments in adolescence and puberty lead to changes in insulin requirements. Relative insulin resistance is due to increased growth hormone. Multiple injection regimens with pen injection devices are often useful.

3. Long-term complications. Screening should include annual retinal examination and urine for microalbuminuria (may be an early predictor of nephropathy). Smoking should be discouraged.

Further reading

Campbell FM. Microalbuminuria and nephropathy in insulin dependent diabetes mellitus. *Archives of Disease in Childhood,* 1995; **73:** 4–7.

Dunger DB. Diabetes in puberty. *Archives of Disease in Childhood,* 1992; **67:** 569–70.

ISPAD and International Diabetes Federation (European Region) Policy Group. *Consensus guidelines for the management of insulin-dependent (type 1) diabetes mellitus (IDDM) in childhood and adolescence 1995. Implementing the St Vincent & Kos Declarations.* London: Freund Publishing House, 1995.

Johnston DI. Management of diabetes mellitus. *Archives of Disease in Childhood,* 1989; **64:** 622–8.

Shield JPH, Baum JD. Prevention of long term complications in diabetes. *Archives of Disease in Childhood,* 1994; **70:** 258–59.
The Diabetes Control and Complications Trial (DCCT) Research Group. The effect of intensive treatment of diabetes on the development and progression of long-term complications in insulin-dependent diabetes mellitus. *New England Journal of Medicine,* 1993; **329:** 977–85.

Related topic of interest

Coma (p. 89)

DISABILITY

It is important to be aware of the terminology used when talking about children with special needs. The WHO has provided useful definitions:

- A *disorder* is a medically definable condition or disease.
- An *impairment* is any loss or abnormality of psychological, physiological or anatomical structure or function.
- A *disability* is any restriction or lack of ability to perform an activity in the manner or within the range considered normal for a human being.
- A *handicap* is the impact of the impairment or the disability on the person's everyday activities.

The Children Act 1989 recognizes that children with disability have special needs and social services, health and education departments have a duty to provide appropriate services for them. There are many aspects of a child's life which may be affected by their disability. Many professionals may be involved, i.e. occupational therapists, physiotherapists, speech therapists, social workers, teachers, orthotists. It is important for these teams to work closely together.

When assessing a child with a disability, in addition to your routine history and examination, the following may need to be considered depending on age and impairment.

Mobility	Physiotherapy has a central role in the prevention of deformity and the promotion of independent mobility. A wide range of aids are available including boots, orthotic supports, walking frames and wheelchairs. Correct seating is paramount for optimal comfort and functioning. Check for contractures, kypho-scoliosis and hip dislocation. The need for home adaptations, e.g. ramps, widened doorways, can be assessed by an occupational therapist.
Feeding, nutrition and growth	As with all children regular assessment of growth and nutrition is important. Feeding problems may arise due to oro-motor dysfunction, movement disorders, communication problems or gastro-oesophageal reflux. Ask advice from speech therapists and dieticians.
Communication	Facilitation of communication should be encouraged at an early age with the involvement of the speech and language team. Alternative communication methods include eye-pointing, signing, communication boards and electronic aids.
Behaviour difficulties	These occur as with other children but may also stem from, or be compounded by, communication problems or frustration with aspects of the disability.
Toileting	Immobility increases the incidence of urinary tract infections and constipation. Where toilet training is a problem the

services of an incontinence team may be useful, in some cicumstances families can apply for financial assistance for disposable nappies.

Education

Special needs nurseries are available for children pre-school. Some children need a statement of educational need which is to ensure appropriate support in school. Although special schools are appropriate for some, if possible, integration into mainstream education is encouraged. All agencies have a duty to cooperate in assessing the needs of the child when they leave school and make the transition to adulthood. Specialist careers advice may be required.

Family lifestyle

It is important to consider social aspects of living with disability. Give advice on family support groups, respite care and benefits such as Disability Living Allowance and grants from the Family Fund.

General health

Immunizations, and concomitant conditions such as asthma, and epilepsy should be considered.

Cerebral palsy

Cerebral palsy (CP) is a permanent, non-progressive disorder of movement and posture secondary to damage of the immature brain. The estimated prevalence is 2–3/1000 live births. Around 40% of children with CP were born prematurely and most commonly they have a hemiplegic or diplegic movement disorder.

Aetiology

- Genetic – congenital cerebral malformations.
- Infection – congenital infection (TORCH), meningitis.
- Vascular – periventricular leukomalacia, intraventricular haemorrhage (particularly associated with prematurity).
- Unknown – no aetiology is found in a significant number of cases.

Classification

There is a trend away from using the traditional classifications. However there is a need to accurately describe a child's particular problem. Two aspects of the condition should be considered:

1. *Abnormality of tone and movement,* e.g. hypotonia, hypertonia, spasticity, rigidity, dyskinesia, athetosis, chorea, dystonia, ataxia.

2. *Distribution of movement disorder,* e.g. hemiplegia, quadriplegia, paraplegia, monoplegia. The clinical pattern

may change with the child's development and using this method of classification allows flexibility.

Children with CP may show delay in other aspects of their development, e.g. language, vision, hearing, social.

Diagnosis

This is often a gradual process based on evolving examination findings. CP may be diagnosed at routine follow-up appointments in high risk groups, at routine developmental screening or if parents identify concerns. Consideration should be made regarding cause, nature and evolution of the disorder.

Investigations

These are primarily of help to identify any underlying cause:

- Chromosomal analysis.
- Urine metabolic screen.
- Congenital infection screen.
- TFT.
- CPK.
- Cranial imaging – MRI, when available, is preferred to CT scan and may identify focal pathology although in the majority of cases mild non specific changes are detected.

Talking to parents

Telling parents that their child has CP needs to be handled sensitively but without delay. Early diagnosis is important for the child in order to implement appropriate management and for the parents to come to terms with the implications. Families will need support and from the outset should be put in touch with social services and voluntary organizations.

Further reading

Hall DMB, Hill PD. *The Child with a Disability*, 2nd edn. Oxford: Blackwell Science, 1996.

Hutchison T. The classification of disability. *Archives of Disease in Childhood,* 1995; **73:** 91–4.

Platt MJ, Pharoah POD. Epidemiology of cerebral palsy. *Current Paediatrics*, 1995; **5:** 151–5.

Rosenbloom L. Diagnosis and management of cerebral palsy. *Archives of Disease in Childhood,* 1995; **72:** 350–4.

Morton RE. Diagnosis and classification of cerebral palsy. *Current Paediatrics*, 1995; **5:** 156–9.

Related topics of interest

Ataxia (p. 42)
Developmental assessment (p. 111)
Developmental delay (p. 115)
Dysmorphology and teratogenesis (p. 128)
Fits, faints and funny turns (p. 144)
Hearing and speech (p. 185)
Vision (p. 374)

DYSMORPHOLOGY AND TERATOGENESIS

Dysmorphology is the study of malformations and birth defects. Abnormal development may be due to a chromosomal abnormality, a single gene defect or a teratogen, or may be multifactorial. Recognition of patterns of multiple congenital abnormalities may help in identifying the aetiology and is important in counselling parents about prognosis, management and risk of recurrence. The majority of single malformations have a multifactorial inheritance and a low recurrence risk. Multiple malformations, particularly when associated with learning difficulties, are more frequently due to a single gene defect or a chromosomal abnormality and the recurrence risk is higher.

Problems

1. Malformation is a primary structural defect occurring in development, e.g. cleft lip or congenital heart defect. Malformation syndromes occur when two or more systems are involved.

2. Disruption or deformation of a normal fetus may occur as a result of amniotic bands or oligohydramnios. Abnormal uterine posture due to neuromuscular disorders may lead to deformities of the legs and feet.

3. Sequence. A single abnormality (malformation, disruption, deformity) initiates a series of events, e.g. Potter's is a malformation sequence of renal agenesis leading to pulmonary hypoplasia, talipes, squashed facies.

4. Association. Certain malformations occur together more often than expected, e.g. CHARGE association, coloboma of the eye, heart defects, choanal atresia, mental retardation, growth retardation and ear abnormalities.

5. Syndrome. A recognized pattern of abnormalities with a uniform cause, e.g. Trisomy 21 (Down's syndrome).

Assessment of a dysmorphic infant

A careful history should include details of the pregnancy, exposure to possible teratogens, parental age, consanguinity and family history. Following examination, all abnormalities should be documented and clinical photographs taken where possible. Further investigations may include chromosomal analysis, DNA studies, metabolic investigations and radiology. Numerous congenital malformations and syndromes have been described, and many are extremely rare. Specialist computer databases are now available to assist in diagnosis.

Miscarriage or stillbirth may be due to congenital malformation, and it is important to examine all abortuses and stillborn infants carefully. If congenital abnormalities are found, cardiac blood samples and skin biopsies can be taken for biochemical and genetic studies to try to identify the defect so that parents can be counselled about the recurrence risk and the availability of prenatal tests in future pregnancies.

Teratogens

Maternal illness, infection or ingestion of certain drugs during early pregnancy can lead to congenital malformation. The most widely known teratogenic drug is the antiemetic thalidomide, which damaged about 10 000 babies worldwide in the early 1960s before it was withdrawn. Other known teratogens include:

- Drugs, e.g. alcohol, anticonvulsants (sodium valproate, phenytoin), anticoagulants (warfarin).
- Maternal disorders, e.g. diabetes, phenylketonuria.
- Intrauterine infection, e.g. toxoplasmosis, rubella, cytomegalovirus.
- Environmental chemicals, e.g. organic solvents.
- Radiation.

Fetal alcohol syndrome

Alcohol is now the commonest teratogen ingested during pregnancy. Even a moderate alcohol intake is associated with an increased risk of spontaneous abortion and mild growth retardation. Fetal alcohol syndrome is seen in babies born to chronic alcoholic mothers. Typical features include a characteristic facial appearance (short palpebral fissures, smooth philtrum, thin upper lip), prenatal and post-natal growth retardation, microcephaly and mild to moderate learning difficulties.

Cleft lip and palate

Cleft lip and/or palate occurs in 1 in 600 live births and is usually an isolated abnormality, but is occasionally part of a chromosomal syndrome or sequence of malformations. There is often a family history, and the risk of recurrence after one affected child can be as great as 1 in 25. Most cases are determined by polygenic inheritance but occasional cases are linked to environmental factors or maternal medication. Affected children encounter both short- and long-term problems which are best managed by a multidisciplinary team.

Problems

- Feeding difficulties.
- Maternal bonding.
- Respiratory problems.

- Speech delay.
- Serous otitis media (glue ear).
- Dental problems.
- Cosmetic appearance.

Aetiology

- Idiopathic.
- Polygenic inheritence; often a positive family history.
- Maternal drugs, e.g. corticosteroids, phenytoin.
- Environmental factors are ill defined.
- Chromosomal abnormalities, e.g. trisomy 13 (Patau's syndrome).
- Pierre Robin sequence. Cleft palate occurs secondary to severe micrognathia.

Normal migration and fusion of mesodermal folds forming the lip, alveolus and anterior hard palate occurs between the fifth and seventh weeks of gestation. Failure of fusion results in unilateral or bilateral clefts. The remainder of the palate fuses in the midline between the ninth and 12th weeks. Tissue migration may be disorganized or obstructed by the tongue, resulting in a midline cleft. Clefts may be identified on antenatal ultrasound.

Clinical features

One-third have a cleft lip only. This is more common in boys (3M:2F), and is more common on the left than the right. One-quarter have a cleft palate only, and this is more common in girls (3F:2M). The remainder have both cleft lip and palate.

Clefts range in severity from a notch in the lip to complete separation of the maxillae. A bifid uvula may indicate the presence of a submucous cleft (poor muscle union in the soft palate), which can lead to difficulties with speech. Clefts may be associated with abnormalities of the cardiovascular, renal, central nervous and gastrointestinal systems, particularly when part of a chromosomal syndrome. Respiratory embarrassment occurs in the Pierre Robin sequence owing to posterior displacement of the tongue secondary to underdevelopment of the mandible. Nursing prone or insertion of a nasopharyngeal airway usually avoids the need for tracheostomy. The respiratory embarrassment resolves spontaneously as the mandible grows, these children usually having a normal profile by 4–6 years of age.

Management

1. Short-term problems

- *Feeding.* Breast-feeding can be successful in some cases. Various special teats are available for bottle-feeding. Orthodontic plates may be helpful.
- *Maternal bonding.* Before and after surgery photographs of a similar cleft may be helpful.

2. Surgery. The precise timing of surgery varies from centre to centre. The lip is closed first (usually by 3 months of age) and the palate is closed later (usually at 6 months). Preoperative orthodontic splints are sometimes used to align the alveolar margins and to reduce the size of the cleft.

3. Longer term problems. These are best managed by a multidisciplinary team. The paediatrician ensures coordination of the team, and monitors growth and development. Surgery is usually undertaken by plastic or maxillofacial surgeons. As the child grows there may need to be revisions to achieve the best cosmetic result. Orthodontic review is important to ensure dental alignment. Audiological assessment is recommended as Eustachian tube obstruction and subsequent serous otitis media is common. Grommets may be needed. Speech delay due to mechanical problems with the palate, exacerbated by glue ear, mean that a speech therapist is a vital member of the team.

Further reading

Habel A, Sell D, Mars M. Management of cleft lip and palate. *Archives of Disease in Childhood,* 1996; **74:** 360–6.

Jones KL. *Smith's Recognizable Patterns of Human Malformation,* 5th edn. Philadelphia, PA: WB Saunders, 1996.

Kingston H. Dysmorphology and teratogenesis. In: *ABC of Clinical Genetics*, 2nd edn. London: BMJ Publishing Group, 1994; 41–6.

Related topics of interest

Chromosomal abnormalities (p. 73)
Congenital infection (p. 93)
Fetal medicine (p. 141)
Hearing and speech (p. 185)

ECZEMA

Atopic eczema affects 3% of children under 5 years old, most commonly from 3 months to 2 years. The skin changes include intraepidermal oedema, which is followed by inflammation and intense itching of the skin. The skin is often erythematous, and may ooze and crust, with later changes of lichenification or alterations of pigmentation. Up to 80% of children affected have a positive family history of atopic conditions. A minor defect of cell-mediated immunity and suppressor T-cell numbers is thought to be a factor in pathogenesis. Rarely, eczema is a feature of another disorder, e.g. Wiskott–Aldrich syndrome, phenylketonuria.

Problems

- Itching.
- Sleep problems.
- Cosmetic disfigurement.
- Secondary infection.
- Failure to thrive.

Clinical history

The child typically presents with patches of dry, scaly, itchy skin which, when scratched, become inflamed and weepy. The face and the limb flexures and the dorsal area of the hands and feet are often involved, but eczema can occur anywhere on the body. It is important to know the full medical history, any known exacerbating factors such as foods, contact with pets or pollen and the family history of atopic disease. It must be established which treatments have previously been used on the skin. It is also useful to establish the nature of the parents' and child's concerns, e.g. sleepless nights from itching, and their expectations from treatment.

Examination

Height and weight should always be documented, and a general physical examination performed. Affected areas of skin may show erythema, vesicles, lichenification or crusting. Painless lymphadenopathy is very common. The skin may exhibit white dermographism, with blanching of the skin after light pressure, and an extra infraorbital fold, the Dennie–Morgan sign, may be seen. A search should be made for signs of infection (pustules, crusting, and weeping).

Management

1. Itching and scratching. Nails should be kept short and clean, and mittens may be helpful at night. Splints are not indicated. Night-time sedatives may be helpful, e.g. trimeprazine, promethazine. Reducing the dryness of the skin will reduce itch.

2. Dryness. Every attempt should be made to keep the skin moist with emollients, e.g. aqueous cream and paraffin-based creams. Emollients need to be applied frequently and regularly. Applying emollient and then bandaging (wet wrapping) is often helpful in severely affected areas and prevents the child from scratching. Some emollients suit certain children better than others so several may need to be tried before the eczema responds. Occasionally children have an adverse reaction to a particular product. Ordinary soap is often drying and irritant and should be avoided. Bath oils and soap substitutes should be used. Washing the hair in the bath should be avoided if possible and a mild shampoo used. A tar-based shampoo is helpful if the scalp is involved. Coal tar or zinc bandages may be used on areas of lichenified eczema.

3. Inflammation. If inflammation is severe, topical treatment with steroid ointments or creams is indicated. Low potency steroid preparations should be used, e.g. 0.5–1% hydrocortisone, the lowest strength being used in facial areas. Occasionally a more potent strength is needed for short periods on selected areas of skin. Side-effects include skin thinning, striae and secondary infection. In uncontrolled cases, oral prednisolone is used. As short stature is not uncommon in severe eczema, effects of uncontrolled skin inflammation must be weighed against steroid side-effects.

4. Infection. Secondary infection may require systemic treatment or local agents, depending on the clinical picture and the organisms cultured. Oral flucloxacillin is usually appropriate. Eczema herpeticum is a severe systemic illness in eczema sufferers which follows a primary infection with herpes simplex. Aggressive supportive therapy, and intravenous acyclovir are indicated.

5. Dietary restriction. For a few children, dietary elimination of dairy products produces an improvement in their eczema. Neither skin tests nor RAST tests are of practical help. More restrictive in-patient elimination diets have also been tried with some improvement for severe disease. Expert dietary advice is essential, as protein, energy, calcium and iron deficiencies may occur.

6. Other treatment measures. Trigger factors should be avoided. There is no convincing evidence that exclusive breast-feeding is protective, although dietary factors in the mother may be relevant. Alternative therapies such as Chinese medicine and acupuncture have been reported to be helpful by some patients.

Irritant contact dermatitis

This looks very like atopic eczema but removal of the irritant cause will cause resolution. A common cause is saliva. Babies and children who dribble develop the rash on the chin and neck. Older children often develop a perioral rash from repeated licking of the lips. Urine is another irritant, leading to nappy rash (see related topic Rashes and blisters, p. 337) and in older children bubble baths are often the culprit. Treatment is to avoid the irritant if possible or in the case of its being saliva or urine, clean and dry the child's skin as soon as possible and apply generous amounts of emollient. *Juvenile plantar dermatosis* is a common form of irritant dermatitis which is characterized by painful, shiny, fissured skin on the bottom of the feet. The cause is hyperhidrosis in occlusive, synthetic footwear, followed by rapid drying. Treatment is use of emollients, applied when shoes are removed and after swimming.

Allergic contact dermatitis

This is caused by a Type IV delayed hypersensitivity response to an allergen which has come into direct contact with the skin, e.g. nickel, cosmetics, plants. Clinically the appearance is that of eczema but the distribution is often diagnostic. Treatment is avoidance of the allergen. Allergy may last many years but is not necessarily lifelong.

Further reading

David TJ. Management of atopic eczema. In: David TJ, ed. *Recent Advances in Paediatrics*, Vol. 12. Edinburgh: Churchill Livingstone, 1994; 187–204.

Related topics of interest

Allergy and anaphylaxis (p. 27)
Asthma (p. 38)
Rashes and blisters (p. 337)

EPIDEMIOLOGY, DEFINITIONS AND STATISTICS

Demography is the study of human populations. Children under 15 years make up approximately one-third of the world's population. One-quarter (~ 350 million) live in developed countries and three-quarters (~ 1050 million) in developing countries. The UK currently has a population of 11 million children, and there are approximately 500 000 births per year. Each family doctor has approximately 2500 patients in his/her practice and, of these, about 450 are under 15 years. With the present birth rate in England and Wales of ~13.5/1000 total population, there will be between 30 and 35 births per practice each year. By far the most common paediatric disorders are those of the respiratory system. Accidents, acute respiratory illness, fevers, convulsions and acute gastrointestinal upsets are the commonest reasons for acute referral to hospital. The Office of Population Censuses and Surveys (OPCS) collects data for England and Wales on births, childhood mortality, communicable diseases, congenital malformations, hospital admissions and other surveys, which it publishes regularly. Some diseases are legally notifiable to the Communicable Disease Surveillance Centre, in particular those that are included in the immunization programme (e.g. mumps, measles, rubella, *Haemophilus influenzae* infection), acute meningitis, food poisoning and dysentery and tuberculosis. The British Paediatric Surveillance Unit (BPSU) was set up in 1986 to enable paediatricians to participate in the epidemiological surveillance of uncommon disorders affecting children. This unit increases awareness of less common disorders and allows a rapid response to public health emergencies. Disorders currently being studied include cerebral oedema following diabetic ketoacidosis, haemolytic uraemic syndrome, hepatitis C infection, Reye's syndrome, medium chain acyl-CoA dehydrogenase deficiency and HIV/AIDS infection.

Mortality rates

The OPCS has defined mortality rates in different age groups. The neonatal, post-neonatal and infant mortality rates are three important indicators of child health. Neonatal and perinatal mortality rates provide an indirect measure of the quality of obstetric and neonatal services. Approximate current rates for England and Wales are given in brackets.

Stillbirth rate (5/1000) — The number of infants born after 26 weeks who show no signs of life per 1000 *total* births.

Perinatal mortality rate (8–9/1000) — The number of stillbirths and deaths in the first week per 1000 *total* births. Principal causes are low birth weight and congenital malformations. The rate is four and a half times higher for multiple births than for singletons.

Neonatal mortality rate (4–5/1000) — The number of deaths in the first 27 days of life per 1000 *live* births. The neonatal mortality rate can be further subdivided into early (deaths in the first 7 days of life) and late (deaths occurring from the 8th to the 27th day inclusive).

Eighty per cent of neonatal deaths occur in the first week, the main causes being congenital abnormality, respiratory distress and prematurity. Neonatal deaths account for 40% of all childhood deaths, the biggest risk factor being low birth weight. Increased rates are also associated with maternal age under 20 years or over 35 years, parity of three or more and lower social class. The place of maternal birth is also a factor, for example mothers born in Pakistan have a higher rate than mothers of the same ethnic group born in this country. Rates vary between different regions of the country with the lowest figure in 1987 in East Anglia, and the highest in Yorkshire, but the relationship with poverty is not exact. Infants classified as illegitimate have a higher rate at about 6/1000.

Post-neonatal mortality rate (3–4/1000)

The number of deaths between 28 days and 1 year of life per 1000 *live* births. The major causes are sudden infant death syndrome (SIDS), congenital abnormalities and respiratory infections. A small number are late deaths due to low birth weight/prematurity. The rate of SIDS was 2/1000 in 1987, but has halved over the last 10 years following changes in sleeping position advice. As with neonatal mortality, deaths in the post-neonatal period are related to age, parity, social class and place of birth of the mother, and birth weight and legal status of the infant. Deaths in this age group show a more pronounced seasonal pattern than at any other time in childhood, with more deaths in the winter, mainly attributable to SIDS and respiratory infections.

Infant mortality rate (IMR 6–7/1000)

The number of deaths in the first year of life per 1000 *live* births. Some Third-World countries have rates in excess of 150/1000. Again, one of the major causes in the UK is congenital abnormality, including congenital heart disease. The IMR has fallen steeply from over 15/1000 in 1975 mainly because of a fall in neonatal deaths.

Mortality in later childhood (~25/100 000 children 1–14 years)

Accidents account for one-quarter of deaths between the ages of 1 and 14 years, with road accidents accounting for the majority. On average, three children die in accidents every day and ~10 000 are permanently disabled each year. Malignancy is the second commonest cause of death in this age group. The remainder include children with inherited disorders (e.g. cystic fibrosis) and acute infections.

Further reading

British Paediatric Surveillance Unit 11th Annual Report (1996–1997). Available from the Royal College of Paediatrics and Child Health Publications Department.

Madeley RJ. Recent trends in infant, neonatal and postneonatal mortality rates. *Current Paediatrics*, 1991; **1:** 49–52.
Platt MJ, Pharoah POD. Child health statistical review, 1996. *Archives of Disease in Childhood,* 1996; **75**: 527–33.
Platt MJ. Child health statistical review, 1997. *Archives of Disease in Childhood,* 1997; **77:** 542–8.

Related topics of interest

Accidents (p. 7)
Prematurity (p. 323)
Sudden infant death syndrome (p. 360)

FAILURE TO THRIVE

Failure to thrive is the term used when a child fails to gain weight at the expected rate. Diagnosis is based on serial measurements and the child's weight is seen to fall across the centiles on a growth chart. The term is usually reserved for growth in pre-school children, particularly under 2 years of age. Growth at this age is almost entirely dependent on nutrition, and the causes of undernutrition may be organic or non-organic. A combination of factors may be responsible for failure to thrive, but many community-based studies have shown that <10% of cases have an organic basis. Approximately 20% of babies who are born small for dates due to intrauterine growth retardation do not show 'catch up' postnatal growth and remain small. However, these children tend to gain weight at an appropriate rate, parallel with but below the normal centiles, so they are not failing to thrive.

Causes

1. Common

- Poor oral intake. Insufficient food may be offered. Bottle feeds may be being made up incorrectly. Breast-feeding techniques may be poor. There may be disordered swallowing or sucking mechanisms, e.g. cerebral palsy, Down's syndrome, cleft palate. Behavioural problems may occur at meal-times.
- Psychosocial deprivation. The influence of lack of nurturing in failure to thrive is difficult to separate from that of undernutrition, but some children fail to thrive in poor social circumstances despite an adequate nutrient intake.

2. Uncommon

- Abnormal nutrient losses

(a) Persistent vomiting, e.g. severe gastro-oesophageal reflux, raised intracranial pressure.

(b) Malabsorption/persistent diarrhoea, e.g. cow's milk intolerance, coeliac disease, cystic fibrosis, chronic infection, e.g. Giardiasis.

- Chronic illness, e.g. infants with cardiovascular or respiratory disease may be too breathless to feed. UTI in the first few months of life may cause failure to thrive.

History

Details of the pregnancy, birth and neonatal period should be noted. Enquiry should be made about symptoms such as vomiting, diarrhoea, dyspnoea, polyuria etc that would suggest chronic illness or abnormal nutrient losses. A full feeding history is vital including the type of feeds offered, the quantity and frequency of feeds, and the timing of introduction of solids. A full family and social history is also very important. Factors such as poverty, maternal health, number of siblings, and parental employment status can all affect the nutrition and nurturing that an infant receives.

Examination

Measurements of weight, length and head circumference should be plotted on a nine-centile growth chart, along with any previous measurements available (e.g. from the parent held record). Correction for prematurity should be made up to the age of 2 years. An assessment of the amount of subcutaneous tissue present is useful – in older children measurements of the mid-upper arm circumference and skinfold thickness (triceps and subscapular folds) can be made. The child should be fully examined to exclude any dysmorphic features, signs of chronic illness, or evidence of a neurological disorder. It is also important to look for any signs of neglect or physical abuse (e.g. poor hygiene, extensive nappy rash, bruising).

Investigations

A trial of feeding to establish whether the child can gain weight if given an adequate dietary intake may be all that is required. Hospital admission is occasionally needed to achieve such an intake. In practice, baseline investigations are often undertaken during this trial of feeding to exclude an organic cause for the failure to thrive.

- FBC. Microcytic anaemia is associated with iron deficiency and coeliac disease. Neutropenia is a feature of Schwachman–Diamond syndrome.
- Iron studies. Ferritin low and total iron binding capacity high in iron deficiency.
- Red cell folate may be low in coeliac disease.
- Renal function tests to exclude chronic renal disease, renal tubular acidosis etc.
- Liver function tests, calcium, phosphate, alkaline phosphatase may be abnormal in severe malabsorption.
- Stool for bacterial and viral culture, microscopy for ova cysts and parasites, reducing substances, fat globules.
- Urine for sugar, protein, culture, and pH.
- Sweat test to exclude cystic fibrosis.
- Antigliadin and antiendomysium antibodies. Proceeding to jejunal biopsy if antibodies are raised or high clinical suspicion of coeliac disease.
- Immunoglobulins.
- Further investigations only if clinically indicated, e.g. thyroid function tests, oesophageal pH monitoring, HIV status.

Management

For a minority of children an underlying organic cause can be identified and treated. For the majority, the approach needs to focus on why the child is being undernourished. A multidisciplinary approach involving paediatrician, health visitor, dietitian, speech therapist, and social worker may be valuable in those who pose the most difficult management problems.

Further reading

Marcovitch H. Failure to thrive. *British Medical Journal,* 1994; **308:** 35–8.
Skuse D. Failure to thrive: current perspectives. *Current Paediatrics,* 1992; **2** (2): 105–10.

Related topics of interest

Child protection (p. 65)
Chronic diarrhoea (p. 77)
Coeliac disease (p. 86)
Cystic fibrosis (p. 107)
Growth assessment (p. 167)
Growth – short and tall stature (p. 171)
Nutrition (p. 303)
Vomiting (p. 377)

FETAL MEDICINE

Routine screening tests are carried out in most pregnancies in the UK, and further tests are available for those at higher risk of a fetal abnormality. Recent advances in antenatal imaging and DNA techniques have widened the range of conditions which can be diagnosed antenatally. Accurate prenatal diagnosis has allowed the advancement of *in vitro* treatment for certain conditions, e.g. rhesus disease and some congenital renal and lung abnormalities. It is also allows delivery of the baby in a centre with facilities for intensive care and neonatal surgery. In severe disorders for which no treatment is available, termination of pregnancy may be indicated, so the parents must be counselled carefully and find this acceptable before extensive investigations are instituted.

Antenatal screening tests

Methods

1. Maternal FBC, blood grouping and rubella titre are carried out at the first antenatal visit. If the mother is rhesus negative the rhesus antibody titre should be monitored. Haemoglobin electrophoresis is indicated in those at high risk of haemoglobinopathy and should be routine in Afro-Caribbeans (15% carry the sickle cell gene).

2. Routine ultrasound (US). Most centres perform an US scan at 16–18 weeks' gestation to confirm dates, locate the placenta and detect structural abnormalities (e.g. neural tube defects, severe skeletal dysplasia, diaphragmatic hernia, renal tract abnormalities). Polyhydramnios may indicate an underlying gastrointestinal atresia, and oligohydramnios is associated with renal abnormalities. More detailed high-resolution anomaly US scans by skilled operators can detect other abnormalities, e.g. various types of congenital heart disease and cleft lip and palate.

3. Maternal serum α–fetoprotein (AFP) is used as a screening test at 16–18 weeks for neural tube defects. Over 80% of open neural tube defects and anencephalies can be detected by a raised AFP, but other causes of a raised level include multiple pregnancy, abdominal wall defects and Turner's syndrome, so further detailed ultrasonography and amniocentesis are indicated. A low serum AFP is associated with an increased risk of Down's syndrome. Many centres have now introduced a 'triple test' screening for Down's syndrome. Risk is estimated from maternal age, low AFP, low serum unconjugated oestriol and high human chorionic gonadotrophin concentrations.

Indications for further investigation

Prenatal investigations are indicated if there is a reliable test available, the disorder is severe and there is an increased risk of fetal abnormality. Factors associated with an increased risk include:

- Raised maternal serum AFP.
- Maternal age over 35 years. Most centres offer amniocentesis to this group because of the increased risk of Down's syndrome.
- Previous affected child, e.g. the recurrence risk is 1 in 4 for an autosomal recessive condition.
- Family history of an inherited condition. Investigation of a family with a single gene defect should ideally be carried out before pregnancy so that detection of biochemical carriers and DNA analysis for genetic markers can be used to estimate the risk of an affected fetus and allow genetic counselling.

Amniocentesis

Amniocentesis is performed at 16–18 weeks. Amniotic fluid is obtained by passing a needle through the abdominal wall and uterus under US guidance. Protein levels or metabolites can be measured in the amniotic fluid, e.g. raised AFP and acetylcholinesterase in neural tube defects, bilirubin in Rhesus disease. This fluid also contains cells that have been shed from the fetal skin, which can be cultured and examined for chromosomal abnormalities, enzyme defects and specific gene defects. Prediction of fetal sex allows abortion of male fetuses in X-linked conditions. In some centres blood samples can be taken directly from the umbilical cord (cordocentesis) for the diagnosis of inborn errors of metabolism, haemoglobinopathies and viral infections. Cordocentesis is also used for blood transfusion in severe rhesus disease.

Problems

- Risk of miscarriage. This is about 1% following amniocentesis and about 2% following cordocentesis, compared with a spontaneous abortion rate at 16–18 weeks of 0.5%.
- Time for results. Culture of amniotic cells and analysis takes 2–3 weeks and this can be an extremely stressful time for couples. If termination of pregnancy is indicated this is relatively late in gestation.
- Small risk of haemorrhage from placenta, cord or uterine vessels, particularly following cordocentesis.
- Small risk of amnionitis.
- Risk of inducing rhesus isoimmunization. Rhesus-negative mothers should be given anti-D.
- Small increase in incidence of postural deformities, e.g. talipes, owing to amniotic fluid leakage.

Chorionic villus sampling (CVS)

Using ultrasound guidance this transcervical technique, performed between 9 and 12 weeks, allows collection of fetally derived chorionic villus material. This procedure is useful in the prenatal diagnosis of chromosomal anomalies, inherited metabolic diseases and conditions amenable to DNA analysis. The major advantage over amniocentesis is that it provides results sooner (usually within 24 hours), allowing earlier termination. The risk of miscarriage is higher than amniocentesis at 2%. CVS should therefore only be recommended for pregnancies with a high risk of abnormality. It has been reported that early CVS may cause limb and facial deformities; however this is yet to be validated.

Prenatal therapy

Routine antenatal screening allows early detection of many fetal anomalies which may be amenable to treatment, e.g. haemolytic disease and congenital heart, lung and renal disease. Fetal anomalies can have an adverse affect on the mother causing hypertension, oedema and pulmonary failure. Any *in utero* intervention is not without risks and these must be clearly explained to the parents.

Fetal arrythmias, which can cause hydrops or fetal death, may respond if the mother is treated with anti-arrythmic agents (e.g. digoxin or flecainide). More invasive interventions include:

- Needle aspiration, e.g. in severe Rhesus haemolytic disease exchange transfusion can be performed via the umbilical cord.
- Feto-amniotic shunting. Insertion of stents to decompress fluid collections and cystic structures, e.g. urinary tract obstruction or pleural effusions.
- Fetal endoscopy. Procedures may be diagnostic or interventional.
- Open fetal surgery. Highly specialized operations are attempted in some units but hold a high risk of fetal mortality. Most forms of fetal surgery are still in their experimental stages. Specific conditions which may be amenable to intervention include congenital diaphragmatic hernia, congenital cystic adenomatoid malformation, abdominal wall defects, sacrococcygeal teratoma, fetal obstructive uropathy, spina bifida, and cleft lip and palate.

Further reading

Kimber C, Spitz L, Cuschieri A. Current state of antenatal in utero surgical interventions. *Archives of Disease in Childhood,* 1997; **76:** F134–9.

Lees M, Winter R. Advances in genetics. *Archives of Disease in Childhood,* 1996; **75:** 346–50.

Sharland G. Changing impact of fetal diagnosis of congenital heart disease. *Archives of Disease in Childhood,* 1997; **77:** F1–3.

Related topics of interest

Chromosomal abnormalities (p. 73)
Gene defects (p. 160)
Inborn errors of metabolism (p. 215)

FITS, FAINTS AND FUNNY TURNS

Children often present to the doctor having had an unexplained episode of collapse, reduced level of consciousness, or abnormal movement or behaviour. The most important part of the assessment is a history from an eye witness. Important signs to enquire about include colour, particularly of lips and tongue, incontinence in older children, type of abnormal movements (ask the witness to demonstrate if possible) length of episode, precipitating factors, and post-ictal symptoms. Ask about family history, neonatal history and past medical history. Does the child have behavioural or learning problems? It is extremely important to diagnose epilepsy correctly to prevent unnecessary restriction on the child and to obtain appropriate treatment. Babies may present with unexplained apnoea with or without abnormal movement and the differential diagnosis is very different from that in older children.

Infants

1. Convulsions are usually caused by infection or metabolic derangement (see related topic Neonatal convulsions, p. 272).

2. Infantile spasms. Also known as West syndrome, the repetitive flexor and/or extensor spasms start between the ages of 4 and 7 months. The child has a number of spasms in quick succession followed usually by crying. Early recognition leads to treatment which may improve the prognosis. EEG shows a characteristic chaotic pattern known as hypsarrhythmia. In 70% there are associated developmental problems or a demonstrable brain abnormality, such as tuberous sclerosis, and they are then said to be 'symptomatic'. Symptomatic spasms are less responsive to treatment and carry a worse developmental prognosis than those occurring in an otherwise normal child. Treatment is with steroids or vigabatrin which should be commenced as soon as possible after diagnosis.

3. Gastro-oesophageal reflux may cause the child to become apnoeic for a short time. The baby has usually been noted to vomit or regurgitate and may arch the back and appear to be in pain.

4. Respiratory disease, e.g. acute bronchiolitis may lead to apnoea. Diagnosis is usually obvious.

5. Münchausen by proxy may be suspected in a baby with recurrent apnoeic or convulsive episodes where no cause is found.

Older children: febrile seizures

These are convulsions occurring with fever in otherwise normal children between the ages of 6 months and 6 years. The convulsion may be simple, i.e. a generalized convulsion of less than 15 minutes duration, occurring only once during a febrile illness in the absence of focal signs, or may be complex, i.e. a focal or prolonged convulsion, often repeated within the same illness, or leaving residual neurological signs (Todd's paresis). Recurrence occurs in 30%. There is an increased risk of non-febrile seizures in later life if the child has pre-existing neuro-developmental problems, complex febrile convulsions occur or if there is a family history of epilepsy. Aims of management are to diagnose and treat the cause of the fever (e.g. meningitis, UTI), assess the risk factors for recurrence and counsel the parents on first aid management of fever and convulsions. The carers of children who have recurrent or prolonged seizures may be given rectal diazepam to use in the event of prolonged fitting.

Older children: non-febrile seizures

Problems

- Recurrent seizures.
- Status epilepticus.
- Side-effects of medication.
- Social and educational effects.

Aetiology

- Idiopathic. Accounts for most cases.
- Trauma. Head injury.
- Infection, e.g. meningitis, both complicating acute illness and as a long-term sequelae.
- Vascular, e.g. AV malformation.
- Tumour, either benign or malignant may give rise particularly to focal fits.
- Genetic. A family history of epilepsy increases the risk of developing the condition. Some types of epilepsy are known to be due to a single gene abnormality.
- Metabolic disease. Acute metabolic derangement, e.g. hypoglycaemia or hypernatraemia.
- Degenerative conditions, e.g. leukodystrophies.
- Cerebral malformations, e.g. neuronal migration disorders, neurocutaneous syndromes.

Epileptic seizures may be generalized or partial, with or without secondary generalization.

Generalized seizures

1. Absence epilepsy occurs most commonly in females aged 6–8 years. Each episode lasts 5–20 seconds but may occur more than 10 times a day. Deteriorating school performance may be an early feature. Hyperventilation may induce an attack and this can be used diagnostically. EEG shows characteristic 3/second spike and wave discharges during an attack. Response to sodium valproate is usually good. Spontaneous resolution by puberty is usual.

2. *Tonic-clonic epilepsy* usually presents between the ages of 5 and 10 but can start at any age. 50% of the children will have one seizure and never have another, so anticonvulsant medication is not usually indicated following the first attack. Remission rates with carbamazepine or sodium valproate therapy monotherapy are 80–90%.

3. *Myoclonic epilepsy*. Sudden involuntary contraction occurs in a muscle or group of muscles, often with retained conscious level.

Partial seizures

1. *Simple partial seizures* produce tonic or clonic movements such as forced deviation of the head and eyes to one side during which the child remains fully conscious.

2. *Complex partial seizures* most commonly arising from the frontal or temporal lobes, account for 25% of childhood epilepsy. There may be an associated aura. Stereotyped movements such as lip smacking may occur. There may be secondary generalization. Treatment is with carbamazepine.

Epileptic syndromes

Epilepsy may develop as part of a syndrome with characteristic fits associated with other specific features.

1. *Landau–Kleffner syndrome* is a combination of fits and loss of language in an otherwise normal child, usually of pre-school age. Early onset is associated with a worse prognosis.

2. *Lennox–Gastaut syndrome* is characterized by intractable seizures, often myotonic. There is severe developmental delay and prognosis is poor.

3. *Benign rolandic epilepsy* has a peak onset at 9–10 years. Focal seizures involving the mouth are often noticed as paraesthesia when cleaning the teeth as they typically occur on getting up in the morning. There may be secondary generalization. EEG shows spikes in the centerotemporal area. Treatment is with carbamazepine and most will have spontaneous remission in adolescence.

Investigation

Selected investigations may include:

- U&E, calcium, magnesium and glucose.
- EEG, which may need to be over a prolonged period including during sleep with video recording of the child in difficult cases.

- CT or MRI imaging.
- pH study in infants in whom gastro-oesophageal reflux is a possible diagnosis.

Management

1. Emergency management of a convulsing child involves airway management, detection and treatment of hypoglycaemia and cessation of the fit with drug therapy. A fit lasting more than 30 minutes or more than one fit without recovery in between, is known as status epilepticus and constitutes an emergency. Treatment should involve a graded approach, usually starting with diazepam followed by paraldehyde and then phenytoin. Other drugs such as phenobarbitone and clonazepam may be tried. Paralysis and mechnical ventilation may ultimately be required in resistant status.

2. Long term. A firm diagnosis of the type of epilepsy should be made to determine the appropriate treatment. Prophylaxis is usually not indicated for an isolated fit. Monotherapy should be used where possible and will achieve remission in 75% of cases. Patients may find it helpful to get in touch with patient support groups. Children with epilepsy should be encouraged to live as normal a life as possible but should not swim or cycle unaccompanied. Showers are preferable to baths. Employment choices may have to take the condition into account (e.g. jobs involving working at heights or with dangerous machinery may be unsuitable) and adolescents will need information about suitability to drive. There is still considerable stigma attached to epilepsy due to public ignorance and the doctor should be prepared to act as the patient's advocate.

Differential diagnoses

Breath-holding attacks

These occur between the ages of 2 and 4 years, often when the child is provoked. The onset can often be predicted and attacks are stereotypical. The child gives a shrill cry, and following forced expiration, loses consciousness. The child becomes cyanosed and may go on to have a tonic-clonic seizure.

Reflex anoxic seizures (pallid spells)

Similar to the above, young children who have experienced sudden pain may cry out, become very pale and then lose consciousness for a few seconds. They recover spontaneously but may cause considerable parental alarm.

Syncope (faints or vaso-vagal attacks)

These occur most often in female adolescents. Collapse is preceded by visual disturbance and pallor. Heat, prolonged standing, pain and fear may precipitate an attack. The episode lasts a few seconds and there is no drowsiness afterwards. Occasionally, syncope is associated with urinary incontinence. If the child is supported upright during the episode, a seizure may occur secondary to the fall in cerebral blood flow.

Benign paroxysmal vertigo

This is thought to be a migrainous phenomenon which occurs in children under 3 years. The sudden attacks of vertigo may cause them to fall over and are often accompanied by pallor, nystagmus, nausea and vomiting. Attacks can last from a few seconds to several minutes.

Night terrors

These occur predominantly in boys aged betweeen 5 and 7 years. They occur in 1–3% of children at some time. The child wakes in the night, crying in apparent fear, thrashes about and does not recognize his parents. Tachycardia, dilated pupils and hyperventilation may occur. The child does not remember the episode in the morning.

Tics

Boys are more often affected than girls and the onset is usually around 6–9 years. The repetitive movements can be controlled voluntarily for a certain length of time but eventually the child feels the need to perform the movement to release tension. Tics may involve any muscle group including the face. One tic may subside to be replaced by another. They diminish in frequency when the child is concentrating. Onset may be linked to psychological stress or due to drugs, e.g. methylphenidate. Combinations of vocal and motor tics occur in Giles de Tourette syndrome.

Cardiac events

Loss of consciousness may result from a sudden fall in cardiac output and may follow exertion in a child with an underlying abnormality. The resulting hypoxia may cause the child to have a seizure which may confuse the diagnosis. Long QT syndrome, congenital heart block and dysrrhythmias such as paroxysmal SVT are possible causes. The child may describe a history of palpitations or there may be a family history of sudden death. If the diagnosis is suspected, the parent should be asked to take the pulse during an attack. Investigations include 12 lead ECG, 24 hour ECG monitoring and echocardiography. Diagnosis and appropriate treatment may prevent a potentially fatal episode.

Further reading

Neville BGR. Epilepsy in Childhood. *British Medical Journal,* 1997; **315:** 924–30.
O'Donohoe NV. Delineation of epileptic syndromes. *Current Paediatrics,* 1992; **2:** 68–72.
O'Donohoe NV. The EEG and neuroimaging in the management of the epilepsies. *Archives of Disease in Childhood,* 1995; **73:** 552–7.
Rutter N, Metcalf DH. Febrile convulsions – what do parents do? *British Medical Journal,* 1978; **2:** 1345–6.
Taylor DC. A psychiatric perspective of epilepsy. *Archives of Disease in Childhood,* 1997; **77** (1): 86–8.
Verity CM. The place of the EEG and imaging in the management of seizures. *Archives of Disease in Childhood,* 1995; **73:** 557–62.
Wallace SJ. Convulsions and funny turns. *Current Paediatrics,* 1992; **2:** 63–7.

Related topics of interest

Arrhythmias (p. 35)
Developmental delay (p. 115)
Neonatal convulsions (p. 272)
Neurocutaneous syndromes (p. 293)

FLOPPY INFANT

Hypotonia in infancy may be due to a paralytic or a non-paralytic disorder. Paralytic conditions cause hypotonia with weakness and may affect the anterior horn cells, nerve fibres, neuromuscular junctions or muscles. Non-paralytic conditions cause hypotonia without significant weakness. The commonest cause of a floppy baby is perinatal asphyxia. The paralytic causes of floppiness are rare, and many are genetically determined, the commonest being spinal muscular atrophy.

1. Paralytic

- Spinal cord disorders. Trauma (e.g. birth injury), tumours.
- Anterior horn cell disease, e.g. spinal muscular atrophy, poliomyelitis.
- Peripheral neuropathy. Very rare in infancy.
- Neuromuscular disorder, e.g. neonatal or congenital myasthenia gravis.
- Congenital myopathy. Structural (e.g. central core disease, muscular dystrophy, myotonic dystrophy) or metabolic (glycogen and lipid storage disorders, periodic paralysis).

2. Non-paralytic

- Disorders affecting the CNS, e.g. birth asphyxia, hypotonic cerebral palsy, Down's syndrome, metabolic disorders (e.g. aminoacidurias).
- Connective tissue disorders, e.g. Ehlers–Danlos.
- Prader–Willi syndrome.
- Metabolic and endocrine disorders, e.g. hypercalcaemia, hypothyroidism.
- Benign congenital hypotonia.

Clinical features

Hypotonia at birth is usually due to severe hypoxia, but is occasionally due to drugs taken by the mother, e.g. diazepam. Severely hypotonic infants lie in the characteristic frog-like position, and on ventral suspension the four limbs hang down and the infant is unable to hold his head up. The head lags on pulling to the sitting position. There may be deformity of the chest and a 'see-saw' respiratory pattern. Infants with cerebral palsy may go through a hypotonic phase before becoming spastic. Benign congenital hypotonia is an idiopathic, non-progressive condition which tends to improve with age, and is a diagnosis of exclusion.

Investigation

- U&Es.
- Thyroid function.

- Serum calcium.
- Chromosomes.
- Investigations for inborn errors of metabolism.
- Brain imaging (e.g. CT or MRI scan). May be evidence of hypoxic damage, e.g. atrophy, cysts.
- Neurophysiology.
- Muscle biopsy.

Spinal muscular atrophy (SMA)

There are three main types of SMA which are due to progressive apoptosis of anterior horn cells. The gene has been located on chromosome 5. Type I (Werdnig–Hoffmann disease) presents in the first few weeks of life with weakness and wasting of the muscles. Fasciculation is seen, particularly in the tongue. There may have been decreased fetal movements and the infant may be profoundly floppy at birth. The facial and bulbar muscles are unaffected so the infant has an alert expression and is able to swallow normally. It is an autosomal recessive condition with a prevalence of 1 in 20 000 births. It is rapidly progressive, with the majority dying of respiratory failure within 18 months. Type II is also autosomal recessive and is a more chronic condition which usually presents between 3 and 12 months of age. It causes severe muscle wasting, contractures and scoliosis, and the majority of affected children die by the age of 10 years. Children with type III (juvenile) SMA develop normally until about 2 years of age, when they develop limb girdle weakness, a waddling gait, and gradual loss of ability to walk. Progression of weakness is episodic and survival into adult life is usual.

Further reading

Roland EH. Muscle disorders in the newborn. In: Roberton NRC, ed. *Textbook of Neonatology*, 2nd edn. Edinburgh: Churchill Livingsone, 1992; 1103–14.

Related topics of interest

Inborn errors of metabolism (p. 215)
Muscle and neuromuscular disorders (p. 269)
Neonatal convulsions (p. 272)

GASTROENTERITIS

Acute gastroenteritis remains a significant paediatric problem, accounting for 5 million deaths annually in the developing world in the under-5 age group, where it often occurs against a background of malnutrition. In Western nations, mortality is now minimal, but gastroenteritis remains an important cause of morbidity, and a common reason for paediatric hospital admissions (second only to respiratory illness). The promotion of adequate fluid balance, good nutritional status and the avoidance of unnecessary drug therapies should be the priorities of all health workers.

Problems

- Dehydration.
- Metabolic disturbances.
- Oliguria/acute renal failure.
- Haemolytic uraemic syndrome.
- Septicaemia.
- Protracted diarrhoea.
- Malnutrition.

Aetiology/pathogenesis

A pathogen may be identified in up to 80% of cases using modern techniques.

1. Viral

- Rotavirus (commonest in UK).
- Enteric adenovirus.
- Small round viruses (astro calici).
- Norwalk.

Rotavirus infection occurs in seasonal outbreaks (December to February), the virus attacking and killing the mature enterocyte, which is then shed from the small intestinal villus. The increased production of immature crypt-like cells with villus shortening then decreases the absorptive and disaccharidase activity of the brush border.

2. Bacterial

- *Campylobacter jejuni* (commonest invasive pathogen in UK).
- *Shigella* spp.
- *Salmonella* spp.
- *E. coli.*
- *Vibrio cholera.*
- *Yersinia enterocolitica.*

Various mechanisms account for bacterial pathogenicity, and several mechanisms may be involved simultaneously:

(a) Mucosal invasion, e.g. *Campylobacter jejuni, Shigella* spp.
(b) Production of cytotoxins which alter mucosal surface properties, e.g. enteropathogenic *E. coli.*
(c) Production of enterotoxins which alter enterocyte salt and water balance, e.g. *Vibrio cholera*, enterotoxigenic *E. coli, Shigella* spp.
(d) Adherence to enterocyte surface, destroying the microvilli, e.g. enteropathogenic and enterohaemorrhagic *E. coli.*

3. Parasitic
- *Giardia lamblia.*
- *Cryptosporidium.*
- *Entamoeba histolytica.*

Again, several mechanisms of pathogenicity may be involved, e.g. parasitic enterotoxin production, altered motility.

Clinical features

A prodromal illness is uncommon, but more likely in viral infection. Vomiting may precede the onset of watery diarrhoea by up to 48 hours. Abdominal cramps may be a feature. Blood and mucus in the stools, with associated fever, suggest an invasive organism. As fluid losses from the gastrointestinal tract increase, dehydration occurs (see features below). Convulsions may occur from pyrexia or metabolic disturbances. Assessment of the abdomen is vital, as blood in the stool, with persistent vomiting, may also be the presenting symptoms of a surgical condition such as an intussusception.

Features of dehydration
- <5% (mild) — Not unwell, dry mucus membranes, thirsty.
- 5–10% (moderate) — Lethargic – sunken fontanelle, sunken eyes, reduced skin turgor, oliguria.
- >10% (severe) — Shocked – hypotension, peri-pheral shut-down.

Investigation

- Weight. Accurate weighing is critical for calculating fluid requirements and assessing the success of rehydration.
- U&E, creatinine, glucose. No biochemical tests are needed in mild cases.

- Urinary urea, creatinine, sodium. Consider these in incipient renal failure.
- Stool. Culture, electron microscopy, enzyme-linked immunosorbent assay (ELISA). Pathogens can be identified, occasionally indicating the need for specific antimicrobial therapy
- Urine, blood, CSF. Consider culture if systemic sepsis is suspected.

Management

The aims should be:

1. Prevention and correction of dehydration. Gastroenteritis can be managed with oral rehydration in the majority of cases, even if the child is moderately dehydrated. Fluids should be offered little and often. Oral rehydration solutions (ORS) are available which contain sodium, chloride and glucose in ratios which promote glucose and amino acid coupled sodium absorption across the enterocyte.The WHO ORS, which is used in areas where cholera is prevalent, has a higher sodium concentration (90 mmol/l) than that of solutions commercially available in the UK (e.g. Dioralyte™ Rhone-Poulenc Rorer, 60 mmol/l of sodium) to replace the high sodium losses in cholera stools.

Fluid requirements over the first 24 hours can be calculated by assessing the volume required to rehydrate the child (the deficit volume) and giving this in addition to maintenance fluids.

The deficit volume (ml) = % dehydration × weight (kg) × 10

(i.e. a 15 kg child who is 5% dehydrated has a deficit volume of 750 ml). Fluid to replace significant ongoing losses (e.g. vomiting, diarrhoea) should also be given. If there is shock, coma, ileus or stool losses are excessive, intravenous therapy is indicated. If shocked, the child should be resuscitated with 20 ml/kg of colloid or normal saline over 30 minutes.

2. Promotion of adequate nutrition. Breast-feeding should continue uninterrupted throughout the illness. For bottle-fed infants, traditional guidelines have recommended a slow re-introduction of formula milk after rehydration in an attempt to decrease the likelihood of protracted diarrhoea ('regrading' through one-quarter, half, three-quarters, full strength feeds over 12–72 hours). However, the incidence of lactose intolerance and cow's milk allergy appears to be declining, and routine 'regrading', certainly in the older infant, is no longer indicated.

3. Avoidance of metabolic disturbance. In moderate and severe gastroenteritis, electrolyte disturbances may occur, particularly hyponatraemia, hypokalaemia, and acidosis. Prerenal failure may occur. Once shock has been corrected, intravenous rehydration should continue with 0.18% saline 4% dextrose (or 0.45% saline 2.5% dextrose if sodium < 130 mmol/l). Potassium should be added to the fluid once urine output is established. Hypernatraemic dehydration (sodium >150 mmol/l) is uncommon but clinical assessment of dehydration is more difficult. The skin may have a doughy consistency and neurological features (e.g. irritability) may be prominent. The serum sodium level should be corrected slowly over 2–3 days to avoid CNS disturbance. Acidosis normally self-corrects with improved tissue perfusion.

4. Appropriate use of drugs. Antibiotics should not be used routinely, but may have a specific role for certain pathogens, e.g. metronidazole for giardiasis. Antidiarrhoeal agents should not be used – they do not reduce fluid losses and may have serious side-effects, e.g. paralytic ileus has been described with loperamide, respiratory depression with diphenoxylate.

Further reading

Turnberg L. Cellular basis of diarrhoea. *Journal of the Royal College of Physicians,* 1991; **25:** 53–62.

Walker-Smith JA. Management of infantile gastroenteritis. *Archives of Disease in Childhood,* 1990; **65:** 917–8.

Related topics of interest

Chronic diarrhoea (p. 77)
Haemolytic uraemic syndrome (p. 179)
Nutrition (p. 303)

GASTROINTESTINAL HAEMORRHAGE

Gastrointestinal haemorrhage is always a worrying symptom, but the commonest presentation in childhood is rectal bleeding due to an anal fissure, which is benign and easily treated. However, less common and more serious causes should be excluded, e.g. intussusception, necrotizing enterocolitis, inflammatory bowel disease. Bleeding may arise from a localized lesion anywhere along the GI tract or it may occur as part of a generalized bleeding disorder (e.g. haemorrhagic disease of the newborn, thrombocytopenia). Occasionally the bleeding is artefactual, e.g. Münchausen syndrome by proxy, swallowed maternal blood from cracked nipples. Common causes of blood-streaked vomitus include swallowed blood or a Mallory–Weiss tear. More significant haematemesis or melaena in childhood is uncommon.

Presentation

- Rectal bleeding.
- Melaena.
- Haematemesis.
- Iron deficiency anaemia (occult blood loss).
- Hypovolaemic shock.

Aetiology

1. *Upper tract bleeding*

- Swallowed blood, e.g. from epistaxis, maternal cracked nipple, during delivery.
- Mallory–Weiss tear.
- Gastritis, gastric ulceration. Often due to drugs, e.g. steroids, NSAIDs, salicylates.
- Oesophagitis. May be secondary to gastro-oesophageal reflux or hiatus hernia.
- Iron poisoning.
- Less common:
  - Oesophageal varices (e.g. portal hypertension in cystic fibrosis).
  - Duodenal ulceration.
  - Volvulus.
  - Meckel's diverticulum.

2. *Lower tract bleeding*

- Anal fissure (usually associated with constipation).
- Infection, e.g. salmonella, campylobacter dysentery.
- Cow's milk allergy (may cause a colitis).
- Trauma (foreign body, sexual abuse).
- Inflammatory bowel disease. Crohn's disease, ulcerative colitis.
- Necrotizing enterocolitis (see related topic Neonatal surgery, p. 285).

- Intussusception.
- Other:
  - Rectal prolapse, haemorrhoids.
  - Duplications, polyp.
  - Rare, e.g. Peutz–Jegher's syndrome, familial adenomatous polyposis coli, angiodysplasia.

3. Other

- Bleeding disorder, e.g. haemorrhagic disease of the newborn (HDN), thrombocytopenia, coagulation defect (inherited or acquired).
- Vasculitis, e.g. Henoch–Schonlein purpura.
- Hereditary haemorrhagic telangiectasia.
- Münchausen syndrome by proxy.

Clinical assessment

In acute large bleeds the child may become rapidly hypovolaemic and resuscitation should always precede investigation.

History

(a) Newborn and early infancy: swallowed blood during delivery is the commonest cause of blood in the vomit of a newborn infant. The Apt's test will distinguish between maternal and neonatal blood (fetal haemoglobin is more resistant to alkali). Haemorrhagic disease of the newborn and necrotizing enterocolitis are important causes of rectal bleeding to consider in the neonatal period.

(b) Later infancy and childhood: in the older child, the history should include enquiry about:

- Rectal bleeding. The colour (bright red, melaena) and amount of blood loss.
- Haematemesis. Can be confused with haemoptysis.
- Associated symptoms, e.g.
  - Constipation.
  - Recurrent vomiting leading to a Mallory–Weiss tear.
  - Epistaxis.
  - Symptoms suggestive of inflammatory bowel disease, e.g. diarrhoea, abdominal pain, weight loss (see related topic Inflammatory bowel disease, p. 221).
- Drug ingestion.
- Recent travel or infectious disease contact.
- Chronic illness, e.g. $\alpha 1$ anti-trypsin deficiency, cystic fibrosis.
- Family history, e.g. familial adenomatous polyposis coli.

On examination

- Signs of hypovolaemia (tachycardia, poor capillary refill etc.).
- Anal fissure, evidence of constipation.
- Rectal examination for polyps, inspection of stool on glove (blood and mucous suggesting inflammatory bowel disease, red currant jelly stool in intussusception).
- Other sites of blood loss, e.g. umbilical in HDN.
- Signs of intestinal obstruction – abdominal distension/tenderness, abnormal bowel sounds (e.g. volvulus), palpable mass (e.g. intussusception).
- Evidence of chronic liver disease (spider naevi, palmar erythema, hepatomegaly).
- Stigmata of rare conditions, e.g. perioral pigmentation in Peutz–Jegher's syndrome, telangiectasia in hereditary haemorrhagic telangiectasia.

Investigations

- FBC. Hypochromic, microcytic (or normocytic) anaemia suggests chronic blood loss.
- Coagulation studies.
- Blood group and save serum for cross match.
- Stool MC&S, ova, cysts and parasites if rectal bleeding.
- Further investigations may be indicated depending on the clinical presentation, e.g.

  Abdominal X-ray. Intussusception, volvulus, ulcerative colitis (toxic dilatation).

  Abdominal US.

  Barium studies: polyps, intussusception, inflammatory bowel disease.

  Endoscopy.

  Meckel's scan: technetium-99 pertechnetate.

  Angiography (rarely needed).

Management

Clearly this will depend on the identified cause, e.g. local anaesthetic creams and correction of constipation for an anal fissure, barium/air enema reduction or surgical intervention for an intussusception.

Children with bleeding oesophageal varices should be stabilized before being transferred to a centre with appropriate expertise. Matched whole blood or packed cells with fresh-frozen plasma should be transfused to achieve a normal blood pressure and adequate tissue perfusion. Overtransfusion may distend varices and worsen bleeding. Bleeding may cease spontaneously as the blood pressure falls, but other measures to control the variceal bleeding may be indicated (e.g. intravenous vasopressin, compression with a Sengstaken–Blakemore tube, endoscopic injection sclerotherapy, rarely surgical porto-systemic shunts). Acute hepatic encephalopathy may be precipitated by increased absorption of ammonia from the bowel. Measures to reduce this risk include regular aspiration of blood from the stomach via a wide-bore nasogastric tube, lactulose and neomycin (reduce colonic pH, reduce ammonia reabsorption, encourage bowel emptying).

Further reading

Raine PAM. Investigation of rectal bleeding. *Archives of Disease in Childhood,* 1991; **66:** 279–80.

Related topics of interest

Anaemia (p. 31)
Bleeding disorders (p. 53)
Cystic fibrosis (p. 107)
Inflammatory bowel disease (p. 221)
Liver disease (p. 244)
Purpura and bruising (p. 330)

GENE DEFECTS

Disorders caused by a defect in a single gene follow a pattern first described by Mendel (Mendelian inheritance). With modern molecular genetic techniques genes are being identified for many diseases, at least 5000 genes have now been recognized. DNA probes have enabled analysis of mutations and tracking of gene inheritance through families. Advanced genetic analysis has revealed that not all inheritance follows Mendelian lines. Non-Mendelian mechanisms including imprinting, mosaicism and mitochondrial disorders. The risks of having an affected child can now be determined much more accurately and antenatal diagnosis is available for a wide range of conditions.

Mendelian inheritance

Autosomal dominant (AD) inheritance

The abnormal gene is expressed in the heteozygote. Therefore each child of an affected and a normal individual will have a 50:50 chance of being affected. Non-affected offspring do not transmit the disorder. AD traits affect both males and females, and the disorder can often be traced back through generations. The frequency with which new mutations occur varies, for example new mutations account for most cases of achondroplasia. Phenotypic expression may vary, producing variations in severity of the condition within the same family. Some AD conditions are sex-influenced (more commonly expressed in one sex), e.g. male pattern baldness.

Examples of AD inheritance

- Huntington's chorea.
- Tuberous sclerosis.
- Congenital spherocytosis.
- Neurofibromatosis.
- Myotonic dystrophy.

Autosomal recessive (AR) inheritance

AR disorders are expressed in individuals who are homozygous for the affected gene, and can occur in both sexes. Both the parents of an affected child must be heterozygotes and are usually unaffected. With rare recessive traits the parents are often related (consanguineous). The risk of recurrence after one child with a recessive disorder is 1 in 4 for each successive child.

Examples of AR inheritance

- Majority of inborn errors of metabolism (e.g. phenylketonuria, galactosaemia, Tay–Sachs disease).

- Cystic fibrosis.
- Sickle cell disease.
- Ataxia telangiectasia.

In some conditions it is possible to be heterozygous for two mutant alleles, e.g. an individual who is heterozygous for both HbS and HbC has a haemoglobinopathy intermediate in severity between sickle cell anaemia and HbC disease.

Sex-linked recessive inheritance

There are no structural genes on the Y chromosome other than those determining sexual development so sex-linked conditions are all X-linked. Males are affected and females are carriers. A carrier female will transmit the gene to half her sons and half her daughters. An affected male will transmit the gene to all his daughters and none of his sons. A female can be affected in the following uncommon circumstances:

- In common X-linked conditions, an affected male and a female carrier can produce a daughter with two mutant alleles, e.g. red–green colour blindness.
- If an X-linked condition occurs in Turner's syndrome (XO), but this is very uncommon.
- Random inactivation of one X chromosome (lyonization) occurs in early embryogenesis and usually results in half the cells in the female having one X inactivated and half having the other X inactivated. Occasionally, by chance, the normal allele is inactivated in more cells than the mutant allele, resulting in partial expression of the mutant gene, e.g. ~ 5% of female carriers of Duchenne muscular dystrophy show some muscle weakness.

Identification of carriers has important implications for genetic counselling for all female family members.

Examples of X-linked recessive conditions

- Chronic granulomatous disease.
- Haemophilia.
- Muscular dystrophy (Duchenne's, Becker's).
- Colour blindness.
- Glucose-6-phosphate dehydrogenase deficiency.

Sex-linked dominant inheritance

The pedigree pattern should not be confused with that of an AD condition. An affected male transmits the disorder to all his daughters and none of his sons. Offspring of an affected female will all have a 50:50 chance of being affected.

Examples of X-linked dominant conditions

- Vitamin D-resistant rickets.
- Oral–facial–digital sydrome.
- Incontinentia pigmenti – lethal in males.
- Ornithine carbamoyl transferase deficiency – lethal in males.

Non-Mendelian mechanisms

Imprinting

This occurs when genes function differently if they are maternally or paternally derived. The best clinical example is the deletion on chromosome 15 in Prader–Willi and Angelman's syndromes. In Prader–Willi syndrome (neonatal hypotonia, initial feeding difficulties and subsequent obesity, small hands and feet, characteristic facies), the deletion is on the paternal chromosome. In Angelman's syndrome (mental retardation, epilepsy, absent speech, ataxia) the deletion is on the maternal chromosome. Some children with Prader–Willi do not have a chromosome deletion but have two maternally derived chromosomes, *uniparental disomy*. This is less common in Angelman's. Imprinting has also been implicated in Wilms' tumour, Beckwith–Wiedemann syndrome and some familial cancers.

Unstable mutations

Unstable mutations, involving trinucleotide repeats, can be inherited Mendelian fashion. Instability of the mutation usually generates larger expansions in offspring. This is called *anticipation*, where the disorder becomes more severe in successive generations, e.g. myotonic dystrophy, fragile X and Huntington's chorea.

Mitochondrial disorders

Not all DNA is within the cell nucleus; mitochondria have their own DNA. Some diseases may be caused by mutations of mitochondrial DNA, e.g. MELAS (mitochondrial, encephalomyopathy, lactic acidosis and stroke-like episodes), MERRF (myoclonus epilepsy and ragged red fibres), Leber's optic atrophy.

Techniques of DNA analysis

DNA analysis allows both carrier detection (X-linked recessive and presymptomatic AD disorders) and prenatal diagnosis. DNA can be extracted from any tissue with nucleated cells, e.g. blood, buccal mucosa and chorionic villus samples. Restriction enzymes split the

DNA at specific sites producing fragments. This DNA can be amplified using polymerase chain reaction (PCR) or cloning, to allow rapid results from small samples. Linkage analysis can be used to map a gene. Gene probes can then be used to detect genome sequences. Fluorescence *in situ* hybridization (FISH) is a technique that detects specific DNA sequences and chromosomal micro-deletions using a fluorescently labelled probe.

Further reading

Lees M, Winter R. Advances in genetics. *Archives of Disease in Childhood,* 1996; **75:** 346–50.

Meeks M, Gardiner M. Molecular genetics for the paediatrician. *Current Paediatrics,* 1996; **6:** 51–5.

Meeks M, Gardiner M. Molecular genetics for the paediatrician: clinical aspects. *Current Paediatics,* 1996; **6:** 125–30.

Related topics of interest

Chromosomal abnormalities (p. 73)
Dysmorphology and teratogenesis (p. 128)
Fetal medicine (p. 141)
Sickle cell anaemia and thalassaemia syndromes (p. 348)

GLOMERULONEPHRITIS

Glomerulonephritis (GMN) is inflammation and proliferation of cells within the renal glomerulus which may occur as a primary condition or associated with a systemic disorder. The majority of cases are immunologically mediated. GMN may present with asymptomatic haematuria, acute nephritic syndrome or a mixed picture of nephritis and nephrosis.

Problems

- Haematuria.
- Hypertension.
- Renal failure.

Aetiology and pathology

In the majority of cases the damage is immunologically mediated, either by deposition of immune complexes within the glomerulus or by interaction of autoantibodies with the glomerular basement membrane. This leads to activation of the complement system and release of cytokines which attract other mediators of glomerular damage, such as neutrophils. Damage may be limited to the kidneys or be part of a systemic disorder. In a few cases the pathogenesis is unknown.

1. *Primary GMN*

- Immune complex GMN
  - Post-infectious acute nephritis (the majority are post-streptococcal).
  - Mesangial IgA nephropathy (Berger's disease).
  - Membranous and membranoproliferative GMN.
- Anti-glomerular basement membrane antibody-mediated GMN, e.g. Goodpasture's disease.
- Pathogenesis unknown.

2. *GMN associated with systemic disorders*

- Immunologically mediated
  - Henoch–Schönlein purpura (renal involvement in 25–50%).
  - Systemic lupus erythematosus and other connective tissue disorders.
  - Vasculitic conditions, e.g. polyarteritis nodosa.
  - Infections, e.g. subacute bacterial endocarditis, shunt nephritis, malaria.
- Hereditary, e.g. Alport's syndrome (GMN associated with sensorineural deafness).
- Other, e.g. diabetes.

Light microscopic changes have led to the description of many categories of GMN, e.g. focal, diffuse, segmental, proliferative, membranous, sclerotic. Immune complexes may be identified by electron microscopy or by immunofluorescence microscopy. Crescent formation represents the end-stage of many disease processes.

Acute nephritic syndrome (acute post-infectious GMN)

This typically occurs 7–14 days after a group A β-haemolytic streptococcal throat infection but can follow other streptococcal infections (e.g. skin) or infections with other organisms, e.g. *Staphylococcus, Salmonella, Mycoplasma,* and viruses (coxsackie, echo, influenza). It can occur at any age but predominantly affects school-age children.

Clinical features

- Dark 'smoky' urine.
- Oliguria.
- Non-specific malaise.
- Hypertension (occasionally acute causing encephalopathy and seizures).
- Fluid retention (usually causing only a mild degree of oedema but if severe can result in heart failure).

Investigation

- Urinalysis. Gross haematuria, granular and red cell casts, variable proteinuria. If proteinuria is heavy, hypoalbuminaemia may occur and the patient will develop the clinical picture of the nephrotic syndrome.
- Plasma U&E, creatinine, calcium, phosphate, bicarbonate. Degree of renal failure may be minimal to severe.
- Evidence of recent streptococcal infection. Throat swab, blood for anti-streptolysin O (ASO) and anti-DNA antibody titres. ASO may not rise, particularly after skin infections.
- Complement screen and immunoglobulins. Low C3 and C4 during acute phase, return to normal within 8 weeks.
- Autoantibody screen, e.g. antinuclear factor positive in lupus nephritis.

Management

Acute GMN is usually mild and requires no specific treatment other than monitoring. There is no real evidence that bed rest is of benefit. Strict fluid balance with daily weighing will limit the risk of fluid overload. Dialysis is rarely needed. Antihypertensive treatment may be required if the blood pressure is not controlled by fluid restriction. Although it does not seem to alter the course of acute GMN, a 10-day course of penicillin is usually given to limit the spread of nephritogenic strains. Renal biopsy is not indicated unless renal function rapidly deteriorates after the acute phase or renal failure persists for several weeks suggesting a cause other than post-infectious. The child can be discharged home once the renal function is seen to be improving. Outpatient follow-up should continue until urinalysis, blood pressure and renal function are normal.

Outcome

Complete recovery occurs in over 95% of children with post-streptococcal GMN. Second attacks are rare. Renal function usually returns to normal within 10–14 days, but microscopic haematuria may persist for 1–2 years. In a few children the disease is fulminant with rapid progression to renal failure. In others there is slow deterioration of renal function over several months, leading to chronic or end-stage renal failure.

Further reading

MacDonel, Barakat AY. Glomerular disease. In: Baraket AY, ed. *Renal Disease in Children; Clinical Evaluation and Diagnosis.* New York: Springer Verlag, 1989; 171–84.

Related topics of interest

Acute renal failure (p. 15)
Chronic renal failure (p. 82)
Haematuria (p. 176)
Nephrotic syndrome (p. 289)

GROWTH ASSESSMENT

Growth assessment is fundamental to all areas of paediatrics and any child who has a chronic illness should be regularly measured to ensure growth is maintained. Growth monitoring is a vital part of child health surveillance. Poor growth may result from many disease processes but may be the earliest sign of endocrine abnormality. Ideally, poor growth should be detected before the child falls below the 0.4th centile.

Normal growth

Growth from conception into infancy is almost entirely dependent on nutrition. During infancy, growth is rapid and rapidly decelerating. Growth hormone (GH) receptors become detectable towards the end of the first year of life, and the slowly decelerating phase of growth during childhood is under GH control. During childhood, height increases by 5 to 7.5 cm/year. The pubertal growth spurt is controlled by both GH and sex steroids, and reaches a peak of between 7 and 12 cm/year.

Pulsatile GH is secreted by the anterior pituitary particularly at night. Secretion is stimulated by growth hormone releasing hormone (GHRH) and inhibited by somatostatin. These are secreted by the hypothalamus under the influence of many factors including neurotransmitters, glucose, amino acids, lipids, insulin-like growth factor 1 (IGF-1), sleep, and temperature.

Growth assessment

1. Height. Accuracy of measurement is very important. Anthropometric equipment for standing height and infant length should be regularly calibrated. If poor growth is suspected, serial height measurements should be made over a minimum period of 3 months. Sitting height should be measured, using a sitting height table, if there is concern regarding disproportionate growth of limbs and spine (e.g. skeletal dysplasia, post-radiotherapy).

2. Weight. Infants should be weighed naked and older children should wear minimum clothing. Assessment of the amount of subcutaneous fat is useful in nutritional problems and calipers are available for measuring skinfold thickness.

3. Head (occipito-frontal) circumference. Head and brain growth is very rapid in the first year of life (approximately 1 cm/month) and then slower during the second year (approximately 2 cm/year). Head growth continues more slowly after the anterior fontanelle closes.

4. Pubertal staging. Growth rate must be related to pubertal stage (see Growth velocity charts below).

5. Parental heights. The target centile range for a child's height can be calculated from the parents' heights. Correction should be made for the sex of the child by adding 14 cm to the mother's height for a boy, or subtracting 14 cm from the father's height for a girl. The arithmetic mean of the adjusted parental heights gives the mid-parental height (MPH). The MPH ± 8.5 cm for girls or ± 10 cm for boys gives the expected adult height range with 95% confidence limits.

6. Bone age X-ray. The bones of the left hand and wrist are used as a standard to assess skeletal maturity. An estimate of final height can be calculated from the chronological age, bone age, and current height.

Growth charts

1. The Tanner–Whitehouse charts. These were first published in 1966 and have been used for 30 years. These charts are now out-dated for several reasons:

- They were derived from data from only a relatively small number of children living in the south east of England, so were not nationally representative.
- There has been a trend towards increasing final height and earlier maturity over the last few decades.
- Weight gain during infancy is now more rapid due to changes in feeding practices.

2. 1990 nine-centile charts. The Tanner–Whitehouse charts have now been replaced by the 1990 nine-centile charts, which were derived from over 25 000 measurements made in seven growth surveys between 1978 and 1990. Some of these surveys were sponsored by the clothes manufacturing industry who were concerned that their standard clothing sizes, based on the old data, were incorrect, e.g. clothes designed for the 6–8-year-old age group were being worn by 4–6-year-olds.

The nine-centile charts have the following advantages:

- Current growth patterns are described more precisely.
- The interval between each pair of centile lines is 2/3 of a standard deviation so that crossing a channel between two lines has the same significance wherever the child is on the chart.

- There are nine centiles instead of the previous seven. Only 1 in 250 children will fall below the lowest line (0.4th centile) compared with 1 in 33 who fell below the old 3rd centile.
- The 'step' at age 2 years when standing height replaces supine height is eliminated.

3. Growth velocity charts. The child's height is measured on two occasions preferably 6–12 months apart. The growth rate (cm/year) is plotted against the age of the child midway between the two measurements. Most children grow at or around the 50th centile rate. A child who consistently grows at the 25th centile velocity will be short, whereas one who consistently grows with a 75th centile velocity will grow tall.

Growth velocity charts should be regarded as probability charts. The probability of two successive annual velocities falling on the 25th centile in a normal child is only $0.25 \times 0.25 = 0.0625$, i.e. only 6.25% of healthy children will grow as slowly as this over a 2 year period. A child must grow at a velocity above the 25th centile to maintain their centile on a 9-centile chart. Growth of less than 4 cm/year or a child growing between this rate and the 25th velocity centile for 2 years requires investigation.

The growth rate must also be related to pubertal stage. A prepubertal child of 12 years grows at approximately 5 cm/year. If puberty is delayed, the growth velocity will continue to decline by approximately 1 cm/year, so that a boy not entering the puberty growth spurt until 16 years will be growing extremely slowly and may even appear to stop growing.

4. Body mass index (BMI) charts.

$$\text{BMI} = \text{wt (kg)}/\ \text{ht}^2\ \text{(m)}$$

BMI has been used as a measure of fatness or obesity. BMI reference curves for British children from birth to 23 years are now available. They may be useful in childhood but they should be used with caution in infancy. There is no evidence that infant BMI is predictive of later BMI.

5. Conditional reference charts. Crossing of the weight centiles in the early months of life can be normal, as an infant finds his/her genetically programmed centile (normal catch-up or catch-down growth). Conditional reference charts may be used to assess whether a given centile shift is abnormal. However, the correct use and interpretation of these charts is complex and they are not widely used.

Growth monitoring

The working party on child health surveillance (see Further reading) makes the following recommendations regarding height monitoring in pre-school children:

- All staff involved with growth monitoring should be trained in measurement techniques and interpretation.
- Equipment used should be regularly calibrated.
- Correction for gestation should be made up to the age of 2 years.
- Length should be measured at birth if the infant is of low birth weight (<2.5 kg) or any abnormality is suspected.
- Length should be recorded at the 6-week examination if the infant was of low birth weight, an abnormality is known or suspected, or if their are concerns regarding feeding. This should be repeated at 12–16 weeks if there is a specific indication.
- Height should be routinely recorded at 18–24 months, 3.5 years and school entry.

Indications for referral to a paediatrician

- > 99.6th or < 0.4th centile.
- Under 5 years and crosses two centile channels within 18–24 months.
- Over 5 years and crosses one centile channel
- Consider referral if between 98th–99.6th or 0.4th–2nd, particularly if there is a discrepancy between the parental height centile and the child's height centile.

Further reading

Cole TJ. Conditional reference charts to assess weight gain in British infants. *Archives of Disease in Childhood,* 1995; **73:** 8–16.

Cole TJ, Freeman JV, Preece MA. Body mass index reference curves for the UK, 1990. *Archives of Disease in Childhood,* 1995; **73:** 25–9.

Freeman JV, Cole TJ, Chinn S, Jones PRM, White EM, Preece MA. Cross sectional stature and weight reference curves for the UK, 1990. *Archives of Disease in Childhood,* 1995; **73:** 17–24.

Hall DM, ed. *Health for All Children.* Report of the Third Joint Working Party on Child Health Surveillance, 3rd edn. Oxford: Oxford University Press, 1996.

Related topic of interest

Growth – short stature, tall stature (p. 171)

GROWTH – SHORT STATURE, TALL STATURE

Growth monitoring is a routine part of child health surveillance. Any child who is short (< 0.4th centile), tall (>99.6th centile) or is growing at an inappropriate rate (under 5 years and crosses two centile channels within 18–24 months or over 5 years and crosses one centile channel) should be referred to a paediatrician for further assessment. Referral should also be considered if a child's height lies between the 98th–99.6th or the 0.4th–2nd centiles, particularly if there is a discrepancy between the parental height centiles and the child's height centile. Tall stature is a much less common presenting problem than short stature, and is usually familial.

Short stature

Children of short stature can be divided into two main groups – those who are small but are growing at an appropriate rate and those who are small and are growing slowly. If no disease is identified and the growth velocity is normal ('short normal' child), it is doubtful whether any treatment can make a substantial difference to the final height. If the growth velocity is low, investigation depends on the age of the child. In the pre-school child, short stature and a low growth velocity are usually associated with poor weight gain (failure to thrive) and the cause is likely to be nutritional. In older children, poor growth may be due to chronic illness (e.g. poorly controlled asthma) but Turner's syndrome, endocrine disease and skeletal dysplasias should also be considered. Constitutional delay in growth and puberty (CDGP) is particularly common in boys and there is often a family history of delayed puberty.

Aetiology

1. *Normal growth velocity*

- Constitutional short stature.
- Low birth weight. IUGR, Silver–Russell syndrome.
- CDGP. Although slow, the growth rate is normal for the pubertal stage.

2. *Low growth velocity*

- Undernutrition.
- Psychosocial deprivation.
- Chronic illness, e.g. renal, cardiovascular, respiratory disease.
- Malabsorption e.g. Crohn's disease, coeliac disease.
- Syndromes, e.g. Turner's, Prader–Willi.
- Skeletal dysplasias – disproportionate body/limbs.
- Endocrine disease – GH insufficiency, panhypopituitarism, hypothyroidism, Cushing's syndrome (usually iatrogenic).

Assessment of a child with short stature

(See also related topic Growth assessment, p. 167)

1. History and clinical examination

- Accurate growth assessment is essential (standing/sitting heights, weight, head circumference, pubertal staging, parental heights) and all measurements should be plotted on a nine-centile growth chart.
- Evidence of chronic illness, malabsorption, or malnutrition may be identified prompting appropriate investigations (e.g. antigliadin antibodies, sweat test, renal function tests).
- Features of hypothyroidism include lethargy, constipation, dry skin, and a goitre.
- Typical features of Turner's syndrome may be present (e.g. neck webbing, widely spaced nipples) but the absence of the typical phenotype does not exclude the syndrome.
- Children with GH insufficiency are said to have a characteristic appearance (truncal obesity, central crowding of facial features, immature facial appearance).
- Symptoms and signs of raised intracranial pressure should be excluded although hypothalamic and pituitary tumours are rare.

2. Investigations – if the history and examination are normal, initial investigations should include thyroid function and bone age X-ray. Blood should also be sent for karyotype in girls to exclude Turner's syndrome.

3. Growth velocity – if history, examination and baseline investigations are all normal, growth velocity should be measured over a minimum of 6 months (preferably one year). A poor growth velocity may lead to further investigation for growth hormone insufficiency.

It is particularly important to relate growth velocity to pubertal stage in a child of pubertal age. Growth during childhood is slowly decelerating. During normal puberty an increase in sex steroid secretion is associated with increased amplitude of pulsatile GH secretion. If puberty is delayed, the growth velocity will continue to decline by approximately 1 cm/year. This means that a boy not entering the puberty growth spurt until 16 years will be growing extremely slowly and may even appear to stop growing, but his growth velocity is appropriate for his pubertal stage. The bone age is delayed and there is a normal height prognosis. Treatment with sex steroids will stimulate both puberty and growth.

If there are signs of puberty but there is no pubertal growth spurt, the growth velocity is low for pubertal stage and GH insufficiency is likely.

Growth hormone insufficiency

1. Congenital

- Idiopathic GHRH deficiency.
- GH gene deletion (very rare).
- Developmental abnormalities, e.g. midline brain defects.

2. Acquired

- Tumours of hypothalamus or pituitary.
- Cranial irradiation.
- Transient insufficiency – low sex hormone concentrations, psychosocial deprivation.

Tests of GH secretion. Random GH levels are rarely of use due to the pulsatile pattern of secretion. 24 hour urinary GH requires an ultrasensitive GH assay to detect the low levels associated with GH insufficiency. GH provocation tests (e.g. insulin, clonidine, glucagon or GHRH stimulation) may be indicated, although their use and interpretation is controversial (see Further reading). Children of pubertal age need priming with sex steroids prior to provocation tests. 12 or 24 hour profiles of GH secretion remain a research investigation at present but abnormalities of pulsatility may be important. Insulin-like growth factor 1 (IGF-1) is GH dependent and levels are low in GH insufficiency. Levels are also low in young children and are affected by liver disease and hypothyroidism.

Management of GH insufficiency. Pituitary derived GH was available in limited supplies from 1958 to 1985 but was withdrawn because of the risks of the transmission of Creutzfeld–Jacob disease. Biosynthetic GH is now available for use in GH insufficiency and is given by daily subcutaneous injection. It has been used in many other conditions, e.g. renal failure, Turner's syndrome, and skeletal dysplasias with some increase in growth velocity but the effect on the final height of these children is still unclear.

Tall stature

Aetiology

- Constitutional, familial.
- True precocious puberty.
- Thyrotoxicosis.
- Excessive androgen secretion (adrenal tumour, congenital adrenal hyperplasia.)
- GH excess (gigantism). Rare, e.g. pituitary adenoma.
- Others, e.g. Marfan's syndrome, homocystinuria, chromosomal abnormalities (e.g. Klinefelter's syndrome (XXY)).

Assessment of a child with tall stature

Thyrotoxicosis, and precocious puberty (true and false) should be excluded by history, examination, and appropriate investigations. It is often difficult to distinguish between a normal tall child and a child with gigantism, but an abnormal GH profile or a raised IGF-1 in the presence of a growth velocity above the 90th centile, or a greater than expected height for the family should be indications to consider pituitary imaging. GH suppression tests used in the diagnosis of acromegaly in adults are rarely useful in children.

Management

Prevention of excessive height is better than trying to lose height already gained. Children with excessive predicted adult heights are currently treated with sex steroids to induce early puberty, but the long-term effects of early exposure, particularly to oestrogen, are unclear. Reduction of endogenous GH secretion by anticholinergic agents or somatostatin are areas of research interest.

Further reading

Brook CGD. Growth. In: *A Guide to the Practice of Paediatric Endocrinology*, Cambridge University Press, 1993; 18–54.

Brook CGD, Hindmarsh PC. Tests for growth hormone secretion. *Archives of Disease in Childhood,* 1991; **66:** 85–7.

Hindmarsh PC, Swift PGF. An assessment of growth hormone provocation tests. *Archives of Disease in Childhood,* 1995; **72:** 362–8.

Shah A, Stanhope R, Matthew. Hazards of pharmacological tests of growth hormone secretion in childhood. *British Medical Journal,* 1992; **304:** 173–4.

Related topics of interest

Chromosomal abnormalities (p. 73)
Failure to thrive (p. 138)
Growth assessment (p. 167)
Puberty – precocious and delayed (p. 326)
Thyroid disorders (p. 363)

HAEMATURIA

Haematuria may occur as an isolated symptom or as part of a systemic disorder. It may be visible to the naked eye (frank or macroscopic haematuria) or be detected only on microscopic analysis of the urine. The source of the blood may be anywhere from glomerulus to urethra, but most cases in childhood are due to UTI or primary glomerular disease.

Causes

- Urinary tract infection (UTI).
- Glomerulonephritis (post-streptococcal, Henoch–Schönlein purpura, familial).
- IgA nephropathy.
- Acute haemorrhagic cystitis. Viral (adenovirus 11 and 21), drugs (cyclophosphamide).
- Calculus.
- Trauma.
- Exercise-induced. Usually after severe exercise and resolves within 48 hours.
- Tumours. Wilms' tumour (uncommon presentation), bladder tumours (rare in children).
- Subacute bacterial endocarditis.
- Infections, e.g. tuberculosis, schistosomiasis.
- Coagulopathies.
- Sickle cell disease. Sickling within the renal medulla leads to local papillary infarcts.
- Renal vein thrombosis. Gross haematuria and palpable renal mass in a newborn infant.
- Factitious haematuria. As part of the Munchausen by proxy spectrum.

Clinical features

The urine is usually pink or brown in colour because of the presence of the oxidized haem pigment. In post-streptococcal GMN the urine is often described as smoky. If the urine is bright red with or without clots then a lower urinary tract source should be suspected. Haematuria may be an isolated finding or be associated with symptoms of a systemic disorder, e.g. Henoch–Schönlein purpura (rash, joint pains). Hypertension and oliguria are features of acute GMN. Frequency and dysuria suggest a UTI which may be accompanied by microscopic haematuria, but presentation with frank haematuria is rare. Loin pain or renal colic suggests the presence of a calculus. SBE, sickle cell disease and coagulation disorders are infrequent causes, but haematuria is rarely the presenting symptom.

Other causes of dark urine should be excluded:

- Bile pigments.
- Haemoglobinuria, myoglobinuria.
- Foods, e.g. beetroot.
- Drugs, e.g. rifampicin.
- Blood from other sources, e.g. menstrual, perianal.
- Urate crystals may appear pink in the nappy of young infants.

Investigation

- *Urinary dipsticks* are very sensitive and are therefore not very reliable. They are also positive for myoglobin and free haemoglobin.
- *Urine microscopy* should always be performed to confirm the presence of red cells (a fresh specimen is important since red cells lyse on standing). The presence of red cell casts indicates an intrarenal cause (either glomerular or tubular) and the red cells may be misshapen owing to distortion as they pass through the glomerular capillary wall. Glomerular casts indicate a glomerular cause. Pyuria and bacteriuria point to an infective cause which should be confirmed by culture. Microscopy may identify the ova of schistosoma if there has been recent travel to the tropics.
- *Other tests* depend on the history, examination and urinalysis:

  Urine culture will confirm a bacterial infection and lead to further appropriate investigations.

  Full blood count, film and coagulation tests. To exclude coagulopathies and sickle cell disease.

  Investigations for glomerulonephritis (see related topic Glomerulonephritis, p. 164).

  Radiology. An abdominal US scan may identify a renal mass, evidence of obstruction or a renal tract calculus. Calculi may be seen on a plain abdominal radiography but an intravenous urogram may be needed to confirm the site of obstruction. Bladder causes of haematuria are very rare in childhood and cystoscopy is seldom indicated.

IgA nephropathy

This is the commonest cause of recurrent asymptomatic haematuria and was first described by Berger in 1968. It presents in later childhood or early adult life with persistent microscopic haematuria and episodes of macroscopic haematuria associated with upper respiratory tract infections.

It was originally regarded as a benign disease but it is now recognized to have a slowly progressive course in some cases, leading to hypertension, proteinuria and eventual chronic renal failure. Occasionally the disease is fulminant, with rapid progression to renal failure. The aetiology is unclear but diffuse mesangial deposits of IgA are seen on immunofluorescent microscopy. It is more common in southern Europe, South-East Asia and Japan, and it is twice as common in males.

Calculi and nephrocalcinosis

Urolithiasis (calculi in the renal tract) and nephrocalcinosis (deposition of calcium in the renal parenchyma) are uncommon in children. Calculi are associated with stasis (e.g. neuropathic bladder), UTIs (especially with *Proteus* spp.), idiopathic hypercalciuria (normal serum calcium) and cystinuria. Nephrocalcinosis is associated with renal tubular acidosis, particularly the distal type.

Further reading

White RHR. The investigation of haematuria. *Archives of Disease in Childhood,* 1989; **64:** 159–65.

Related topics of interest

Glomerulonephritis (p. 164)
Urinary tract infection (p. 370)

HAEMOLYTIC URAEMIC SYNDROME

Haemolytic uraemic syndrome (HUS) is an uncommon but serious condition with an incidence of at least 75 cases per year in the UK. The incidence has risen abruptly since the early 1980s, but this may be because of improved reporting. HUS is characterized by microangiopathic anaemia, thrombocytopenia and acute renal failure. Over 50% of patients require dialysis for acute renal failure and the mortality in the acute phase is 10–15%. The majority of cases are associated with a prodromal diarrhoeal illness (D+), but rare cases are idiopathic, inherited or drug associated (D−).

Problems

- Haemolytic anaemia.
- Thrombocytopenia.
- Renal failure.
- Hypertension.
- Neurological impairment.

Aetiology and pathology

1. *Typical HUS (post-diarrhoeal, epidemic, D+)* is associated with infections, especially verotoxin-producing *E. coli*, but is also described following viral infections (e.g. coxsackie), shigella dysentery and *Streptococcus pneumoniae*. The renal damage is primarily glomerular with a thrombotic microangiopathy causing multisystem disease. Endothelial injury may be mediated by activated neutrophils, or by the direct effect of endotoxin or verotoxin.

2. *Atypical HUS (sporadic, D−)* is rare and may be idiopathic, inherited or associated with drugs such as mitomycin C, crack cocaine, quinine. The renal damage is arteriolar with intimal and subintimal oedema, necrosis and proliferation.

Clinical features

1. *Typical HUS (D+)*. The majority of cases of HUS are D+. The diagnosis should be considered in any child who develops pallor, oliguria or haematuria following a diarrhoeal illness, particularly if the diarrhoea is bloody. It occurs in summer epidemics, typically in infants and young children, and is equally common in boys and girls. Bruising and petechiae occur secondary to thrombocytopenia, and jaundice may develop. Hypertension, if present, is usually mild. CNS involvement (e.g. convulsions) is rare and the long-term prognosis is good with supportive treatment (90% survival). Recurrences are unusual.

2. *Atypical HUS (D−)*. This is uncommon and tends to occur in older children. There is no seasonal variation in incidence and there is usually no prodromal diarrhoea. Hypertension is

severe, CNS involvement is common and the prognosis is poor. It can recur in transplanted kidneys.

Investigation

- Full blood count and film. Thrombocytopenia (< 100 x 10^9/l), microangiopathic haemolytic anaemia (Hb < 10 g/dl, distorted and fragmented red cells), neutrophilia (poor prognostic factor if greater than 20 x 10^9/l).
- Fibrin degradation products (FDPs). Raised.
- Urea, creatinine, and electrolytes. Urea typically > 18.
- Stool culture. *E. coli* serotype 0157:H7 is the commonest verotoxin-producing *E. coli* (VTEC) associated with D+ HUS. It may be isolated for many weeks, but the earlier the stool collection the higher the chance of isolation.
- Elastase. Produced by activated neutrophils (higher levels are associated with worse outcome).

Management

1. Anaemia should be corrected with repeated small transfusions of packed cells.

2. Fluid and electrolyte balance. Record strict input and output charts with fluid restriction and daily weights. Dialysis is implemented early for fluid overload and a rising urea or potassium. Peritoneal dialysis is the method of choice.

3. Hypertension should be treated vigorously with antihypertensive agents, fluid restriction and dialysis.

4. Complications include respiratory failure and pancreatitis.

5. Specific therapies. Many have been tried, including heparin infusions, antiplatelet agents such as dipyridamole and infusions of fresh-frozen plasma but their benefit is unproven. Prostaglandin I_2 activity has been noted to be low in the acute phase, which may be the result of impaired synthesis or increased degradation. Interest currently surrounds the use of PGI_2 infusions in the acute phase.

Outcome

In a national study carried out in the UK of children diagnosed as having HUS between 1985 and 1988, Milford *et al.* (1990) identified 298 children. Ninety-five per cent of these were D+, and at follow-up 13% had either died or had significant renal morbidity (hypertension, chronic or end-stage renal failure). Of the children with D^- HUS, 79% were dead, hypertensive or in renal failure. Other studies have shown significant residual nephropathy in as many as one-third of patients 5–10 years after the acute episode. These abnormalities of renal function may be subtle and indicate only abnormal renal functional reserve, but this may have long-term implications. The follow-up of these children should at least include regular monitoring of blood pressure, serum creatinine and urinalysis for protein.

Further reading

Milford DV, Taylor CM, Guttridge B, Smith HR, Scotland SM, Gross RJ, Hall SM, Rowe B, Kleanthous H. Haemolytic uraemic syndrome in the British Isles 1985–8: association with verotoxin producing *Escherichia coli*. 1. Clinical and epidemiological aspects. 2. Microbiological aspects. *Archives of Disease in Childhood*, 1990; **65:** 716–21, 722–7.

Related topics of interest

Acute renal failure (p. 15)
Chronic renal failure (p. 82)

HEADACHE

Headache is a frequent symptom in childhood, and is usually benign and short-lasting. Less frequently it may be a symptom of serious underlying disease such as an intracranial neoplasm or encephalitis. Pain receptors are not present within the brain itself, but are found in the blood vessels at the base of the brain, in the meninges, the paranasal sinuses, teeth, eyes and the muscles of the head, face and neck.

Aetiology

1. Acute headache

- Acute febrile illness.
- Localized infection within the head, e.g. otitis media, sinusitis.
- Acute central nervous system infection, e.g. encephalitis, meningitis.
- Trauma – accidental or non-accidental.
- Hypertension.
- Intracranial haemorrhage, e.g. from a vascular malformation or ruptured aneurysm.
- Physical factors, e.g. hunger, noise.

2. Recurrent headache

- Migraine.
- Raised intracranial pressure, e.g. from neoplasm, hydrocephalus, benign intracranial hypertension.
- Tension.
- Depression or anxiety.
- Epilepsy.
- Metabolic problems, e.g. hypoglycaemia, porphyria.
- Refractive errors and referred ocula pain, e.g. glaucoma, uveitis.
- Systemic inflammatory disease, e.g. Still's disease, systemic lupus erythematosus (SLE).

History

If the headache is acute in onset, the history must elicit any symptoms of meningitis (fever, vomiting, photophobia), a history of recent trauma, or of other acute infection, e.g. otitis media. Paroxysmal headaches with nausea and a preceding aura are suggestive of migraine, and a positive family history is found in up to 90% of cases. Recurrent headaches which are present on morning waking, are accompanied by vomiting or which worsen with straining or coughing are suspicious of an intracerebral mass lesion (displacing or dilating intracranial vessels). Enquiry should be made about the child's gait and any recent personality changes. The social history should enquire about any obvious causes of stress.

Examination

In acute headache, the child's temperature and conscious level should be recorded, and the child should be examined for neck stiffness. An assessment should be made of the child's growth, including head circumference. Examination of the skin may reveal stigmata of the neurocutaneous syndromes, which are associated with intracranial neoplasms. A full neurological examination should be performed, with particular attention to gait, fundoscopy, visual fields and visual acuity. Blood pressure should be measured in all cases. The cranium should be auscultated for bruits, occasionally heard with arteriovenous malformations. There may be evidence of localized pathology in the head and neck, e.g. teeth, sinuses.

Investigation

In some cases, repeated clinical assessment only is required. Selected investigations may include:

- FBC, ESR.
- U&E, glucose.
- Blood culture. In acute febrile illness.
- Skull radiographs exclude fracture. Features of raised intracranial pressure (suture diastasis, increased digital markings), suprasellar calcification (found in craniopharyngioma) may be found, but CT or MRI will be indicated if there is clinical suspicion of raised intracranial pressure.
- CT or MRI scan excludes hydrocephalus or a space-occupying lesion. MRI is the investigation of choice, especially to exclude posterior fossa pathology.
- Cerebral angiography is occasionally needed to demonstrate local blood vessel anatomy prior to surgery.
- EEG. Slow-wave changes in encephalitis, epileptic focus.
- Lumbar puncture may include CSF microscopy, culture and sensitivity, cytospin (if malignancy suspected), virology or a search for acid–alcohol-fast bacilli if tuberculous meningitis is suspected. Lumbar puncture is contraindicated if a mass lesion is suspected, or if there is raised intracranial pressure.

Management

Management depends entirely on the cause of the headache, e.g. appropriate antimicrobial treatment of CNS infection, with management of raised intracranial pressure, neurosurgical intervention for hydrocephalus, arteriovenous malformation, etc. Migraine is normally characterized by nausea, visual disturbance and unilateral paroxysmal headache. Management may be both symptomatic (paracetamol, antiemetic drugs) and prophylactic (regular sleep and meals, avoidance of known food triggers, beta-blockers or pizotifen – an antihistamine and serotonin antagonist). Recurrent tension headaches in the absence of organic pathology need a combined approach of strong reassurance and strategies to reduce stress.

Further reading

Hockaday JM. Management of migraine. *Archives of Disease in Childhood,* 1990; **65:**1174–76.

Wilson J. Headache in childhood. In: Brett EM, ed. *Paediatric Neurology,* 3rd edn. Edinburgh: Churchill Livingstone, 1997; 589–97.

Related topics of interest

Big heads, small heads (p. 49)
Hypertension (p. 199)
Meningitis and encephalitis (p. 265)
Neurocutaneous syndromes (p. 293)

HEARING AND SPEECH

Language development may be affected by environment, intelligence and genetic factors, by auditory input received and by articulatory processes. Hearing loss can be classified into sensorineural or conductive deafness. Sensorineural hearing loss (SNHL) is caused by a lesion in the cochlear or auditory nerve and its central connections. Most cases are congenital; however bacterial meningitis is the most common cause of acquired SNHL. Conductive hearing loss is due to middle ear pathology, usually secretory otitis media. This is a common problem and parental smoking is a risk factor. The number of children with severe hearing loss requiring a hearing aid is 1.3 per 1000.

Important milestones of hearing and language development are:

- 4–6 weeks: smiles, then vocalizes in response to sounds.
- 3–4 months: turns to sounds on a level with the ear.
- 7–8 months: produces a few consonants – ba, da – and imitates sounds of two syllables.
- 12 months: two to three words used with meaning.
- 15 months: jargon speech and many words.
- 21–24 months: puts 2–3 words together into a sentence spontaneously.
- 3 years: asks questions and understands much of adult speech. Vocabulary of 200 words, including pronouns.

Aetiology of deafness

- Perinatal, e.g. hyper-bilirubinaemia, drugs (frusemide, gentamicin), neonatal meningitis, hypoxic ischaemic encephalopathy.
- Genetic, e.g. Treacher Collins, Alport, Usher, Waardenburg. Isolated deafness may also be genetically determined.
- Intrauterine disease. Congenital infection with CMV, rubella, toxoplasma, syphilis and herpes simplex may cause deafness.
- Acquired. Acquired causes include trauma, meningitis and chronic secretory otitis media.
- Other, e.g. mucopolysaccharidosis (e.g. Hunter's syndrome) and Pendred's syndrome (hypothyroidism, autosomal recessive inheritance), long QT interval.

Aetiology of speech delay

- Hearing defects.
- Genetic factors.
- Global developmental delay.
- Environmental factors.
- Neurological disorders.
- Palatal dysfunction.

Clinical assessment

A detailed family history of language development and deafness is needed. The history of the pregnancy, delivery and postnatal period should be noted; any significant illnesses or trauma since birth may also be relevant. Enquiry should be made about the child's preverbal language development and current opportunities for talking with adults and peers. Maternal concerns about the child's hearing should always be taken seriously. Relevant abnormal behaviour, e.g. excessive gesturing, may be reported. A full clinical examination should search for features of syndromes associated with deafness and should include growth measurements and a formal assessment of development.

Hearing assessment

The test must be chosen according to the child's age and intelligence. The child surveillance programme should include enquiry into parental concerns, familial deafness and the child's startle reflex at 6–8 weeks of age, and a distraction hearing test at the age of 7–9 months. Surveillance between 18 months and 4 years is more difficult, relying on assessment of language, with audiology referral if there are doubts.

Evoked oto-acoustic emissions (EOAC) are currently used for screening at-risk neonates. It is a quick, easy and sensitive test and has now been recommended for universal screening.

The distraction test uses frequency-specific stimuli, e.g. the Manchester rattle, and may be used for infants from 7 months old.

Speech tests ('show me the fish') such as the Kendall or McCormick toy tests may be useful for the child below the age of 4 years. Performance tests, requesting a specific response every time a sound is heard, may also be of value.

From 4 years, pure-tone audiometry with headphones can be used, and this method forms the basis for screening hearing at school entry, 'the sweep'.

Other useful investigations are electrocochleography (ECOG) and brain-stem evoked responses – both may be useful if global developmental delay impairs responses in the distraction or performance tests. Tympanometry may be of value in assessing middle ear problems.

Language assessment

Speech and language disorders are common. Difficulties may be detected by parents, health professionals, nursery or playgroup leaders. Formal screening is not required. Language tests must include assessment of comprehension, expression, articulation and symbolic language, and are best performed by a speech therapist. The Reynell developmental language scales include assessment of both comprehension and expression. The Renfrew scheme tests expressive language (naming multiple pictures or telling the story of a picture). The Edinburgh articulation test concentrates on production of consonants. Symbolic language may be tested by the miniature toys test.

Investigation

For 60–80% of deaf children there is an identifiable cause. Investigation is important for genetic counselling and for management of associated problems.

- Serology. Rubella-specific IgM may be present in the neonate, or rubella IgG beyond 6 months of age.
- Urine collection. Test for blood and protein (Alport's syndrome), mucopolysaccharides, viral culture (CMV, rubella).
- Chromosomal analysis.
- Thyroid function (Pendred's syndrome). A perchlorate test should be included.
- ECG. A long QT segment may be present in the syndrome of Jervell and Lange-Nielsen.
- Radiology. Skull radiographs, cranial CT or MRI scan to investigate craniofacial abnormalities and bone dysplasias.
- Ophthalmic assessment. Cataracts and retinopathy in congenital rubella syndrome, heterochromia irides in Waardenburg's syndrome.

Management

1. Hearing deficit. Early diagnosis of a hearing deficit is important because of the social and educational impact of deafness. The aim is to prevent disability and improve outcomes for speech, language and communication. Secretory otitis media can be managed conservatively or surgically, with grommet insertion to ventilate the middle ear. Cochlear implant may be an option for some children with sensorineural deafness.

Communication is of prime importance for a child with a hearing deficit. This may be achieved through speech therapy, learning to lip read, or by using sign language, finger spelling, Makaton or electronic devices. Genetic counselling should be offered where appropriate.

2. Language/communication disorder. Detection at an early age allows assessment to exclude other problems (e.g. cerebral palsy, deafness, learning difficulties), relieves parental anxiety, and allows intervention to improve the disorder. Speech and language disorders are common and most children will improve with supervision. Speech therapists work with parents and nursery or school, to teach the child the components of language that they do not have. Some children have associated cognitive, coordination or behavioural difficulties. Appropriate provision should be made for the education of children with speech and language difficulties, either by adaptation within a mainstream school or by placement in a special school.

Communication disorders – the autistic spectrum disorders

Autism

1. Definition. A specific disorder of communication/behaviour recognized through the classical triad of:

- Impaired social interaction (social isolation).
- Impaired communication.
- Impaired imagination.

This leads to a display of rigid, repetitive behaviour and fixed interests which can adversely affect the child's general development and educational performance.

2. Aetiology. Extensive research has identified no single specific cause. It is likely to be multifactorial and complex in nature. Autism may be associated with another disability, e.g. cerebral palsy, epilepsy, sensory impairment, or learning disability.

3. Epidemiology. The true incidence is uncertain but it is a rare condition affecting approximately 5–10 per 10 000 children. It is more commonly recognized in boys than girls.

4. Associated features include indifference to noise, echolalia, hyperactivity and repetitive movements (e.g. rocking, swinging, arm flapping), outbursts of crying/screaming, lack of fear of danger, and limited body language. Some children have special skills in areas such as music, drawing or calculation.

5. Management. Autistic behaviour is often displayed from very early childhood but may not be recognized as such for some time. Early diagnosis is valued by parents and professionals alike as it allows the introduction of specialist teams and support agencies. As with all children with special needs, diagnosis and management is aided by a multidisciplinary, multiprofessional approach. Practical advice is needed for parents and carers on how to manage the child, who may benefit from highly structured surroundings and well-organized routines. Education must allow flexible solutions. A range of educational provisions and approaches may be required in an attempt to teach communication and socially acceptable behaviours.

Asperger's syndrome

This is recognized as being part of the autistic spectrum. It is considered to be a more mild, and therefore more able, form of autism. These children display the traits of poor sociability, poor communication skills, limited imagination and fixed interests but they have a greater ability with language than those with autism. It is often diagnosed later than autism and may go unrecognized. The prevalence is therefore difficult to estimate but it is probably at least 2–3 times more common than autism. They often have special skills including excellent memory and have a specific interest in certain subjects, e.g. astronomy, computing, board games. These children usually function in a mainstream school although they not infrequently become the focus of bullying because of their poor sociability and communication skills.

Further reading

Baird G. Speech and language problems in pre-school children. *Current Paediatrics,* 1995; **5:** 98–105.

Fonseca SJ, Patton MA. Clinical assessment of deafness. *Current Paediatrics,* 1992; **2:** 229–32.

Frith U, ed. *Autism and Asperger syndrome*. Cambridge: Cambridge University Press, 1991.

Hall DMB, ed. *Health for all Children. A Programme for Child Health Surveillance,* 3rd edn. Oxford: Oxford University Press, 1996; Ch. 10 and 12.

Richardson M. Otoacoustic emissions. *Archives of Disease in Childhood,* 1995; **73:** 284–6.

Related topics of interest

Developmental assessment (p. 111)
Developmental delay (p. 115)
Learning disability (p. 236)
Prematurity (p. 323)
Vision (p. 374)

HEART FAILURE

Inability of the heart to maintain cardiac output in childhood is usually associated with congenital heart disease which causes either pressure or volume overload. Signs and symptoms almost always develop in the first year of life, with biventricular failure resulting in pulmonary venous and hepatic congestion. Occasionally there is a non-cardiac cause such as fluid overload or anaemia. Heart failure is uncommon in older children. Specific disease of the heart muscle (infective, metabolic, drugs) may impair cardiac function resulting in a dilated cardiomyopathy. Pericarditis may result in an effusion or fibrosis which can impede cardiac function. Management of heart failure is aimed at removing treatable causes, reducing sodium and water load, improving myocardial contractility and general supportive measures such as maintaining good nutrition.

Problems

- Breathlessness.
- Sweating.
- Failure to thrive.
- Shock.

1. Presenting in the first week of life

- Severe left ventricular outflow tract obstruction, e.g. interrupted aortic arch, severe coarctation of the aorta, critical aortic stenosis.
- Hypoplastic left heart.
- Endocardial fibroelastosis.
- Myopathy (Pompe's, viral).
- Volume overload, e.g. cranial arteriovenous fistula.

2. Presenting in infancy

(a) Non-cardiac

- Fluid overload.
- Anaemia.
- Septicaemia.

(b) Cardiac

- Pressure overload, e.g. coarctation of the aorta.
- Volume overload, e.g. large VSD, PDA.
- Myocardial disease, e.g. myocarditis, metabolic defect, ischaemia (e.g. asphyxia).
- Arrhythmias, e.g. supraventricular tachycardia.
- Endocardial fibroelastosis.

3. Presenting in later childhood

- Systemic hypertension, e.g. renal disease.
- Pulmonary hypertension, (e.g. idiopathic, CHD with increased pulmonary blood flow or pulmonary venous obstruction, chronic lung disease (e.g. cystic fibrosis)).

- Myocarditis (viral especially Coxsackie and echovirus, rheumatic fever).
- Cardiomyopathy (including drug toxicity, e.g. anthracyclines).

Clinical features

Infants present with breathlessness and sweating particularly on exertion (feeding, crying). They take longer to complete a feed and failure to thrive is common. Examination reveals tachycardia, tachypnoea and hepatomegaly. There may be a murmur due to tricuspid/mitral valve incompetence, a congenital heart defect, or anaemia and a gallop rhythm may be heard. If heart failure is due to a heart defect (e.g. large VSD) symptoms usually develop over the first 6 weeks of life as pulmonary vascular resistance falls and left to right shunting increases. Hypotension occurs if heart failure is severe. Cyanosis develops if there is marked pulmonary oedema. Auscultation over the anterior fontanelle will reveal a bruit in the presence of an intracranial arteriovenous fistula. Basal crepitations and peripheral oedema do not usually occur in young children although there may be some facial puffiness. In neonates, if the heart failure has been present antenatally, there may be ascites, pleural and pericardial effusions and generalized oedema (hydrops fetalis). Older children exhibit clinical features of right or left heart failure as seen in adults (raised jugular venous pressure (JVP), hepatomegaly, peripheral oedema, etc.).

Investigation

- CXR. Cardiomegaly, pulmonary plethora.
- ECG. Arrhythmias, evidence of ventricular strain or ischaemia.
- Echocardiography provides a measure of left ventricular function (e.g. fractional shortening) and identifies congenital heart defects.
- Other investigations to identify cause, e.g.
  - Viral titres (especially Coxsackie, echovirus).
  - Thyroid function tests.
  - Urine and plasma amino/organic acids (inborn errors of metabolism).
  - Urinary glycosaminoglycans (mucopolysaccharidosis).
  - Creatine kinase (myopathy).

Management

1. Oxygen. Supplemental oxygen is given via head box or face mask to maintain arterial saturations.

2. Diuretics remain the mainstay of treatment. Frusemide is the most widely used, with spironolactone added for its potassium-sparing properties. Fluid restriction may be of some benefit.

3. *Treat anaemia.* Small transfusions of packed cells with diuretic cover to prevent worsening of fluid overload.

4. *Digoxin* is used for its positive inotropic effect but controversy surrounds its value, particularly in situations of volume overload, e.g. VSD.

5. *Vasodilators,* e.g. captopril, are particularly useful in conditions in which there is poor left ventricular function, such as dilated cardiomyopathy.

6. *Nutritional support.* Heart failure leads to increased nutritional requirements owing to a raised metabolic rate. If the patient is very breathless, nasogastric feeds should be introduced, and calorie supplements should be considered at an early stage.

7. *Positive inotropes,* e.g. dopamine, are used in the intensive care setting to improve myocardial contractility.

8. *Surgery.* If heart failure remains poorly controlled or the child is severely failing to thrive, surgical correction of structural heart defects (e.g. large VSD) or pulmonary artery banding to reduce pulmonary blood flow may be necessary.

Pericarditis

In the developing world, pericarditis is most commonly secondary to a pulmonary infection (e.g. *Staphylococcus aureus*, *Haemophilus influenzae*, pneumococcus, tuberculosis) or rheumatic fever. In the UK these causes are rare. Pericarditis may occur as part of a systemic viral infection often in association with myocarditis. Other causes in childhood include leukaemic infiltration, uraemia, post-cardiac surgery (Dressler's syndrome), SLE and post-irradiation. Clinical features include retrosternal pain, fever, dyspnoea, cough, muffled heart sounds and a pericardial rub. Inflammation may lead to the development of a pericardial effusion with subsequent cardiac tamponade (raised JVP, hepatomegaly, pulsus paradoxus). The CXR may show an enlarged globular heart and ECG findings include concave ST elevation and small voltage QRS complexes. Investigations include echocardiography, blood cultures, viral titres, Mantoux test and culture of pericardial fluid (obtained by pericardiocentesis). Treatment is supportive, antibiotics or antituberculous drugs if an infective cause is identified with or without drainage of the pericardial effusion. With chronic inflammation (e.g. tuberculosis) the pericardium may become scarred causing a constrictive pericarditis (ascites, hepatomegaly).

Further reading

Cardiac emergencies. In: Advanced Life Support Group. *Advanced Paediatric Life Support*, 2nd edn. London: BMJ Publications, 1997; 106–10.

Related topics of interest

Arrhythmias (p. 35)
Cyanotic congenital heart disease (p. 104)
Heart murmurs (p. 194)
Shock (p. 344)

HEART MURMURS

Heart murmurs are commonly heard during childhood particularly when the child is pyrexial and tachycardic. Most are innocent flow murmurs and the child should be re-examined when well to ensure that the murmur resolves. If the murmur persists, features such as a loud, long, or diastolic murmur, a thrill, or abnormal heart sounds suggest underlying congenital heart disease (CHD). A murmur that is soft, short, systolic, and varies with the position of the child is likely to be innocent. A venous hum is a continuous murmur best heard in the supraclavicular region which varies with the position of the child.

Assessment of a child with a heart murmur

History

Important aspects of the history include:

- Known predisposing factors, e.g. intercurrent illness, prematurity, Down's syndrome.
- Family history of illness, e.g. maternal diabetes, Marfan's syndrome.
- Previous child with CHD – the risk of a subsequent child being affected is increased three times.
- Symptoms such as poor feeding, sweating, failure to thrive, hypercyanotic spells.

Examination

Any child with a heart murmur should be carefully examined with particular attention to the following features:

- Presence or absence of cyanosis (see also related topic Cyanotic congenital heart disease, p. 104).
- Character and timing of the murmur (site, systolic/diastolic, loud/soft, thrill/heave).
- Abnormal heart sounds, e.g.
  - the second sound (S2) is usually single in cyanotic CHD.
  - fixed splitting of S2 suggests an atrial septal defect.
  - a loud pulmonary component of S2 is associated with pulmonary hypertension.
  - an ejection click may be heard in aortic stenosis.
- Evidence of heart failure (tachycardia, tachypnoea, hepatomegaly, sweating) – see related topic Heart failure (p. 190).
- Presence of dysmorphic features (e.g. Turner's syndrome, Noonan's syndrome).
- Presence of non-cardiac anomalies, e.g. cleft lip and palate, renal tract abnormalities, limb abnormalities.
- Evidence of poor growth – the height, weight and head circumference should be plotted on a growth chart.

Investigations

A child with an innocent sounding murmur who has no associated problems (such as failure to thrive, dysmorphic features) does not usually require any investigations. If congenital heart disease is suspected, investigations may include CXR, ECG, transcutaneous oxygen saturation, hyperoxia test, and karyotype. Referral to a cardiologist for further investigation (e.g. echocardiogram, cardiac catheterization) may be considered if these investigations are abnormal or if the child is symptomatic.

Congenital heart disease

Congenital heart disease (CHD) is the commonest serious congenital abnormality occurring in 8 per 1000 live births; 10–15% have an associated non-cardiac anomaly. Acyanotic lesions account for the majority of defects (more than 70%) and early death is uncommon. Cyanotic lesions account for only about 25% of CHD cases, but many are life-threatening in the first few weeks of life. Even with surgery, 15–20% of these affected will die in the first year of life.

Aetiology

- Idiopathic / multifactorial inheritance.
- Chromosomal abnormalities.
  50% of children with Down's syndrome have cardiac defects (particularly septal defects).
  10% of girls with Turner's syndrome have coarctation.
  Cardiac defects are common in trisomy 18 (Edward's), trisomy 13 (Patau's), and 22q-.
- Teratogens, e.g. congenital rubella, alcohol.
- Maternal conditions, e.g. diabetes.
- Single gene defects, e.g. Marfan's, Noonan's.
- Associated conditions, e.g. Cornelia de Lange syndrome (VSD).

Complications

- Heart failure.
- Failure to thrive.
- Arrhythmias.
- Subacute bacterial endocarditis (SBE).
- Sudden death.
- Pulmonary hypertension.
- Polycythaemia, thromboembolic events and hypercyanotic spells in cyanotic CHD.

Acyanotic congenital heart defects

1. Ventricular septal defect (VSD). This is the commonest heart defect and it usually presents with an asymptomatic murmur. The murmur may not be heard at birth but becomes audible over the first few weeks of life as the pulmonary vascular resistance falls and left to right shunting through the defect increases. Larger defects may present with heart failure as shunting increases. The murmur is typically pan-systolic, loudest at the lower left sternal edge, and often associated with a thrill. More than 50% close spontaneously. Progressive shortening of the murmur and an increasingly loud pulmonary component of the 2nd heart sound are evidence of pulmonary hypertension, which may develop if the left to right shunt is large. Eventual reversal of the shunt leads to cyanosis (Eisenmenger syndrome).

- CXR – normal, or cardiomegaly and pulmonary plethora.
- ECG – normal, or biventricular hypertrophy. RVH increases as pulmonary hypertension develops.

2. *Atrial septal defect (ASD).* An ASD usually presents with an asymptomatic ejection systolic murmur in the pulmonary area with fixed splitting of the second heart sound. This murmur is due to increased flow over the pulmonary valve and there may be a diastolic murmur in the tricuspid area. Spontaneous closure is very unusual and surgical closure is usually required. Pulmonary hypertension or heart failure may develop in adult life. SBE is very rare. The majority are secundum defects due to failure of closure of the foramen ovale. Primum defects are due to failure of development of septum primum.

- CXR – normal, or cardiomegaly with prominent right atrium and pulmonary arteries.
- ECG – left axis deviation in primum defects.
  normal or right axis deviation in secundum defects.
  incomplete right bundle branch block.

3. *Atrioventricular septal defect (AVSD).* Also known as an atrioventricular canal defect or endocardial cushion defect, this defect is particularly associated with Down's syndrome but it may occur as an isolated defect. Complete or partial absence of the septum at the atrioventricular junction is associated with abnormalities of the atrioventricular valves. Failure to thrive, heart failure and repeated chest infections are common. There is usually a pan-systolic murmur at the lower left sternal edge with a palpable thrill. A systolic murmur at the apex with radiation to the axilla will be heard in the presence of mitral regurgitation. A mid-diastolic murmur may also be heard representing excessive flow across the tricuspid valve.

- CXR – cardiomegaly, pulmonary plethora.
- ECG – left axis deviation producing a superior axis, prolonged PR interval, partial right bundle branch block, RVH with or without LVH.

4. Pulmonary stenosis (PS). This presents with an asymptomatic ejection systolic murmur in the pulmonary area, radiating to the back and often associated with a thrill. The second heart sound is normal (cf. ASD).

- CXR – normal, or post stenotic dilatation of the pulmonary artery.
- ECG – RVH increases with severity.

5. Aortic stenosis (AS). AS often presents with an asymptomatic murmur, but if severe, can cause heart failure or sudden death. There is an ejection systolic murmur in the aortic area radiating to the carotids. An ejection click may be heard.

- CXR – normal, or post stenotic dilatation of the aorta.
- ECG – LVH and LV strain increases with severity.

6. Patent ductus arteriosus (PDA). Classically described as causing a continuous machinery murmur which extends through systole and the second heart sound into diastole. It is best heard under the left clavicle and radiates through to the back. The peripheral pulses are full and collapsing, with easily palpable foot pulses. It is common in premature infants who may present with heart failure. In older children it is usually asymptomatic.

- CXR – normal unless very large left to right shunt.
- EGG – as CXR.

7. Coarctation of the aorta. Coarctation usually presents with hypertension in the arms, with or without heart failure but occasionally it presents simply with an asymptomatic systolic murmur. This murmur may be due to flow through the coarctation or through collaterals, or it may be due to an associated VSD.

Management of a child with acyanotic CHD

1. Medical. The majority of children with asymptomatic murmurs do not require any specific treatment. They should be monitored for signs of failure to thrive, ventricular hypertrophy, heart failure and pulmonary hypertension. Parents should be advised about antibiotic prophylaxis against SBE, and about the importance of immunizations. Most children will limit their own exercise and the only condition in which strenuous exercise should be avoided is moderate to severe aortic stenosis due to the risk of sudden death. Adequate nutrition is important particularly if the child is in heart failure as calorie requirements will be increased.

2. *Surgical.* Septal defects which will not close spontaneously are closed surgically. Reduction of pulmonary blood flow by pulmonary artery banding is sometimes necessary with large defects to reduce symptoms of heart failure and to prevent the development of pulmonary hypertension. The defect is then repaired at a second operation months to several years later, when the child is bigger.

If outflow obstruction (e.g. AS, PS, coarctation) is marked with increasing ventricular hypertrophy or heart failure, repair is indicated. Balloon angioplasty is becoming increasingly popular, particularly for coarctation, but the obstruction often recurs.

Related topics of interest

Cyanotic congenital heart disease (p. 104)
Heart failure (p. 190)
Hypertension (p. 199)

HYPERTENSION

Blood pressure increases with age and there is no precise definition of hypertension, but a child with a blood pressure greater than the 95th centile for age may be considered to have significant hypertension. Severe hypertension has been defined as a blood pressure greater than the 99th centile for age. Hypertension should not be diagnosed until an abnormal blood pressure has been confirmed on several occasions. Mild, asymptomatic hypertension, particularly in older children, is usually primary or essential. These children may be at increased risk of ischaemic heart disease and cerebrovascular disease in adult life. The majority of children with severe symptomatic hypertension have an underlying cause, most commonly renal parenchymal disease.

Problems

- Heart failure.
- Acute hypertensive encephalopathy.
- Increased risk of ischaemic heart disease and cerebrovascular disease in adult life.

Aetiology

1. Primary (essential).

2. Secondary

(a) Renal (95% of secondary hypertension)

- Chronic GMN.
- Reflux nephropathy.
- Haemolytic uraemic syndrome.

(b) Vascular

- Coarctation of the aorta.
- Renal artery stenosis.
- Renal vein thrombosis.

(c) Endocrine

- Cushing's syndrome.
- Primary hyperaldosteronism (Conn's).
- Congenital adrenal hyperplasia.
- Neuroblastoma.

(d) Other

- Intracranial tumours.
- Post head injury (cerebral oedema, intracranial haemorrhage).
- Drugs, e.g. steroids.
- Lead poisoning.
- Porphyria.

Clinical features

Hypertension is often asymptomatic and detected only on routine examination. Blood pressure measurement is an essential part of the examination of any child with renal, cardiac or endocrine disease. Three or more readings should be taken with a cuff whose bladder width is at least 75% of the upper arm length. A cuff that is too small will give a spuriously elevated blood pressure. In infants and small children the Doppler method is recommended.

There may be a history of genitourinary symptoms suggesting a renal cause. The child should be examined for evidence of abdominal masses, endocrine disease, coarctation, renal bruits (renal artery stenosis), raised intracranial pressure and Turner's syndrome.

Coarctation presents with hypertension in the arms, with or without heart failure. Absent femoral pulses or radio-femoral delay may be the only signs, or a systolic murmur may be heard. The CXR may show cardiomegaly but is often normal. Rib notching due to collaterals is sometimes seen in older children. Left ventricular hypertrophy and optic fundi changes develop in long-standing hypertension. Symptoms only occur as a result of the complications of hypertension i.e. raised intracranial pressure (vomiting, headaches, visual disturbance, seizures) or left ventricular failure (dyspnoea, cough). Facial palsy is an uncommon presenting feature.

Investigation

- Urinalysis and urine culture.
- U&E and creatinine.
- Renal imaging (US, isotope scanning).
- Urinary catecholamines (VMA, HVA).
- Other tests. Depending on history, examination and preliminary laboratory findings, e.g. plasma renin and aldosterone, cortisol, abdominal angiography, brain imaging.

Management

All patients with essential hypertension should be advised not to smoke, and to lose weight if obese. Girls should be advised against using the contraceptive pill. If the hypertension is secondary, it may be possible to treat the cause (e.g. repair of coarctation, relief of renal artery stenosis). If borderline, the hypertension should be monitored and drug treatment may not be necessary. If the blood pressure is undoubtedly high or if there are signs or symptoms the hypertension should be treated with hypotensive drugs (diuretics, beta-blockers, vasodilators, angiotensin-converting enzyme inhibitors).

Acute hypertensive encephalopathy

Acute hypertension is most commonly seen in glomerulonephritis, haemolytic uraemic syndrome or following a head injury. Encephalopathy may rapidly develop, with vomiting, headaches, neurological signs (e.g. visual symptoms, facial palsy), impaired consciousness and seizures. It is an emergency requiring controlled blood pressure reduction with i.v. sodium nitroprusside or labetalol.

Further reading

Deal JE, Barratt TM, Dillon MJ. Management of hypertensive emergencies. *Archives of Disease in Childhood*, 1992; **67:** 1089–92.

de Swiet M, Dillon MJ, Littler W *et al.* Measurement of blood pressure in children. Recommendations of a working party of the British Hypertension Society. *British Medical Journal,* 1989; **299:** 497.

Report of the Second Task Force on Blood Pressure Control in Children. *Pediatrics,* 1987; **79:** 1–25.

Related topics of interest

Adrenal disorders (p. 23)
Coma (p. 89)
Glomerulonephritis (p. 164)
Heart murmurs (p. 194)

HYPOGLYCAEMIA

Blood glucose concentration is normally maintained within narrow limits by homeostatic regulation of glucose production and utilization. Hypoglycaemia is a common problem in the newborn period, being particularly associated with prematurity and small size. It is less common in infancy and childhood, but may be the first indication of metabolic or endocrine dysfunction. The exact incidence is difficult to ascertain as there is no consensus over the definition of hypoglycaemia, with glucose concentrations ranging from < 1 mmol/l to < 4 mmol/l in various textbooks. Repeated hypoglycaemia is a recognized cause of neurological damage, but the level at which this occurs is unclear. Asymptomatic hypoglycaemia has been associated with abnormal sensory evoked responses at levels below 2.6 mmol/l.

Aetiology

Hypoglycaemia may result from either inadequate glucose production or excessive glucose consumption. In the neonatal period this may be transient or persistent.

1. Neonatal period and infancy

(a) Transient

- Decreased production. Poor oral intake, prematurity, small for dates.
- Increased utilization. Hyperinsulinism (infant of a diabetic mother, rhesus disease, maternal beta-blocker therapy, idiopathic).
- Both decreased production and increased utilization. Fetal distress, hypothermia, sepsis, cyanotic CHD.

(b) Persistent

- Decreased production. Inborn errors of metabolism (e.g. glycogen storage disorders, fatty acid oxidation defects), hormone deficiencies (e.g. hypopituitarism, adrenal insufficiency).
- Increased utilization. Hyperinsulinism (nesidioblastosis, Beckwith–Wiedemann syndrome).

2. Childhood

- Decreased production. Liver disease (e.g. Reye's syndrome), toxins (e.g. alcohol), hormone deficiencies (e.g. growth hormone, cortisol), ketotic hypoglycaemia (accelerated starvation).
- Increased utilization. Hyperinsulinism (islet cell tumour, exogenous insulin excess in diabetes mellitus).

Clinical features

Symptoms occur as a result of the lack of glucose available for CNS metabolism and increased catecholamine secretion in response to hypoglycaemia. In the neonatal period features include irritability, jitteriness, apnoea, hypotonia and convulsions, although many infants are asymptomatic. In the older child features include lack of energy, tremor, headache, hunger, pallor, sweating, tachycardia, mental confusion, visual disturbance, behavioural abnormalities, seizures and coma. Hypoglycaemia in childhood usually occurs after a fast (e.g. overnight), but hyperinsulinism may precipitate hypoglycaemia after meals. Features such as hepatomegaly, cataracts and metabolic acidosis suggest an inborn error of metabolism. Short stature, micropenis or electrolyte disturbances suggest an endocrine disorder.

Transient neonatal hypoglycaemia

Infants who are small for gestational age (SGA) have reduced glycogen stores which are rapidly used up after birth, and the blood glucose will fall over the first few hours of life. The risk of hypoglycaemia recedes once oral feeding is fully established, but there are a group of underweight children, particularly under the age of 3 years, who remain prone to ketotic hypoglycaemia owing to reduced gluconeogenic reserve. Premature infants are vulnerable to hypoglycaemia because of their limited glycogen reserves and immaturity of the gluconeogenic and glycogenolytic pathways. Birth asphyxia leads to depletion of glycogen reserves as a result of catecholamine and glucagon release. There may also be transient hyperinsulinism due to pancreatic ischaemia.

The transient hyperinsulinism of the infant of a diabetic mother usually resolves within the first week of life. The hyperinsulinism of Beckwith–Wiedemann syndrome may be transient or prolonged, occasionally persisting into adult life.

Persistent hyperinsulinism

Anatomical abnormalities of the pancreas (nesidioblastosis and islet cell adenomas) are the commonest causes of prolonged severe hypoglycaemia in infancy. Infants with nesidioblastosis are large for gestational age (LGA) and look similar to infants of diabetic mothers at birth. Hyperinsulinism is due to inappropriate pancreatic endocrine development, resulting in an excess of β-cells.

Investigation of hypoglycaemia

It is vital that investigations are performed when the child is hypoglycaemic.

- Blood glucose.
- Blood insulin. If high or normal despite hypoglycaemia, this confirms hyperinsulinism.
- Urinary ketones. Hyperinsulinism causes non-ketotic hypoglycaemia. Hypoglycaemia with ketosis is a feature of hormone and enzyme deficiencies.
- Other investigations as indicated (e.g. growth hormone, cortisol, amino acids, free fatty acids, lactate) for metabolic disorders or hormone deficiencies.

Management

1. Oral carbohydrate. Monitoring of blood glucose in high-risk neonates (small for gestational age, infants of diabetic mothers, etc.) and early introduction of feeds may avoid the need for i.v. dextrose.

2. Intravenous dextrose. Glucose utilization in normal infants is 5–7 mg/kg/min and in adults is 2 mg/kg/min. A child who needs more than these levels to maintain blood glucose has hypoglycaemia due to excessive utilization. Levels of 15–20 mg/kg/min are frequently needed to maintain normoglycaemia in the presence of hyperinsulinism.

3. Glucagon. Can be given intramuscularly or subcutaneously if i.v. access is difficult. It is useful in diabetics who are unable to take carbohydrate orally, but in other conditions it may lead to rebound hypoglycaemia by stimulating hyperinsulinism.

4. Diazoxide. Inhibits glucose-stimulated insulin release and is potentiated by simultaneous administration of a thiazide diuretic. It may be sufficient to control hypoglycaemia in Beckwith–Wiedemann syndrome.

5. Somatostatin long-acting analogues. May be useful in nesidioblastosis.

6. Surgery. Partial or total pancreatectomy may be indicated for nesidioblastosis and insulinoma.

7. Specific treatments, e.g. hormone replacement, dietary management of inborn errors of metabolism.

Further reading

Hawdon JM, Ward Platt MP, Aynsley-Green A. Prevention and management of neonatal hypoglycaemia. *Archives of Disease in Childhood,* 1994; **70:** F60–64.

Koh THHG, Aynsley-Green A, Tarbit M, Eyre JA. Neural dysfunction during hypoglycaemia. *Archives of Disease in Childhood,* 1988; **63:** 1353–8.

LaFranchi S. Hypoglycemia in infancy and childhood. In: Mahoney CP, ed. *Pediatric and Adolescent Endocrinology. Pediatric Clinics of North America,* 1987; **34**(4): 961–82.

Lucas A, Morley R, Cole TJ. Adverse neurodevelopmental outcome of moderate neonatal hypoglycaemia. *British Medical Journal,* 1988; **297:** 1304–8.

Related topics of interest

Diabetes mellitus (p. 119)
Small for dates, large for dates (p. 352)

IMMUNIZATION

Immunization may be achieved actively or passively. Active immunization is the basis of the routine childhood vaccination programme, using inactivated or live attenuated organisms or their products to stimulate antibody production. Protection by actively produced antibody or antitoxin will then last for months or years, with booster doses reinforcing immunity. Passive immunity is achieved by the injection of human immunoglobulin, providing immediate, but only temporary protection.

Routine vaccination of children ensures the best possible protection from serious infectious disease, but relies on a positive, well-informed approach by all health care workers to achieve optimum results.

UK routine vaccination programme (1996)

The Department of Health have a standard immunization programme outlined below.

- Diphtheria, tetanus, pertussis (DTP), Hib and oral polio vaccines are given at 2 months, 3 months and 4 months. This accelerated schedule was introduced in 1990 to follow the WHO guidelines, providing earlier protection against pertussis and allowing less opportunity for inter-current illnesses, avoiding delay in immunization.
- Measles, mumps and rubella vaccine (MMR) is given at 12–15 months (any age above 12 months).
- Diphtheria, tetanus and polio booster and second MMR vaccine is given prior to school entry, age 3–5 years.
- BCG vaccine is given by certain health authorities to children age 10–14 years and infant BCG is given to high risk groups in the neonatal period.
- Adolescent booster tetanus, low dose diphtheria and polio given age 13–18 years.

Contraindications to immunization

True contraindications to immunization are uncommon and if doubts exist further advice should be sought from a consultant paediatrician, public health physician or district immunization co-ordinator.

General contraindications to immunization are:

- An acute illness (not a minor infection without pyrexia) at the time of vaccination. Delay immunization until well.
- A severe local reaction to a previous dose of vaccine, i.e. extensive erythema and swelling of most of the circumference of the upper arm, or most of the anterolateral surface of the thigh.
- A severe systemic reaction to a previous dose of vaccine, i.e. fever of 39.5°C or above within 48 hours of

vaccination; anaphylaxis; prolonged inconsolable screaming, convulsion or encephalopathy within 72 hours of vaccination.
- Live vaccine (polio, MMR and BCG) should not be administered to immunocompromised or those on high dose steroid treatment (2 mg/kg/day).

The following are *not* contraindications to immunization:

- Family history of any adverse reaction following immunization.
- Previous history of pertussis, measles, rubella or mumps infection.
- Prematurity: immunization should be given at actual not corrected age.
- Stable neurological conditions, e.g. Down's syndrome or cerebral palsy.
- Contact with an infectious disease.
- Asthma, eczema, hay fever or 'snuffles'.
- Treatment with antibiotics or locally acting (topical or inhaled) steroid.
- Child's mother pregnant.
- Child being breast fed.
- History of jaundice after birth.
- Child under a certain weight.
- Over the age recommended in immunization schedule.
- 'Replacement' corticosteroids, e.g. congenital adrenal hyperplasia.

Individual vaccines

1. *Pertussis.* Pertussis is a killed vaccine given in combination with diphtheria, tetanus and more recently also Hib. Children with a history of febrile fits or a family history of epilepsy can safely be immunized, after counselling and reassuring the parents accordingly.

Immunization for children with uncertain or evolving neurological conditions may need careful discussion with the consultant paediatrician, vaccination may be deferred or acellular pertussis vaccine offered.

2. *MMR.* This combined vaccine of live attenuated measles, mumps and rubella should be given irrespective of a previous history of the three illnesses. Specific contraindications are:

- Immunosuppression secondary to disease or drugs, including high dose steroids.
- Immunization with another live vaccine (usually BCG) in the previous 3 weeks.

(a) MMR and egg allergy: MMR was previously contraindicated for those with egg allergy. There is now increasing evidence that MMR vaccine can safely be given to a child who has had previous anaphylaxis to egg. If there is concern, paediatric advice should be sought and the vaccine given as a day case in hospital.

(b) Second MMR: A second dose of MMR prior to school entry was introduced in 1996. The aim is to prevent reaccumulation of sufficiently susceptible children to sustain a future epidemic. Schoolgirl single rubella vaccination has now been discontinued.

3. Haemophilus influenza type b. (Hib). The Hib bacterium is an important cause of morbidity and mortality affecting primarily the pre-school age group, causing meningitis, epiglottitis and septicaemia. Routine vaccination was introduced in the UK in 1992/93, leading to a dramatic decline in reported cases of invasive disease. Hib vaccine can be combined with DTP vaccine and given as one injection.

4. Polio. Live oral polio vaccine is routinely used in the UK, and contains live attenuated strains of polio vaccine. Inactivated polio vaccine is available as an intramuscular preparation, for those children in whom live vaccine is contraindicated. Symptoms of diarrhoea and vomiting are contraindications.

5. BCG. It remains national policy to immunize schoolchildren between ages of 10 and 14 years against tuberculosis, in addition to selective immunization of babies and children in high risk groups. Notifications of tuberculosis were on the decline until 1987, since which time there has been a slow increase in reported cases. Incidence varies widely between geographical areas and ethnic groups and is generally higher in inner city areas and in groups of populations originating from high risk areas (Indian sub-continent and Africa).

6. Other vaccines. Certain vaccines are recommended for high risk groups or for foreign travel. These include influenza, pneumococcus, hepatitis A, hepatitis B, meningococcus groups a and c and typhoid (see Further reading).

Vaccine controversies

From time to time controversy is raised regarding the safety of vaccines, especially when an alteration is made to the immunization schedule. True severe adverse reactions to vaccines are rare. As yet there is no clinically proven evidence to support the alleged link of MMR vaccine with Crohn's disease or autism. Health professionals must aim to promote the positive public health aspects of vaccination.

Providing adequate information to parents enables them to make an informed decision regarding vaccination for their child.

Further reading

Campbell AGM. New vaccines on the horizon. *Current Paediatrics*, 1995; **5:** 140–2.
Department of Health. *Immunisation against Infectious Disease*. London: HMSO, 1996.

Related topics of interest

Meningitis and encephalitis (p. 265)
Rashes and blisters (p. 337)

IMMUNODEFICIENCY

Recurrent minor infections are very common during early childhood due to increasing contact with other children and immaturity of the immune response. However, immunodeficiency should be considered if infections are unusually frequent or severe, are due to unusual organisms, or are associated with failure to thrive. Immunodeficiency may be congenital or acquired (e.g. HIV infection, drugs). Apart from selective IgA deficiency, congenital immunodeficiency disorders are rare. Transient hypogammaglobulinaemia may occur during infancy due to delayed maturation of immunoglobulin production. Spontaneous recovery occurs within the first 12–18 months of life.

Aetiology

1. Congenital

- Antibody deficiency (defect of humoral immunity) e.g. X-linked agammaglobulinaemia, IgG subclass deficiency, selective IgA deficiency. Chronic sinopulmonary infections, meningitis, septicaemia and osteomyelitis caused by encapsulated bacterial pathogens (*Pneumococcus*, *Haemophilus*) are common.
- Defects of cell-mediated immunity, e.g. DiGeorge syndrome, Wiskott–Aldrich syndrome, Nezelof syndrome, ataxia telangiectasia. These are less common than defects of antibody production. Fungal, viral (CMV, adenovirus), parasitic, mycobacterial and opportunistic (e.g. *Pneumocystis carinii*) infections are typical.
- Phagocyte dysfunction, e.g. chronic granulomatous disease, Job syndrome, Chediak–Higashi syndrome, cyclical neutropenia. A large number of phagocyte defects have been described. Staphylococcal and fungal infections commonly affect the skin, mucous membranes, liver and bone causing suppurative lymphadenopathy, osteomyelitis, hepatic abscesses and purulent skin lesions.
- Defects of complement function, e.g. C3 deficiency (leads to severe pyogenic infections), C6,C7,C8 deficiency (associated with recurrent Neisserial infection).
- Combined defects of humoral and cell-mediated immunity, e.g. severe combined immunodeficiency (SCID).

2. Acquired

- Infection (HIV).
- Drugs, e.g. steroids, chemotherapy – mainly affect cell mediated immunity.
- Irradiation.
- Hodgkins' disease.

- Immunoglobulin loss, e.g. protein-losing enteropathy, nephrotic syndrome.
- Uraemia.
- Malnutrition.
- Splenectomy – especially prone to infection with encapsulated organisms.

Investigation of suspected immunodeficiency

Some investigations are readily available, but others are only performed in specialized laboratories. Discussion with a paediatric immunologist in complex cases will help the clinician decide which investigations are appropriate.

- FBC, film – lymphopenia typical in SCID, neutropenia in Schwachman syndrome, cyclical neutropenia.
- Microbiology to identify parasitic, bacterial, fungal and viral pathogens.
- Immunoglobulin levels (total and IgG subclasses).
- Complement levels.
- Specific antibody measurement, e.g. to immunization antigens (tetanus toxoid, Hib) or blood group antigens (isohaemagglutinins).
- HIV serology.
- Lymphocyte numbers and function tests, e.g. CD4/CD8 ratios, nitrogen phytohaemagglutinin test which measures T-cell proliferation.
- Tests of chemotaxis and opsonization, e.g. nitroblue tetrazolium dye reduction test is an *in vitro* measure of granulocyte function.

General management of a child with immunodeficiency

1. Treat infections promptly with narrow-spectrum agents whenever possible, together with physiotherapy for chest infections.

2. Prophylactic antibiotics may increase the risk of resistant organisms, but are useful in some patients, e.g. cotrimoxazole to prevent *Pneumocystis carinii* pneumonia (PCP) in those with AIDS.

3. Pooled human immunoglobulin infusions may be given to patients with antibody deficiency every 2–4 weeks depending on serum levels and clinical response. Consider giving immunoglobulin in other immunodeficiencies if in contact with chickenpox (zoster immune globulin with or without acyclovir) or measles.

4. *Avoid live vaccines* particularly in those with cell-mediated immunodeficiency.

5. *Irradiate blood products* before transfusion to prevent graft-versus-host disease in cellular immunodeficiency.

6. *Human recombinant interferon* has been used to improve phagocyte bactericidal activity in some disorders. Granulocyte colony stimulating factor may be helpful in neutropenia, e.g. post-chemotherapy.

7. *Bone marrow transplantation* is the treatment of choice for patients with SCID or DiGeorge syndrome.

8. *Detection of carriers and prenatal diagnosis* is available for some disorders

Specific conditions

1. *Selective IgA deficiency*. This is by far the most common immunodeficiency (incidence approximately 1 in 500 of the population). Many patients are asymptomatic, but there is an increased incidence of associated IgG subclass deficiency and autoimmune diseases. Symptoms include recurrent otitis media and chest infections which should be treated with antibiotics with or without physio. In severe cases immunoglobulin infusions may be considered.

2. *IgG subclass deficiency*. There are four IgG subclasses. IgG1 and 3 fix complement and are involved in the protein antigen response (e.g. toxoids). IgG2 is involved in the carbohydrate antigen response (e.g. encapsulated Hib, pneumococcus). IgG4 is less well characterized. IgG2 deficiency is the commonest in childhood. It normally accounts for ~25% of the total serum IgG and deficiency is three times more common in boys than girls. Presenting features include recurrent severe upper repiratory tract infections (otitis media, sinusitis, tonsillitis), bronchopulmonary infections, bronchiectasis, and severe atopy (associated particularly with IgG3 deficiency).

3. *X-linked agammaglobulinaemia (Bruton type)*. This is a rare condition due to a mutation in the cytoplasmic signal transducing molecule on the long arm of the X chromosome. Affected males are usually asymptomatic until the age of about 6–9 months as placentally transferred immunoglobulins provide protection. Presenting features

include recurrent pyogenic infections, chronic lung disease, diarrhoea, or failure to thrive. Levels of circulating B cells and immunoglobulins A, M, G and D are absent or low. Antibody response to previous immunizations is absent. Treatment is with immunoglobulin infusions and prompt treatment of infections.

4. *Severe combined immunodeficiency.* There is failure of both cellular and humoral immunity. Inheritance may be autosomal or X-linked recessive. Presentation with diarrhoea, failure to thrive, pneumonia and mucocutaneous candidiasis occurs in the first few months of life. There may be a family history of an unexplained infant death. Graft-versus-host disease may be triggered by blood transfusions or by transplacental passage of maternal lymphocytes. Lymphoid hypoplasia with absent thymus and tonsils is a feature. Some infants can be shown to have abnormalities of adenosine deaminase enzyme activity, and enzyme replacement with bovine extracted enzyme can be helpful. Bone marrow transplantation provides the only cure.

5. *DiGeorge syndrome.* T-cell dysfunction is associated with congenital heart disease (particularly interrupted aortic arch), thymic aplasia, hypocalcaemia (due to absent parathyroid glands), and abnormal facies.

6. *Wiskott–Aldrich syndrome.* X-linked recessive condition in which lymphopenia and defective T-cell function are associated which eczema and thrombocytopenia. Levels of IgA and IgE are usually raised, with low IgM and normal IgG. The majority die of overwhelming sepsis in childhood although bone marrow transplantation may offer a cure.

7. *Chronic granulomatous disease.* The first of the neutrophil dysfunction disorders to be described. It is an X-linked recessive condition in which neutrophils can engulf bacteria normally but are unable to produce antimicrobial oxidant factors to kill them. The white cell count and immunoglobulin levels are normal. It is diagnosed by the nitroblue tetrazolium dye reduction test.

8. *Acquired immunodeficiency syndrome (AIDS).* This results from infection with the human immunodeficiency virus (HIV). Transmission may be parenteral (from infected

blood products, i.v. drug abuse), vertical (from an infected mother), or sexual (heterosexual, homosexual, sexual abuse). The latent period between infection and symptoms is longer for parenterally acquired infection than for those who are vertically infected. Over 75% of those who are vertically infected will have symptoms by the age of 2 years. Presentation may be with severe recurrent infections, failure to thrive, opportunistic infections (e.g. PCP), HIV encephalopathy, lymphocytic interstitial pneumonitis (a slowly progressive chronic lung disease), or malignancy (e.g. lymphomas, Kaposi's sarcoma rare in children). Diagnosis may be difficult in the first year of life due to persistence of maternal antibodies. PCR to detect and amplify HIV genetic material, high levels of IgG, IgM, and IgA, and low CD4 numbers with reversed CD4:CD8 subsets may be helpful diagnostic indicators. Management involves the prevention and early aggressive treatment of infections, PCP prophylaxis with cotrimoxazole or nebulized pentamidine, and specific antiretroviral treatments, e.g. AZT (3′-azido-3′-deoxythymidine).

Further reading

Gibb D, Newell ML. HIV infection in children. *Archives of Disease in Childhood,* 1992; **67:** 138–41.

Haeney M. Clinical aspects of antibody deficiency. *Hospital Update.* February 1990: 122–134.

Roberton D. Basic investigation of children with recurrent infections. *Current Paediatrics,* 1993; **3** (1): 6–9.

Sharland M, Gibb D, Tudor-Williams G, Walters S, Novelli V. Paediatric HIV infection. *Archives of Disease in Childhood,* 1997; **76:** 293–6.

Strobel S. Nonmalignant disorders of lymphocytes: primary and acquired immunodeficiency diseases. In: Lilleyman JS, Hann IM, eds. *Paediatric Haematology.* Edinburgh: Churchill Livingstone, 1992; 273–327.

Related topics of interest

Failure to thrive (p. 138)
Immunization (p. 206)
Lumps in the neck (p. 251)

INBORN ERRORS OF METABOLISM

An error may occur in any metabolic pathway due to a genetically inherited enzyme defect. A characteristic phenotype results and many of the defects can now be identified by enzyme assays or by DNA technology. Most are recessively inherited and the majority are uncommon, but they may cause severe neurological impairment and are often fatal. An enzyme deficiency results in organ damage by:

- accumulation of the enzyme substrate, e.g. hyperphenylalaninaemia in phenylketonuria (PKU), glycogen due to defects of the glycogen degradation pathway.
- overproduction of other metabolites by metabolism of the substrate via alternative pathways, e.g. metabolic acidosis and hyperammonaemia in urea cycle disorders.
- lack of production of the normal metabolites, e.g. hypoglycaemia in disorders of fatty acid oxidation.

Treatment by induction of enzyme activity, biochemical correction with special diets, or bone marrow or organ (e.g. liver) transplantation may improve symptoms and allow normal development in some cases. Identification of the defect is important not only for treatment, but also for genetic counselling.

Presentation

Metabolic disorders can present at any age. Most being inherited as autosomal recessive conditions, they are more common in consanguineous marriages. There may be a family history of the condition or a history of a previous stillbirth or infant death. Onset may be insidious (failure to thrive, developmental delay) or acute (hypoglycaemia, fits, encephalopathy).

1. Neonatal period and early infancy. Typical presenting features include:

- Acute encephalopathy (hypotonia, drowsiness, fits, vomiting, hypoglycaemia, and metabolic acidosis). These infants are often initially thought to be septicaemic. Symptoms improve on stopping feeds and giving i.v. fluids, but worsen again on reintroduction of feeds.
- Sudden unexpected infant death.
- Failure to thrive.
- Prolonged jaundice. Galactosaemia presents with hypoglycaemia, cataracts, jaundice and moderate to severe liver disease in the neonatal period. It is due to galactose-1-phosphate uridyl transferase (G1PUT) deficiency. Urine tests positive for reducing sugars (Clinitest) but negative for glucose (Clinistix). Treatment is with a lactose and galactose-free diet. It is a rare condition (incidence < 1 in 50 000 live births).

- Dysmorphic features, e.g. Zellweger syndrome – a peroxisomal disorder causing typical craniofacial features, fits, hypotonia, hepatomegaly.
- Cataracts.
- Peculiar smell. Disorders of the metabolism of branched chain amino acids (leucine, isoleucine, and valine) present with metabolic acidosis and characteristic excretion of urinary organic acids (organic aciduria), some of which have distinctive odours, e.g. maple syrup urine disease.
- Detected by screening. Phenylketonuria has an incidence of about 1 in 10 000 births and neonatal screening is routinely performed in the UK (Guthrie test). Phenylalanine accumulates due to absent phenylalanine hydroxylase activity. This has early adverse effects on the developing CNS leading to severe mental retardation. Affected children are typically fair-haired, blue-eyed and often have eczema. Treatment with a low phenylalanine diet can prevent mental retardation if commenced in the first 2–3 weeks of life.

2. *Later infancy and childhood*

- Episodic vomiting, lethargy, hypoglycaemia, metabolic acidosis.
- Convulsions and acute encephalopathy.
- Hepatocellular damage, e.g. tyrosinaemia, haemochromatosis, Wilson's disease.
- Visceromegaly, e.g. glycogen storage disease Type I (von Gierke's disease) – glucose-6-phosphate deficiency results in hepatomegaly, enlarged kidneys, short stature and truncal obesity. Recurrent hypoglycaemia is a major problem.
- Cardiomyopathy, e.g. glycogen storage disease Type II (Pompe's disease) in which acid maltase deficiency results in cardiomyopathy.
- Muscle weakness or cramps, myoglobinuria, e.g. glycogen storage disease Type V (McArdle's disease) in which myophosphorylase deficiency causes muscle cramps.
- Developmental delay or regression, e.g. sphingolipidoses – lysosomal storage disorders leading to intracellular deposition of sphingolipids in many tissues (Tay-Sachs disease, metachromatic leucodystrophy, Gaucher disease, Krabbe disease, Niemann–Pick disease). Disorders of purine metabolism (Lesch–Nyhan syndrome).

Peroxisomal disorders (X-linked adrenoleucodystrophy, Zellweger syndrome).

- Dysmorphic features, e.g. mucopolysaccharidoses – deficiency of specific lysosomal enzymes results in accumulation of partially degraded glycosaminoglycans (GAGS = dermatan sulphate, heparan sulphate, keratan sulphate) in many tissues. GAGS are also found in the urine. The commonest are Hurler's syndrome (MPS I), Hunter's syndrome (MPS II – X-linked), Sanfilippo's syndrome (MPS III), and Morquio's syndrome (MPS IV). Features vary from type to type but may include coarse facial features, corneal clouding, airway problems, learning difficulties, joint stiffness, skeletal dysplasia, cardiac disease (cardiomyopathy, mitral/aortic valve thickening) and cervical myelopathy (see Further reading).

Acute metabolic encephalopathy

Inborn errors of metabolism may precipitate acute encephalopathy by causing disturbance of glucose metabolism, metabolic acidosis, hyperammonaemia, or liver dysfunction. The child may present in the neonatal period or may be completely well for months or years until a stressful event (e.g. prolonged fasting, infection) triggers an acute metabolic encephalopathy which mimics Reye's syndrome (see below).

Investigations

- Blood glucose.
- Acid-base status.
- Liver function tests with clotting studies.
- Plasma ammonia – normally < 50 μmol/l but will rise in any unwell child. Encephalopathy may occur at a level > 100 μmol/l, but it is usually over 200 μmol/l.
- Urinary ketones.
- Lactate and pyruvate. Pyruvate is the end point of anaerobic glycolysis and is the starting-point of gluconeogenesis. Lactate arises from normal anaerobic glycolysis and under normal conditions is in equilibrium with pyruvate (L:P = 15-25:1). The lactate:pyruvate ratio in urine, plasma, and CSF increases in hypoxaemia, and in inherited disorders of the respiratory chain. Other findings include hypoglycaemia, metabolic acidosis, and abnormal plasma and urinary amino acids. Examples include hereditary lactic acidosis, and pyruvate dehydrogenase deficiency.
- Store frozen plasma, urine, with or without CSF for further diagnostic tests, e.g. urinary amino and organic

acids, plasma amino acids. Definitive diagnosis may require enzyme measurement in cultured skin fibroblasts or DNA analysis (e.g. MCAD deficiency).

Causes of hyperammonaemia

These include:

- Amino acid disorders, e.g. methylmalonic acidaemia, propionic acidaemia.
- Disorders of fatty acid metabolism, e.g. carnitine deficiency and medium chain acyl-CoA dehydrogenase (MCAD) deficiency. Fatty acids are metabolized by beta-oxidation within mitochondria. Carnitine is required for transport of long chain fatty acids into mitochondria. Defects result in hypoglycaemia, abnormal urinary organic acids, and hyperammonaemia.
- Urea cycle defects, e.g. citrullinaemia, and ornithine trancarbamylase (OTC) deficiency. Defects may occur at any step in the metabolism of waste nitrogen to urea. Encephalopathy is associated with respiratory alkalosis and metabolic acidosis, very marked hyperammonaemia, and abnormal urine and plasma amino acids especially glutamine. OTC deficiency is an X-linked recessive condition and raised urinary orotic acid is typical.
- Reye's syndrome.
- Liver failure.
- Proteus urinary tract infection.
- Drugs (e.g. asparaginase, sodium valproate).

Management of acute metabolic encephalopathy

1. Correct hypoglycaemia with dextrose infusion, ensure high energy intake to restrict catabolism, and exclude protein.

2. Treat shock and maintain fluid balance.

3. Sterilize gut with oral antibiotics and laxatives to reduce enterohepatic recirculation of nitrogen.

4. Treat raised intracranial pressure due to cerebral oedema, and control seizures.

5. Specific therapies to remove toxins, e.g. L-arginine enhances the urea cycle, and sodium benzoate or sodium phenylbutyrate improve ammonia excretion. Dialysis is sometimes used to remove toxins and maintain fluid balance.

Outcome

The outcome of acute metabolic encephalopathy is usually poor so it is important to recognize inborn errors of metabolism before this occurs.

Reye's syndrome

Reye's syndrome is an acute encephalopathy associated with fatty degeneration of the liver. Treatment is supportive and the mortality is high. The aetiology is obscure but there is a possible association with aspirin ingestion, varicella and influenza B infections. Aspirin is no longer recommended for children under the age of 12 years except in special circumstances (e.g. juvenile chronic arthritis).

Investigations

- Hyperammonaemia.
- Hypoglycaemia.
- FBC – raised WBC.
- Liver function tests – raised bilirubin, and transaminases (AST, ALT).
- Prolonged PT.

General management of inborn errors of metabolism

1. Nutrition. Reduce dietary intake of enzyme substrate with exclusion diets (e.g. PKU) and replace essential nutrients. Ensure a regular carbohydrate intake in conditions prone to hypoglycaemia, e.g. type I glycogen storage disease may need overnight feeds. Enhance excretion of metabolites, e.g. ammonia. Some conditions are vitamin responsive.

2. Emergency regimens to prevent acute encephalopathy. During intercurrent illness change diet to high carbohydrate intake e.g. soluble glucose polymer drinks, to prevent decompensation and encephalopathy. If vomiting, refusing to drink, or becoming encephalopathic change to i.v. dextrose.

3. Enzyme replacement therapy. Bone marrow and organ transplantation have been used in some conditions (e.g. Hurler's syndrome, some urea cycle defects).

4. Genetic counselling and antenatal diagnosis. One in four recurrence risk if autosomal recessive. Enzyme assays or DNA analysis may be possible on amniotic cells or chorionic villous samples.

5. Multidisciplinary management of associated problems, e.g. developmental delay, cardiac disease.

Further reading

Dixon MA, Leonard JV. Intercurrent illness in inborn errors of intermediary metabolism. *Archives of Disease in Childhood,* 1992; **67:** 1387–91.

Green A, Hall SM. Investigation of metabolic disorders resembling Reye's syndrome. *Archives of Disease in Childhood,* 1992; **67:** 1313–17.

Hardie JRM, Newton LH, Bruce JC, Glasgow JFT, Mowat AP, Stephenson JBP, Hall SM. The changing clinical pattern of Reye's syndrome 1982–90. *Archives of Disease in Childhood,* 1996; **74:** 400–5.
Kelly DA. Organ transplantation for inherited metabolic disease. *Archives of Disease in Childhood,* 1994; **71:** 181–3.
Morris AAM, Leonard JV. Early recognition of metabolic decompensation. *Archives of Disease in Childhood,* 1997; **76:** 555–6.
Touma EH, Charpentier C. Medium chain acyl-CoA dehydrogenase deficiency. *Archives of Disease in Childhood,* 1992; **67:** 142–5.
Wraith JE. Diagnosis and management of inborn errors of metabolism. *Archives of Disease in Childhood,* 1989; **64:** 1410–15.
Wraith JE. The mucopolysaccharidoses: a clinical review and guide to management. *Archives of Disease in Childhood,* 1995; **72:** 263–7.

Related topics of interest

Coma (p. 89)
Developmental delay (p. 115)

INFLAMMATORY BOWEL DISEASE

Inflammatory bowel disease is uncommon in childhood and usually presents in late childhood or adolescence. Crohn's disease is more common than ulcerative colitis (UC) and there is often delay in diagnosis due to the non-specific nature of the initial symptoms (e.g. recurrent abdominal pain, weight loss, growth failure). Simple screening blood tests such as full blood count, albumin and inflammatory markers (CRP, ESR) may help identify those who require further investigation. UC usually presents with bloody diarrhoea or rectal bleeding due to proctosigmoiditis. Infective causes of acute or chronic colitis should be excluded. Colitis does occur in infancy and early childhood but is now thought to be more often due to food allergy (particularly cow's milk intolerance) than true inflammatory bowel disease. Treatment is with dietary exclusion and the intolerance usually resolves with time.

Problems

- Abdominal pain.
- Chronic diarrhoea.
- Growth failure.
- Delayed puberty.
- Anaemia.
- Extraintestinal manifestations, e.g. arthritis, renal disease, ocular complications, hepatobiliary disease, finger clubbing.
- Psychosocial disruption.
- Risk of malignancy.

Aetiology

Many factors have been implicated in the pathogenesis of inflammatory bowel disease but the aetiology remains unclear. A positive family history does seem to be a consistent risk factor. These individuals may have a genetic predisposition which leads to an altered immunological response within the intestinal mucosa. Repeated episodes of infantile gastroenteritis or food allergy have been suggested to increase the risk of later inflammatory bowel disease and breast feeding may have a protective effect. Specific infective agents including *Mycobacterium paratuberculosis* have received interest as possible aetiological agents. Recent research has suggested a link between exposure to the measles virus (*in utero* infection or by immunization) and the later development of Crohn's disease, but this has not been substantiated. Some studies have suggested that stressful life events such as parental death or divorce may be risk factors, but this has not been confirmed by other studies. In adults, UC is more common in non-smokers, whereas Crohn's disease seems to be more common in smokers.

Crohn's disease

Pathology

Crohn's disease can affect any part of the GI tract, the terminal ileum and proximal colon being the most common sites. The disease is patchy with normal bowel found between affected areas. Inflammation is transmural and histologically there are typical non-caseating granulomas. Ulceration and fissuring may give the mucosa a cobblestone appearance. Fibrous stricture formation may occur.

Clinical features

There has been a rapid increase in the incidence of Crohn's disease since the 1950s. The prevalence is now ~10 per 100 000 childhood population per year. Typical features include colicky abdominal pain, intermittent diarrhoea (± blood and mucous), weight loss, oral ulceration, perianal skin tags or fissuring, anaemia, general malaise and fever. However, the early symptoms are often non-specific and the disease may present with growth failure or delayed puberty with few or no gastrointestinal symptoms; the diagnosis should therefore be considered in adolescents who present with apparent anorexia nervosa. Extraintestinal manifestations include arthralgia, arthritis, uveitis, clubbing, erythema nodosum, and liver dysfunction.

Routine blood tests may reveal anaemia, a raised platelet count, hypoalbuminaemia, and raised inflammatory markers (e.g. erythrocyte sedimentation rate, C reactive protein). Diagnosis depends on endoscopy and biopsy. White cell scans offer a non-invasive screening technique (see Further reading) and contrast radiology (barium meal and follow through) may also be useful.

Management

High dose steroids have been the mainstay of treatment for many years to induce remission but they have significant side-effects. Topical preparations (e.g. budesonide or prednisolone enemas) may be used for localized rectal disease. Elemental diets are now thought to be as effective as steroids at inducing remission, and they are given orally or by nasogastric tube. Their mechanism of action is unclear, but they avoid the risks of further growth retardation that are associated with steroids. Aminosalicylates (e.g. sulphasalazine, mesalazine, olsalazine) may be used to induce remission but are more effective in preventing recurrence. Immunosuppressive agents such as azathioprine and cyclosporin are sometimes used in resistant disease and may facilitate a reduction in steroid dose in those with steroid dependent disease. Antibiotics including metronidazole may also be used. Intensive nutritional management is vital to correct growth failure. Surgery may be considered for some children, e.g. for localized disease, failure of medical treatment, obstruction. As with any chronic illness, Crohn's disease may have a significant psychosocial impact on the child and the family.

Prognosis

The disease usually follows a remitting and relapsing course. There is an increased risk of malignancy with long-standing disease affecting the colon.

Ulcerative colitis (UC)

Pathology

There is inflammation of the mucosa of part or all of the large intestine (most commonly the rectum and distal colon). The inflammation is continuous rather than patchy, with the mucosa becoming friable and ulcerated. Typical histological features include inflammatory infiltration and crypt abscesses. Acute dilatation of the colon (toxic megacolon) may precede perforation.

Clinical features

Unlike Crohn's disease, the prevalence of UC has remained relatively static at ~ 6 per 100 000 childhood population per year. The mean age of onset is 10 years. Diarrhoea (± blood and mucous) is the commonest presenting feature and the onset is usually sudden. Other features include lower abdominal pain, weight loss and tenesmus. Extraintestinal manifestations similar to those found in Crohn's disease may occur.

Hypochromic anaemia, hypoproteinaemia and raised inflammatory markers reflect disease activity. After exclusion of infective causes of bloody diarrhoea (e.g. *Salmonella*, *Shigella*, *Campylobacter*, *Yersinia*, *Entamoeba*), diagnosis is confirmed by rectosigmoidoscopy and biopsy. Abdominal X-ray may be useful to look for colonic dilatation. Barium enema may show loss of the normal colonic haustrations but is rarely indicated since the advent of endoscopy.

Management

Treatment options to induce and maintain remission include steroids (oral or topical), aminosalicylates, and immunosuppressive agents. Unlike Crohn's disease, elemental feeds alone do not induce remission, but nutritional management is very important to ensure adequate growth is maintained. Severe, fulminating colitis is a medical emergency requiring intravenous resuscitation, antibiotics, hydrocortisone and parenteral nutrition.

Total colectomy may be considered for some children, e.g. intractable disease, toxic megacolon, colonic haemorrhage or perforation. Restorative proctocolectomy with an ileal reservoir offers an alternative to an ileostomy but complications include excessive stool frequency, faecal incontinence, and pouchitis.

Prognosis

Most will experience at least one relapse after initial treatment and the disease often follows an acute course in childhood. Isolated proctosigmoiditis or distal colitis has the best prognosis, but the risk of extension of disease is higher in children than adults. There is an increased risk of colorectal adenocarcinoma in adult life so regular colonoscopy is recommended.

Further reading

Booth IW. Chronic inflammatory bowel disease. *Archives of Disease in Childhood,* 1991; **66:** 742–4.

Kirschner BS. Ulcerative colitis in children. In: Lebenthal E, ed. *The Pediatric Clinics of North America. Pediatric Gastroenterology I.* Philadelphia: WB Saunders, 1996; **43**(1): 235–54.

Hyams JS. Crohn's disease in children. In: Lebenthal E, ed. *The Pediatric Clinics of North America. Pediatric Gastroenterology I.* Philadelphia: WB Saunders, 1996; **43**(1): 255–77.

Jobling JC, Lindley KJ, Yousef Y, Gordon I, Milla PJ. Investigating inflammatory bowel disease – white cell scanning, radiology, and colonoscopy. *Archives of Disease in Childhood,* 1996; **74:** 22–6.

Walker-Smith JA. Management of growth failure in Crohn's disease. *Archives of Disease in Childhood,* 1996; **75:** 351–4.

Related topics of interest

Abdominal pain – recurrent (p. 4)
Chronic diarrhoea (p. 77)
Gastrointestinal haemorrhage (p. 156)

JAUNDICE

Jaundice is clinically detectable when the serum bilirubin exceeds 85 μmol/l and, in the older infant or child, often indicates serious underlying pathology. Jaundice is said to be conjugated if the conjugated fraction of the total bilirubin is more than 15%. Bilirubin will then be present in the urine, which will be dark, and absent in the stool, which will be pale in colour. Neonatal jaundice is discussed in a separate chapter.

Causes of unconjugated hyperbilirubinaemia

1. Haemolysis. This causes a large bilirubin load which the liver is unable to metabolize fast enough. It may be secondary to:

- Drugs, e.g. Vitamin K.
- Infection, e.g. mycoplasma, haemolytic–uraemic syndrome.
- Congenital red cell membrane defects, e.g. spherocytosis.
- Congenital red cell enzyme defects, e.g. G6PD.

2. Hereditary enzyme deficiencies, e.g. Gilbert's syndrome, Crigler–Najjar syndrome.

Causes of conjugated hyperbilirubinaemia

- Hepatocellular disease, e.g. viral hepatitis, Wilson's disease, α_1-antitrypsin deficiency.
- Extrahepatic biliary obstruction, e.g. gallstones, biliary atresia.
- Intrahepatic biliary hypoplasia, e.g. Alagille syndrome.
- Enzyme deficiencies, e.g. Rotor, Dubin–Johnson.
- Systemic disease, e.g. bacterial sepsis, right heart failure.

Clinical assessment

The history should always elicit whether there is a family history of liver disease, jaundice or consanguinity and race should be noted. There may be a recent history of anaesthetic, contact with infectious disease, blood transfusion or foreign travel. Jaundice can be seen in the conjunctivae and the skin. Further examination may reveal pyrexia, hepatic tenderness or enlargement, splenomegaly or stigmata of chronic liver disease. Stool and urine should always be inspected personally by the doctor.

Investigation

- FBC, reticulocyte count, film and Coomb's test.
- Coagulation screen.
- Liver function tests including total and conjugated bilirubin, albumin, globulin and liver enzymes.
- Blood culture; viral serology.
- Urine for presence of bile; viral and bacterial culture.

- Abdominal ultrasound to assess liver size and texture, portal and hepatic venous flow, presence of biliary obstruction, ascites. Other imaging with CT and MRI, isotope scans and, rarely, ERCP may be appropriate.
- Other tests as appropriate clinically, e.g. serum copper and caeruloplasmin, α_1-antitrypsin phenotype.

Viral hepatitis

The commonest cause of viral hepatitis in the UK is hepatitis A. Hepatitis B has a high prevalence in South-East Asia and Africa. Hepatitis A and E are spread by the faeco-oral route and B, C and G are blood-borne. Other causes include Epstein–Barr virus, herpes virus, CMV and adenovirus.

Hepatitis A

Hepatitis A is an RNA virus spread by the faecal-oral route, particularly in situations of poor sanitation. The incubation period is 15–40 days and jaundice may be preceded by nausea, vomiting, pyrexia, diarrhoea and abdominal pain. It may be asymptomatic in children. Prevalence of immunity in the population is around 40%. Diagnosis is confirmed by detection of IgM antibodies to hepatitis A. Complications are a prolonged cholestatic phase, fulminant hepatic failure and, rarely, bone marrow aplasia. There is no chronic carrier state. There is no specific treatment – antiemetics should be avoided because of impaired hepatic metabolism and severe vomiting may be a warning sign of fulminant hepatic failure. Protection can be provided by vaccination.

Hepatitis B

This DNA virus may be spread perinatally from a mother who is acutely infected or who is carrying 'e' antigen for hepatitis B. In this situation there is an 86% risk of perinatal transmission. This may not cause acute infection in the neonate but the risk of chronic carriage is high. It may also be transmitted via infected blood products, intravenous drug abuse or occasionally via saliva from a human bite. The incubation period is 3–6 months. Infection may cause acute hepatitis, fulminant hepatic failure or asymptomatic chronic carriage. Other features include papular dermatitis (Gianotti–Crosti syndrome) chronic or persistent hepatitis, and an increased risk of cirrhosis and hepatocellular carcinoma with chronic carriage. Diagnosis depends on appearance of surface antigen 3–6 weeks after infection. There is a high recurrence rate in transplanted livers but this may nevertheless be indicated in fulminant hepatic failure. Babies whose mothers are infected should be given immunoglobulin as soon after birth as possible and a course of vaccination commenced. Although routine immunization is given in many countries, the UK only vaccinates high risk infants at present.

Hepatitis C

This is an RNA virus which is transmitted parenterally. It accounts for 95% of post transfusion hepatitis in those given blood products before screening was introduced in 1990. Most cases in adults in the UK are due to intravenous drug use. Infection may be asymptomatic, or after an incubation period of 7–8 weeks may cause an acute hepatitis, with chronicity in about 40% of cases, although the data on children are limited. The time course of the disease is very variable. There is a long-term risk of cirrhosis and a risk of hepatocellular carcinoma. The perinatal transmission risk from an infected mother is 5–10% rising to 40% if the mother has concommitent HIV infection. The virus is very diverse genetically and there are high mutation rates. It is therefore difficult to develop a vaccine. Alpha-interferon may help eliminate persistent viraemia and prevent disease progression. Treatment with ribavirin is also the subject of current interest. Recurrence rate in transplanted livers is approaching 100%.

Hepatitis D

This is a defective virus which can only infect in the presence of concurrent hepatitis B infection. It causes the severest liver damage of all the hepatitis viruses.

Hepatitis E

This is similar to hepatitis A in that it is spread by the faecal-oral route and causes a similar clinical picture but more severe. Chronic carriage has not been described. Incubation period is 15–60 days. It has a high mortality rate amongst pregnant women.

Inherited conditions

Gilbert's syndrome

Impaired activity of uridine diphosphate glucuronyl transferase (UDPGT) causes reduced bilirubin clearance. Prevalence is 6% and inheritance is autosomal dominant with variable expression. A mild hyperbilirubinaemia, <70 μmol/l may present after puberty with intercurrent illness or the raised bilirubin may be discovered coincidentally on biochemical testing. There are no other abnormal findings and the condition is entirely benign.

Crigler–Najjar syndrome

This rare condition is caused by a reduced amount or absence of UDPGT. Severe unconjugated bilirubinaemia develops in infancy and may lead to kernicterus. Type I is the more severe and is autosomal recessive. Prolonged phototherapy may be required to control the bilirubin levels. Liver transplantation should be considered. Type II is autosomal dominant with incomplete penetrance, and treatment with phenobarbitone produces a fall in bilirubin.

Alagille syndrome

This syndrome of arteriohepatic dysplasia is autosomal dominant with variable penetrance. As well as intrahepatic duct paucity which leads to cholestatic jaundice and occasionally cirrhosis, affected individuals have unusual facies (broad forehead, widely spaced eyes, pointed chin). Other features which may be present include ocular abnormalities (posterior embryotoxon), vertebral arch defects ('butterfly' vertebrae), peripheral pulmonary stenosis and tubulointerstitial nephropathy.

Wilson's disease

Wilson's disease is caused by defective copper handling by liver cells which accumulates and causes damage to liver, brain and kidney. Liver disease rarely manifests before the age of 5 years and may present as asymptomatic hepatomegaly, subacute or chronic hepatitis or fulminant liver failure. Older children may present first with the neurological and psychiatric symptoms (tremor, dysarthria, behavioural change). Other complications include Fanconi's syndrome with progressive renal failure, Kayser–Fleischer rings, and haemolysis. Sufferers will have low levels of serum copper and caeruloplasmin. Treatment is by decreasing oral copper intake and chelation with penicillamine.

Further reading

Balistreri WF. Metabolic diseases of the liver. In: Behrman RE, Kliegman RM, Arvin A, eds. *Nelson Textbook of Paediatrics*, 15th edn. 1996; 1138–41.

Gregorio GV, Mieli-Vergani G. Hepatitis B infection. *Current Paediatrics*, 1995; **5** (1): 24–7.

Gregorio GV, Mieli-Vergani G, Mowat AP. Viral hepatitis. *Archives of Disease in Childhood*, 1994; **70:** 343–8.

Kelly DA. Hepatitis C infection after blood product transfusion. *Archives of Disease in Childhood*, 1996; **75** (5): 363–5.

Related topics of interest

Liver disease (p. 244)
Neonatal jaundice (p. 276)

JUVENILE CHRONIC ARTHRITIS

Juvenile chronic arthritis (JCA) is relatively uncommon, affecting 1 in 5000 children, but it is an important cause of chronic handicap. Over recent years there has been increasing debate about classification, and in many children the clinical picture changes as the disease progresses. Classification is important however, as it enables the family to be given clearer information about possible complications and prognosis.

Problems

- Joint destruction and deformity, particularly polyarticular JCA.
- Uveitis, particularly ANA-positive pauciarticular JCA.
- Amyloidosis.
- Side-effects of treatment, e.g. steroids, hydroxychloroquine (retinopathy), D-penicillamine (blood dyscrasias, proteinuria).
- Family and social disruption.

Differential diagnosis

- Infection. Septic arthritis (bacterial, tuberculous, viral) or reactive arthritis (rubella, Lyme disease).
- Henoch–Schonlein purpura. Acute joint pain and swelling with characteristic purpuric rash, nephritis and gastrointestinal involvement.
- Gastrointestinal disorders. A seronegative type arthritis may occur in pateints with Crohn's, ulcerative colitis, shigella dysentery and *Yersinia* infection.
- Haematological. Haemophilia may lead to haemarthroses which if recurrent may cause permanent joint damage.
- Rheumatic fever.
- Trauma. Accidental, non-accidental.
- Connective tissue disease. Systemic lupus erythematosus, dermatomyositis.

Clinical features

JCA causes pain, swelling and stiffness of one or more joints. Diagnosis depends on three criteria:

- Onset under 16 years.
- Arthritis of one or more joints for a minimum of 3 months.
- Exclusion of other diseases.

Current classification divides JCA into six main groups which have different natural histories:

1. Early onset pauciarticular (50%) involves four joints or less. The usual age of onset is 1–5 years and it is more common in girls. There are usually no systemic symptoms. If the onset is monoarticular, the knee is most frequently affected. The cervical spine, jaw, and the small joints of the hands and feet are rarely affected. Joint disease is rarely progressive and usually resolves by the age of 16 years. Chronic iridocyclitis (uveitis) is a major problem and ophthalmic review is essential (increased risk if ANA positive).

Investigations: positive antinuclear antibody (70%), negative rheumatoid factor (RhF), association with HLA DRw5/8.

2. *Late onset pauciarticular arthritis* is a group of conditions also known as the spondyloarthropathies. They affect mostly boys over 9 years who are often HLA B27 positive. Sacroiliitis may occur although often late in the disease and there is a high incidence of enthesopathies (inflammation of the junction between tendon or fascia and bone) at the heel, feet and knees. There may be a family history of sero-negative arthritis. Acute uveitis occurs in around 10%. Juvenile ankylosing spondylitis (associated with anterior uveitis, HLA B27) follows a similar course to that in adults. SEA (seronegative enthesopathy and arthropathy) syndrome is thought by some to be the commonest sub-group of spondyloarthropathy. Others in this group include arthritis associated with inflammatory bowel disease and Reiter's syndrome.

Investigations: ANA and RhF negative.

3. *Psoriatic arthropathy* may occur before the onset of the rash but the typical nail-pitting and a family history of psoriasis is often the clue to diagnosis. It is often classified with the spondyloarthropathies but is different in that sufferers are more likely to be girls and there is asymmetrical small joint involvement and dactylitis.

4. *Systemic onset (Still's disease).* Arthritis may be delayed for weeks or even months, and the major features at the onset are systemic (intermittent high fever, splenomegaly, rash, lymphadenopathy). Onset is usually under 5 years of age and it is equally common in boys and girls. It may take many weeks to make the correct diagnosis, which depends on clinical features and exclusion of infection (viral, bacterial, mycoplasma) and neoplastic disorders (leukaemia, neuroblastoma). Pericarditis is relatively common, and

hepatitis and myocarditis are less common complications. The arthritis is characteristically relapsing and remitting. Amyloidosis may develop usually presenting with proteinuria.

Investigations: ANA and RhF negative, raised ESR, raised WBC, raised platelets, anaemia.

5. Polyarticular RhF negative. Five or more joints are involved, commonly the knees, ankles, small joints of the hands and feet, the jaw, and cervical spine. Joint swelling and stiffness may be painful or relatively pain-free. Onset can occur at any time from 1–15 years. Joint involvement usually follows a chronic, progressive course. Involvement of the temporomandibular joints can produce micrognathia. Systemic features are minimal but there may be a low grade fever, weight loss, and anaemia. Uveitis is rarely a feature.

Investigations: ANA usually negative, RhF negative.

6. Polyarticular RhF positive. This is similar to adult rheumatoid arthritis. It accounts for the smallest proportion (about 5%) of all JCA. It is more common in girls and tends to affect children over 8 years. Arthritis tends to follow a progressive and severe course and so second line drugs often need to be started early. Symmetrical involvement of small and large joints is seen. Rheumatoid nodules may develop. Uveitis does not occur.

Management

Effective management depends on a multidisciplinary approach (paediatrician, rheumatologist, GP, orthopaedic surgeon, ophthalmologist, physiotherapist, occupational therapist, social worker, school). Treatment is supportive, to relieve symptoms and maintain function, but is not curative.

1. Analgesics, e.g. NSAIDs, may control the inflammation but do not influence the outcome of the disease.

2. Corticosteroids are indicated in acute systemic involvement, severe joint disease refractory to other drugs, and uveitis. Intra-articular steroid injections may be useful for large joints. They do not alter the long term outcome of the disease.

3. Disease-modifying agents, e.g. hydroxychloroquine, D-penicillamine, methotrexate. Used in progressive polyarticular JCA. Sulphasalazine is used in the spondyloarthropathies.

4. *Physiotherapy and splinting,* to maintain function and prevent contractures. Splints may be either for rest (night splints) or for activities (working splints). They may relieve pain in an acutely inflamed joint. Gait retraining, serial casting and orthotics may also be required.

5. *Surgery,* e.g. soft tissue release, joint replacement.

Further reading

Fink CW, Fernandez-Vina M, Stastny P. Clinical and genetic evidence that juvenile arthritis is not a single disease. *Pediatric Clinics of North America*, 1995; **42** (5): 1155–67.

Malleson PN. Management of childhood arthritis. Part 2: chronic arthritis. *Archives of Disease in Childhood*, 1997; **76:** 541–4.

Murray K, Thompson SD, Glass DN. Pathogenesis of juvenile chronic arthritis: genetic and environmental factors. *Archives of Disease in Childhood*, 1997; **77:** 530–4.

Related topics of interest

Limping (p. 239)
Purpura and bruising (p. 330)

KAWASAKI DISEASE

Kawasaki disease (mucocutaneous lymph node syndrome) is a systemic vasculitis of early childhood, with a prevalence of 3.4 per 100 000 children under 5 years in the British Isles. Oriental races are more at risk than Caucasian (80 000 reported cases in Japan), and although epidemiological studies are highly suggestive of an infective aetiology no definite pathogen has yet been established. Sudden death from coronary complications occurs in at least 2% of cases, and although specific therapy with aspirin and intravenous immunoglobulin may reduce coronary artery abnormalities, treatment must be given during the initial 10 days of the illness to be of benefit. Prompt diagnosis is therefore essential.

Epidemiology

- Eighty per cent of patients are under 4 years old.
- Spring and summer outbreaks occur in the UK, winter and spring outbreaks in Japan.
- Incidence peaks every 3 years.
- Male:female ratio 1.5:1.
- No genetic links, but racial predisposition (Orientals).

Pathogenesis

There is a vasculitis of small and medium-sized arteries throughout the body. Damaged vessels may develop aneurysms and thrombosis, and may heal with fibrosis and calcification, initiating premature atherosclerosis. The mechanism of endothelial injury is unclear but may be an abnormal reaction to a common infective agent.

Clinical features

Diagnosis is established by the presence of characteristic clinical criteria and the exclusion of conditions which may mimic Kawasaki disease. There is no single or specific diagnostic test. The criteria are:

(a) Fever for 5 or more days; plus
(b) Presence of four of the following five conditions:

- Bilateral conjunctival injection.
- Change in the mucous membranes of the upper respiratory tract, e.g. injected pharynx, dry, cracked lips or strawberry tongue.
- Change in the peripheral extremities, e.g. oedema, erythema or desquamation.
- Polymorphous rash.
- Cervical lymphadenopathy; and

(c) Exclusion of staphylococcal and streptococcal infection, measles, drug reaction, juvenile rheumatoid arthritis, etc.

In the presence of coronary artery aneurysms, fever plus three of the five criteria in (b) is sufficient for diagnosis.

Fever is usually high, spiking and prolonged, lasting for 1–2 weeks before subsiding or persisting as a low-grade fever for a further 2–3 weeks. The characteristic desquamation of the fingers and toes is not seen until 10–20 days after the onset of the fever. The rash may be extremely variable, with urticarial, maculopapular or multiforme-type lesions of various distributions around the body. Perineal desquamation may also be seen.

Other features may be seen, such as irritability, arthritis, aseptic meningitis, hepatitis and hydropic gall bladder.

Cardiovascular complications occur in 20–30% of patients. Myocarditis, pericarditis, arrhythmias and cardiac failure may occur in the first 10 days of the illness. Arteritis of the coronary vessels may lead to aneurysm formation, with a peak frequency 4 weeks after the onset of symptoms. Sudden death may occur from massive myocardial infarction or haemopericardium after aneurysmal rupture between 2 and 12 weeks after the disease onset.

Investigations

- FBC. Normochromic normocytic anaemia and polymorphonuclear leucocytosis are common in the first week. The platelet count is often normal in the first week, but rises to very high peaks of 800 up to 2 000 x 10^9 by the third week.
- Acute-phase proteins. Raised ESR, CRP.
- Microbiology. Exclude other possible causes, e.g. by throat swab, blood cultures and viral titres.
- ECG.
- Chest radiograph.
- Echocardiogram. Full assessment should be performed by an experienced paediatric cardiologist in order to detect coronary aneurysms.

Treatment

Once the diagnosis is established, treatment should commence without delay.

High-dose intravenous immunoglobulin should be given at a dose of 2 g/kg over 12–18 hours. High fluid volumes may be needed, and careful monitoring is essential if there is already evidence of cardiac involvement. Doses of 400 mg/kg/day for 4–5 days appear to be less effective.

High-dose aspirin (30 mg/kg/day) should commence immediately, and be continued until the fever has resolved. A lower dose (3–5 mg/kg/day) should then continue.

If the initial cardiac echo was abnormal, repeated assessments should be made at weekly intervals, with the addition of dipyridamole or prostacyclin if there are coronary aneurysms. If initial cardiac echo was normal, repeat assessment may be made at 6 weeks, as late aneurysm formation may still occur. If coronary artery abnormalities do occur, long-term follow-up with continuing low-dose aspirin therapy is advised.

Further reading

Dhillon R, Newton L, Rudd PT. Management of Kawasaki disease in the British Isles. *Archives of Disease in Childhood,* 1993; **69:** 631–8.

Levin M, Tizard EJ, Dillon MJ. Kawasaki disease: recent advances. *Archives of Disease in Childhood,* 1991; **66:** 1369–72.

Nadel S, Levin M. Kawasaki disease. In: David TJ, ed. *Recent Advances in Paediatrics,* Vol. 11. Edinburgh: Churchill Livingstone, 1993; 103–6.

Related topic of interest

Pyrexia of unknown origin (p. 334)

LEARNING DISABILITY

Definition

There is wide variation in the terminology used to describe children with limited intellectual capacity, for example mental handicap, mental retardation, educational subnormality. *Learning disability* is the most acceptable term currently used in the UK.

This 'umbrella' term covers a wide range of problems, of variable aetiologies, which may present at different ages. For simplification, learning disability can be divided into:

1. General learning disability which is an overall reduction in intellectual capacity. IQ measurement can be used to distinguish between mild learning disability (MLD) IQ 50–70 and severe learning disability (SLD) IQ < 50.

2. Specific learning difficulty which is a deficit in one or more abilities, e.g. Dyslexia or emotional/behavioural difficulties.

It is estimated that up to 20% of all children may at some time require extra help in school.

Severe learning disability (IQ < 50)

The prevalence of SLD in the UK is approximately 3.7 per 1000 children. For these children underlying brain pathology can often be identified from clinical history or examination. SLD may result from intra-uterine, perinatal or postnatal events, e.g. congenital infection, birth asphyxia or meningitis. Chromosomal abnormalities, e.g. Down's or fragile X syndrome, account for approximately 20–25% of cases. A small number of children have a progressive degenerative or metabolic condition. As underlying organic pathology is more likely in SLD these children may have associated physical impairments. Children with severe learning difficulties generally have limited success in academic tasks and as adults are unlikely to lead independent lives.

Mild learning disability (IQ 50–70)

Exact figures for the prevalence of MLD are difficult to achieve as not all these children require extra educational support at school. MLD can result from certain clinical syndromes and disorders and an organic cause should always be considered. However in comparison to SLD, a biological cause is rarely found in children in this IQ range. MLD is more commonly due to a combination of environmental and genetic factors and is more frequently identified in lower socio-economic groups. Children with MLD have general difficulty with academic skills and when they leave school often succeed in more practical professions.

Learning disability may be recognized at any age depending on the severity of the disability; the nature of the underlying cause and at what stage parents or professionals identify concerns with the child's development. Early recognition i.e. pre-school, is useful for liaison with educational services in order for provision to be made prior to school entry.

'Special Educational Needs' – Statementing

Children with a learning disability have special educational needs (SEN). The Education Act 1993 recognizes the importance of identifying these children and emphasizes that all children with SEN require the greatest possible access to a broad balanced education concentrating on strengths rather than deficits. The current aim is for children with SEN to be educated in mainstream school, alongside their peer group, where reasonably practical, taking into account the child and parents' wishes.

Some children will qualify for a statutory assessment leading to a 'Statement of Special Educational Needs'. This allows resources to be specifically directed towards the individual needs of that child. This is a multidisciplinary process in which all professionals involved with that child (paediatrician, therapists, educational psychologist, teacher) make their assessment of that child's areas of strengths and weaknesses and put forward their proposed recommendations for education.

Specific learning disability (dyslexia)

A significant number of children have unexplained difficulties with one or more of the basic learning skills, reading, writing, spelling or arithmetic. One term used for these children is dyslexia. A wide spectrum in the degree of difficulty is recognized.

- Aetiology. Despite extensive research no specific cause has been identified. Likely to be multifactorial.
- Epidemiology. More common in boys than girls, the disorder effects approximately 2–5 % of school children. A family history is common.

The main problems arise from poor visual perception and poor visual-spatial memory, leading to difficulty sequencing left to right; reversal or inversion of letters; mirror writing; difficulties with tables, days of the week and the alphabet. Associated problems include spatial difficulties leading to clumsiness (dyspraxia); a short attention span and emotional difficulties.

Management

When a specific learning difficulty is suspected an assessment will be made by the educational psychologist. Reassurance for parents can bring an immense sense of relief from long-held concerns.

Further reading

Hall DMB, Hill P. *The Child with a Disability*, 2nd edn. Oxford: Blackwell Science, 1996.
Polnay L, Hull D. *Community Paediatrics*, 2nd edn. Edinburgh: Churchill Livingstone, 1993.

Related topics of interest

Chromosomal abnormalities (p. 73)
Developmental assessment (p. 111)
Developmental delay (p. 115)
Disability (p. 124)

LIMPING

Limping or refusal to weight bear usually results from lower limb pain which may arise from a soft tissue, muscle, bone, or joint problem. Joint disorders may be localized to a single joint (monoarthritis) or involve several joints (polyarthritis). All joints should be examined for evidence of pain, swelling, or limitation of movement, and it should be remembered that hip pain is frequently referred to the knee. Limping without pain is less common, e.g. undiagnosed congenital hip dislocation.

Aetiology of a limp

- Soft tissue. Trauma, ingrowing toenail, nail in shoe, inguinal lymphadenitis.
- Muscle. Trauma, myalgia secondary to infection (e.g. viral), muscular dystrophy, early poliomyelitis, cramp.
- Bone. Trauma (accidental, non-accidental), osteomyelitis, tumour (leukaemia, osteosarcoma, neuroblastoma), rickets.
- Joint. Trauma, septic arthritis, haemarthrosis, juvenile chronic arthritis (JCA), tuberculous arthritis, irritable hip, Perthes' disease, slipped femoral epiphysis, Osgood–Schlatter disease, Henoch–Schönlein purpura, rheumatic fever, reactive arthritis (secondary to viral infection), intra-articular fracture, gut arthropathy (ulcerative colitis, Crohn's disease), Lyme disease.

Clinical features

There may be a history of trauma but children frequently sustain bumps and falls which are often insignificant. Although an irritable hip is the most common cause of hip pain or limp in young children, it is vital to exclude septic arthritis and osteomyelitis. Localized bone swelling, tenderness, or heat suggest either osteomyelitis or a fracture. Ankle, knee, and hip joints should be examined for swelling, pain, redness and limitation of movement. In the older child, Perthe's disease and slipped upper femoral epiphysis should be considered. Pain may also be referred to the legs from the abdomen (e.g. psoas spasm in appendicitis) or from the spine. Enlarged inguinal lymph nodes secondary to soft tissue inflammation can cause a child to limp. Evidence of associated conditions may be present, e.g. rash and haematuria in Henoch–Schönlein purpura, or gastrointestinal symptoms in gut arthropathy. Examination of a child with a limp should also include examination of the shoes (protruding nail, excessively tight).

Irritable hip (transient synovitis)

This is the commonest cause of hip pain and limping in childhood. The aetiology is unclear but it may follow a mild upper respiratory tract infection. Peak age is 2–10 years and it is more common in boys. An otherwise well child presents with sudden onset of a limp and pain in one hip or knee. Movements of the hip joint are limited but there is no swelling. Investigations including FBC, ESR, and radiology are usually normal. The condition resolves in 7–10 days and treatment consists of simple analgesia, and bed rest, with traction in some cases. A small proportion (<5%) subsequently develop features of Perthes' disease.

Osteomyelitis

Acute osteomyelitis can occur at any age. Infection is spread either haematogenously from a distant focus or directly from a penetrating injury. Long bone metaphyses are most commonly affected but any bone can be involved. It is particularly severe in the neonatal period when it is frequently multifocal. Chronic osteomyelitis occurs if the acute infection is inadequately treated, or if the organism is of low virulence.

The causative organism is most commonly *Staphylococcus aureus* (> 70%). Other organisms include *Streptococcus*, *Haemophilus influenzae*, enteric and gram negative organisms. In neonates, Group B haemolytic streptococcus and coliforms are important causes. *Candida albicans* can cause disease in the immunosuppressed and those on intravenous feeding. Children with sickle cell disease are susceptible to *Salmonella* osteomyelitis. Chronic osteomyelitis may be caused by *Mycobacterium tuberculosis* and other rare organisms such as actinomycosis.

Clinical features

Onset of acute osteomyelitis is usually sudden. The distant focus from which infecton has spread may be obvious (e.g. umbilical cord or skin sepsis) but it is frequently clinically inapparent. The child rapidly becomes toxic, febrile, and unwell, and is reluctant to move. Vomiting and headache are often prominent features in older children, and neonates may present with circulatory collapse. The affected limb is swollen, red, and painful, and the adjacent joint may contain a sympathetic effusion. Spread of infection into the joint occurs in the neonatal period as vascular connections still exist, but in older children spread is normally prevented by the epiphyseal growth plate. Chronic osteomyelitis usually presents with a grumbling fever associated with bone pain and/or swelling, which must be distinguished from neoplastic conditions.

Differential diagnosis of bone pain

1. Swelling

- Osteomyelitis (acute/chronic).
- Fracture.
- Infantile cortical hyperostosis (Caffey's disease).
- Advanced osteosarcoma.

2. *No swelling*

- Osteomyelitis.
- Benign tumour: osteoid osteoma.
- Malignancy: osteosarcoma, Ewing's sarcoma, neuroblastoma, leukaemia.

Investigations

- FBC – neutrophilia.
- Blood cultures – positive in more than 50% of cases.
- ESR – raised.
- Radiology – no bony changes are seen on X-ray for 5–10 days although there may be some soft tissue swelling. Spotty rarefaction and subperiosteal new bone formation are the first radiological changes.
- Isotope bone scan – a technetium scan may detect an area of osteomyelitis before radiological changes are seen.

Management

1. *Antibiotics* should be started early and should be given in high dose intravenously for at least the first week. They should include anti-staphylococcal cover combined with another antibiotic to cover the main non-staphylococcal infections. Oral antibiotics are then given to complete a 6 week course. Chronic osteomyelitis is treated with a prolonged course of antibiotics (6–12 months).

2. *Surgical drainage* is required if pus collects in the medullary cavity, subperiosteally, or subcutaneously.

3. *Pain relief.* Pain may be very severe and treatment includes analgesics, splinting of the limb, and release of pus that is under tension.

4. *General supportive measures* include rehydration and treatment of anaemia.

5. *Physiotherapy* is employed after the acute phase to prevent contractures and strengthen muscles.

Complications

These include pathological fracture, limb shortening and chronic infection with discharging sinuses. Vertebral osteomyelitis may lead to paravertebral abscess, vertebral collapse and pyogenic meningitis.

Septic arthritis

Occuring mainly in children under 5 years, septic arthrits most commonly affects the large joints. It is caused by similar organisms to those causing osteomyelitis and clinical features are also similar. The affected joint is held in the position of maximum relaxation and is swollen, hot, red, and painful.

Investigations

- FBC and ESR.
- Blood cultures.
- Aspiration of the joint – microscopy, gram stain, and culture.
- Radiology – there may be widening of the joint space. Adjacent osteomyelitis is particularly common in neonates as the primary site of infection is usually bone.

Management

Management is similar to osteomyelitis, with antibiotics given for a minimum of 3 weeks.

Rheumatic fever

Rheumatic fever develops as an abnormal immunological reaction to a β-haemolytic streptococcal throat infection. It usually affects school-age children, with symptoms developing 2–3 weeks after a throat infection. The revised Jones criteria require two major features, or one major and two minor features plus evidence of streptococcal infection, to make the diagnosis.

1. *Major features.* Carditis, migratory polyarthritis, chorea, erythema marginatum, subcutaneous nodules.

2. *Minor features.* Previous rheumatic fever, arthralgia, fever, raised ESR or CRP, leucocytosis, prolonged PR interval on ECG.

3. *Evidence of streptococcal infection.* Raised ASO titre, positive throat swab culture.

Carditis may present with a pericardial rub or effusion (pericarditis), arrthymias or heart failure (myocarditis), or a heart murmur (endocarditis). Up to 50% will have long-term cardiovascular disease (e.g. valvular damage).

Treatment is with bed rest, anti-inflammatory drugs (NSAIDs), and penicillin. Rheumatic fever can recur and prophylactic penicillin should be given until well into adult life.

Perthes' disease

Commoner in boys and with a peak age of 5–10 years, Perthes' disease is a segmental avascular necrosis of the femoral head. Aetiology is unknown. It presents with a limp and limitation of hip abduction with or without pain. The majority are unilateral. Treatment involves ensuring the femoral head is maintained in the acetabulum whilst healing occurs.

Slipped femoral epiphysis

This condition is commoner in boys and is associated with obesity, tall stature and gonadal immaturity. Peak age is 10 to 15 years and 20% are bilateral. Presentation will depend on the degree of slippage but is usually with pain in the hip, thigh, or knee with the leg held in external rotation. X-rays show slippage of the capital epiphysis downwards and backwards. A complication is avascular necrosis due to interruption of the blood supply. Treatment is by pinning but if the slip is severe, osteotomy may be required. The other hip must be watched carefully.

Further reading

Jenkins EA, Hall MA. The limping child. *Current Paediatrics*, 1992; **2:** 223–5.
Nade S. Bone and joint infection in childhood. *Current Paediatrics*, 1996; **6:** 9–15.

Related topics of interest

Bleeding disorders (p. 53)
Juvenile chronic arthritis (p. 229)
Orthopaedic problems in childhood (p. 308)
Purpura and bruising (p. 330)

LIVER DISEASE

Acute liver failure

Acute liver failure may be the first presentation of liver impairment or may occur in a child who is known to have underlying liver disease. The term fulminant hepatic failure is used when the patient has acute liver failure without pre-existing liver disease. It occurs, by definition in association with hepatic encephalopathy. The most common cause is viral hepatitis. There is a particularly high risk with concommitent hepatitis B and D infections. Other causes include toxins such as paracetamol poisoning. There is a high mortality of 65–90%, depending on the degree of encephalopathy.

Problems

- Coagulopathy.
- Hypoglycaemia.
- Cerebral oedema.
- Hypoxia.
- Renal failure.
- Metabolic/acid–base disturbance.
- Sepsis.

Causes

1. Infective. Viral hepatitis (see related topic, Jaundice, p. 225).

2. Drugs and toxins, e.g. paracetamol, halothane, sodium valproate, *Amanita phalloides* (death cap mushroom).

3. Metabolic. Tyrosinaemia, galactosaemia, Wilson's disease, Reye's syndrome.

4. Ischaemic. Budd–Chiari syndrome, post shock or cardiac surgery.

Clinical features

Anorexia, nausea and vomiting are accompanied by behavioural change. There may be a history of hepatitis or of metabolic disease. There may be signs of chronic liver disease. Encephalopathy produces restlessness, aggression and confusion and there may be tachypnoea with deep respirations. Asterixis is a late feature, as are stupor and coma. The degree of coma can be graded 1–4 depending on conscious level, neurological signs and EEG changes.

Investigation

- Liver function tests, ammonia.
- FBC, crossmatch.

- Coagulation screen.
- U&E, glucose, acid-base, calcium, phosphate and magnesium.
- Liver ultrasound.
- Viral serology.
- Blood culture.
- Urine and serum for toxicology.
- Other tests for specific disease, e.g. α_1-antitrypsin, copper and caeruloplasmin.

Management

Management is supportive while waiting for spontaneous recovery of the liver or transplantation. Specialized intensive care is needed. Sedative drugs should be avoided, as they mask encephalopathy, and protein feeds should be stopped. Neomycin and lactulose are give to sterilize the gut and reduce enterohepatic absorption. Coma depth should be monitored. Coagulopathy should be treated with intravenous vitamin K and fresh frozen plasma, in conjunction with H_2 blockers to reduce bleeding from gastric erosions. Cardiorespiratory stability, normoglycaemia and acid–base balance are important, as is preventing raised intracranial pressure.

Chronic liver disease

The hepatocyte has a remarkable ability to regenerate following injury. However, after an acute hepatitis, inflammation may be ongoing (chronic persistent and chronic active hepatitis). Chronic liver damage may also develop insidiously (e.g. metabolic, autoimmune or neoplastic disease, cystic fibrosis) with little or no symptoms initially. The growth of excessive fibrous tissue during healing causes the pathological process known as cirrhosis. Chronic liver failure and cirrhosis may lead to portal hypertension and eventual death.

Problems

- Anorexia and poor nutrition.
- Ascites.
- Altered drug metabolism.
- Bleeding due to decreased clotting factors and thrombocytopenia.
- Renal dysfunction including the hepatorenal syndrome.
- Pruritus secondary to cholestasis.
- Portal hypertension.
- Encephalopathy.
- Acute decompensation. May be provoked by infection or bleeding.

Clinical features

Chronic liver disease may manifest itself in the skin with jaundice, spider naevi and palmar erythema. There may be hepatomegaly although in children with cirrhosis the liver may shrink in size. Splenomegaly may be present with portal hypertension. Ascites may cause the child local discomfort as well as a poor appetite which exacerbates the nutritional problems. In severe disease, the child may have flapping tremor of the hands (asterixis) and signs of neurological impairment due to encephalopathy. Vitamin E deficiency due to chronic cholestasis may also present with neurological problems.

Management

Management consists of monitoring and treating complications. This is best done in conjunction with a specialist liver unit. As with any chronic disease, the social and psychological effects on the child and family must always be considered when drawing up the plan of management. The definitive management in many cases is liver transplantation.

1. Nutrition. It is important that the child maintains an adequate calorie intake and is monitored for hypoglycaemia. Some children may require special diets. Vitamin supplementation is important particularly for fat soluble vitamins. Growth must be monitored.

2. Ascites. Treatment is with diuretics and paracentesis to ease discomfort.

3. Drug metabolism. Drugs which are metabolized by the liver may need to be given in reduced doses or avoided altogether.

4. Cholestasis. Ursodeoxycholic acid may be helpful to maximize bile excretion. Pruritus may be alleviated by cholestyramine.

5. Monitoring. Regular monitoring of liver enzymes, bilirubin, clotting (in particular INR) and platelet count are all necessary to look for signs of disease progression.

Portal hypertension

The normal pressure in the portal venous system is around 7 mmHg and portal hypertension occurs at pressures exceeding about 10 mmHg. Causes may be due to prehepatic, intrahepatic or post hepatic obstruction to blood flow.

Causes

1. Prehepatic. due either to portal vein occlusion or increased blood flow.

(a) Neonates: congenital occlusion of portal vein, occlusion due to umbilical sepsis, or as a complication of umbilical artery catheters.

(b) Older children: intra-abdominal sepsis, inflammatory bowel disease, hypercoagulability states.

2. Hepatic. Cirrhosis of any cause, e.g. cystic fibrosis, congenital hepatic fibrosis.

3. Post-hepatic. Budd–Chiari syndrome (hepatic vein occlusion), constrictive pericarditis, congestive heart failure.

Problems

- Gastrointestinal haemorrhage.
- Hypersplenism, thrombocytopenia.
- Ascites.
- Encephalopathy.
- Septicaemia.

Clinical features

Portal hypertension frequently presents with upper gastrointestinal bleeding from oesophageal varices or from gastritis. There may be stigmata of chronic liver disease. There may also be signs of the underlying disease, e.g. Wilson's disease or constrictive pericarditis.

Investigations

Baseline investigations are as for acute hepatic failure. In addition other investigations may be indicated:

- CXR and echocardiography to exclude constrictive pericarditis.
- Endoscopy to look for site of GI bleeding.
- Liver biopsy.

Management

Management of variceal haemorrhage is described under related topic, Gastrointestinal haemorrhage (p. 156). Treatment options for the portal hypertension include portosystemic shunt surgery or liver transplantation.

Liver transplantation

Patients with chronic liver disease and also selected patients with metabolic disease or fulminant liver failure should be considered early for transplantation. Current 1 year survival figures are 80–90%. Absolute contraindications are metastatic malignancy, permanent neurological deficit and intractable extrahepatic sepsis. Complications are rejection, opportunistic infection (bacterial, fungal, viral and *Pneumocystits carinii*), renal failure and vascular thromboses. Expert initial assessment and care of the child's general condition, especially nutritional status, will minimize post-operative problems.

Further reading

Beath SV, Booth IW, Kelly DA. Nutritional support in liver disease. *Archives of Disease in Childhood*, 1993; **69:** 545–7.

Lee H, Vacanti JP. Liver transplantation and its long-term management in children. *Paediatric Clinics of North America*, 1996, **43:** 99–124.

Related topics of interest

Gastrointestinal haemorrhage (p. 156)
Jaundice (p. 225)
Neonatal jaundice (p. 276)

LUMPS IN THE GROIN

Lumps in the groin can often be diagnosed by careful history and examination taking into account the anatomical landmarks of the area. In boys, a careful examination of the scrotum and testes is essential. In a girl, the finding of bilateral masses in the inguinal canal or bilateral inguinal herniae should lead to investigation to exclude testicular feminization syndrome.

Lumps in the scrotum

1. Hydrocoele is due to a fluid-filled processus vaginalis surrounding the testis. It is common at birth. It is fluctuant and transilluminable and the testis may be difficult to feel. Most resolve by the age of 1 year. Persistence beyond that age may be due to associated hernia.

2. Testicular torsion presents in boys as an acutely painful, swollen testis. It may also present with abdominal pain and vomiting. Immediate surgical correction is required to prevent the testis becoming necrotic and contralateral orchidopexy is usually performed as the other side is at increased risk of torsion in the future.

3. Testicular tumours are very rare in childhood. Germ cell tumours occurring in neonates, present as a painless mass and rarely metastasize. In older boys they may be painful and if the tumour secretes β human chorionic gonadotrophin they may also develop gynaecomastia. Adolescents with tumours often present with metastatic disease. Benign neoplasms include Sertoli cell tumours which occur in babies under 6 months and Leydig cell tumours which typically occur in 4–9-year-olds and are associated with precocious puberty.

4. Cysts of the spermatic cord may occasionally cause problems if they twist, presenting similarly to testicular torsion.

Lumps in the inguinal canal

1. Inguinal herniae are commoner in boys and on the right side. They start as a mass in the inguinal canal which may then extend into the scrotum and 10% are bilateral. The mass is present intermittently and appears when the child cries or strains, disappearing when they are quiet or asleep. The hernia may contain omentum or any intra-abdominal organ such as gut, liver or ovary. An incarcerated hernia is present all the time and is tender. It should be reduced if possible and surgery arranged as soon as possible to prevent strangulation.

This causes interruption of the blood supply and subsequent necrosis of the sac contents.

Herniae are more common in premature infants, those with chronic lung disease (e.g. cystic fibrosis) and connective tissue disease (e.g. Ehlers–Danlos syndrome, mucopolysaccharidoses). In the latter two groups there is also an increased risk of recurrence following repair. Premature babies have a risk of post-operative apnoea and so require careful monitoring.

2. *Undescended testes* may be found in the canal. If they can be milked down into the base of the scrotum then they are retractile and do not require operation. True undescended testes which have not descended by 1 year of age should be brought down operatively.

Lumps in the lateral groin

1. *Lymphadenopathy* may be localized or generalized (see also related topic Lumps in the neck, p. 251). Localized tender enlargement of the inguinal glands may be due to infection anywhere from the perineum to the toes.

2. *Maldescended or ectopic testes* may be found anywhere outside the inguinal canal. They will never naturally descend correctly into the scrotum and so require surgical intervention.

Further reading

Kass EJ, Lundak B. The acute scrotum. *Paediatric Clinics of North America*, 1997; **44** (5): 1251–66.

Skoog SJ. Benign and malignant paediatric scrotal masses. *Paediatric Clinics of North America*, 1997; **44** (5): 1229–50.

Related topics of interest

Lumps in the neck (p. 251)
Newborn examination (p. 296)

LUMPS IN THE NECK

The neck is an anatomically compact area which contains a number of important structures and organs. Diagnosis of abnormalities can often be made by their position relative to anatomical landmarks. When examining a neck lump, depth below the skin, mobility, shape and texture, transilluminability and lumps elsewhere in the body are important pointers in making the diagnosis. Lumps within the skin or sub-cutaneous tissues include sebaceous cysts and lipomata.

Types of lump

1. Thyroglossal cysts are embryological remnants of thyroid tissue but may first present in children and young adults. They are midline swellings which characteristically move upwards on protruding the tongue or swallowing.

2. Thyroid gland may enlarge generally, producing a goitre, or may develop discrete nodules within it. The child should be examined for signs and symptoms of hyperthyroidism (tremor, weight loss, eye signs) and hypothyroidism (constipation, lethargy, weight gain). Solitary nodules are very rare in childhood, causes being benign adenomata, cysts, colloid nodules or carcinoma. Investigation is with thyroid function tests and ultrasound and in the case of a nodule, an isotope scan may be indicated.

3. Branchial cysts and sinuses are embryological remnants of the branchial clefts, most commonly the 2nd. They may present after an upper respiratory tract infection when they may discharge. A cyst presents as a painless swelling at the border of the sternomastoid, but if infected it becomes painful and red.

4. Sternomastoid tumour is thought to be due to trauma to the muscle during delivery. The baby presents with a palpable lump on the sternomastoid associated with shortening of the muscle and a resulting torticollis to that side. If left untreated the child may develop brachycephaly due to lying asymetrically. Treatment is with physiotherapy.

5. Cystic hygroma is a congenital abnormality of lymphatics and is present from birth. It presents as a transilluminable, fluctuant mass. It may contain vascular elements and may be very large. Major complications are cosmetic, infection or trauma.

Lymphadenopathy

Lymph node enlargement can occur in anterior or posterior triangles as well as in the submental and occipital areas. It is extremely common in children particularly associated with acute upper respiratory tract infection. In this case it is usually tender and subsides within a week or two. Where there is swelling which is larger than expected, lasts longer or where the glands are firm, tethered to surrounding structures or where the child has other symptoms, other diagnoses should be considered. Specific enquiry should be made about fevers, rash, respiratory symptoms, weight loss, cat scratches, drugs and foreign travel. Examination should look for lymphadenopathy elsewhere, hepatosplenomegaly and local infection at sites from which lymph drains into the neck.

Generalized lymphadenopathy

1. *Infection* may be bacterial, protozoan (e.g. toxoplasmosis) or mycobacterial, including atypical species. Viruses which may be responsible include measles, rubella, Epstein–Barr, cytomegalovirus and cat scratch fever.

2. *Kawasaki disease* is a condition of unknown aetiology which presents with lymphadenopathy as well as rash, mucous membrane involvement and conjunctivitis (see related topic Kawasaki disease, p. 233).

3. *Malignancy*. Lymphoma, leukaemia, Langerhans cell histiocytosis and metastases from solid tumours.

4. *Eczema*. Children with widespread eczema often have generalized lymphadenopathy, probably due to repeated scratching and infection.

5. *Collagen disorders,* e.g. juvenile rheumatoid arthritis and systemic lupus erythematosus.

6. *Drugs* can occasionally cause lymphadenopathy, e.g. carbamazepine and phenytoin.

7. *Storage disorders,* e.g. Gaucher's disease and Niemann–Pick disease.

Localized lymphadenopathy

1. *Localized pyogenic infection* (e.g. of the throat, or scalp) will cause enlargement of the node group which drains the area.

2. *Malignancy*. Lymphoma may present with localized node enlargement. Metastatic spread may be localized to nodes draining a particular region.

3. *Immunization* may cause localized lymphadenopathy, e.g. BCG.

Investigations

- FBC, film and ESR.
- Bacteriology specimens, e.g. throat swab.
- CXR for hilar lymphadenopathy in lymphoma or sarcoidosis.
- Viral serology.
- Lymph node biopsy if no adequate explanation can be found for the lymphadenopathy. This should be undertaken under general anaesthetic as pre-operative assessment may underestimate the involvement of underlying structures.

Further reading

Morland B. Lymphadenopathy. *Archives of Disease in Childhood*, 1995; **73** (5): 476–9.

Related topics of interest

Kawasaki disease (p. 233)
Lumps in the groin (p. 249)
Malignancy – leukaemia and lymphoma (p. 257)
Pyrexia of unknown origin (p. 334)
Thyroid disorders (p. 363)

MALIGNANCY IN CHILDHOOD

Malignant disease is the second most common cause of death after accidents in children between 1 and 15 years, accounting for 16% of deaths. Nationally, approximately 1200 new cases of leukaemia and cancer are diagnosed each year. With a UK population of ~ 11 million children, this gives a 1 in 600 risk of developing cancer in the first 15 years of life. Overall, cancer is approximately one-third more common in boys. Despite being the second most common cause of death in children, a GP whose list includes 500 children could expect to see only two new cases in 35 years. However, by the year 2000, 1 in 1000 20-year-olds will be a survivor of childhood cancer, so the late effects of both the disease and its treatment are becoming increasingly important.

Problems

- Immunosuppression.
- Treatment tolerability.
- Family and social disruption.
- Late effects.
- Second tumours.

Relative incidences in the UK

1. *Leukaemia* (33%) is the commonest malignancy with 400–450 new cases per year (ALL accounts for 75% of cases).

2. *Brain and spinal cord tumours* (25%) are the second commonest childhood cancers with 300 new cases per year.

3. *Lymphomas* (11%). There are approximately 140 new cases per year, with non-Hodgkin's lymphoma being more common than Hodgkin's lymphoma.

4. *Other solid tumours.* Neuroblastoma (70 cases/year), Wilms' tumour (70 cases/year), retinoblastoma (35 cases/year), and hepatoblastoma (10 cases/year) together account for 15–20% of childhood cancers. There are approximately 60 new bone tumours (osteosarcoma, Ewing's sarcoma) and 50 new soft-tissue sarcomas (rhabdomyosarcoma) per year. Other tumours (e.g. germ cell, thyroid) are very rare.

Aetiology

The causes of childhood cancer are, for the most part, unknown but probably result from the interaction of a number of factors. The UK Co-ordinating Committee on Cancer Research (UKCCR) in collaboration with the UK Children's Cancer Study Group (UKCCSG) set up a case–control study in 1992 to investigate the aetiology of leukaemia. The study will try to establish the role of exposure of the parental germ cells, the fetus and the child to ionizing radiation and certain chemicals. Other possible aetiological factors include exposure to extremely low-frequency electromagnetic fields (e.g. proximity to high-power cables), or an abnormal response to a common infection.

In certain conditions there is a genetic predisposition to malignancy, e.g. chromosomal abnormalities (Down's syndrome), single gene defects (over 25% of children with retinoblastoma have a family history) and DNA repair syndromes (ataxia telangiectasia).

p53 is a tumour-suppressor gene located on chromosome 17. Raised levels and mutations have been found in many tumour types. Li–Fraumeni syndrome is described in families with germline mutations of *p53*, who have a much increased incidence of cancer, particularly breast cancer and soft-tissue sarcomas.

Treatment

Most children with cancer in the UK are now treated within clinical trials coordinated by the Medical Research Council (MRC), UKCCSG or European study groups. Results from these trials are continually evaluated and changes in protocols made to try to maximize survival whilst minimizing late effects. Without these national and international studies the numbers treated in each centre would be too small to detect statistically significant improvements in outcome rapidly. Improved survival has been achieved by the use of more intensive chemotherapy regimens which have been made possible by better supportive care (e.g. early introduction of antibiotics for febrile neutropenia, granulocyte colony-stimulating drugs to improve bone marrow recovery). The introduction of 5-HT_3 inhibitors (e.g. ondansetron) has reduced the severity of nausea and vomiting, and improved treatment tolerability.

Survival

Overall, more than 50% of children with leukaemia and cancer now survive beyond 5 years. For some malignancies (e.g. ALL, NHL, Wilms') the survival rates are now better than 70%, and in these it is important to minimize the late effects of the treatment. In contrast, survival rates for malignancies such as brain tumours and advanced neuroblastoma remain poor despite intensive chemotherapy and radiotherapy.

Late effects

The improved survival from childhood cancer has led to increasing concern about the long-term effects of the disease and its treatment on the survivors. These late effects include:

- Impaired growth and development (particularly following cranial irradiation).

- Increased risk of second tumours.
- Drug effects, e.g. cardiotoxicity secondary to anthracyclines.
- Infertility due to gonadal irradiation or chemotherapy.
- Neuropsychological sequelae which may be subtle defects (e.g. difficulties with mental arithmetic following cranial irradiation) or more pronounced, particularly when treated at a young age.

Treatment strategies must now be evaluated, not only in terms of improved survival, but also in terms of the health status of survivors.

Further reading

Chambers EJ. Radiotherapy in paediatric practice. *Archives of Disease in Childhood,* 1991; **66:** 1090–2.

Goldman A. ABC of palliative care: special problems of children. *British Medical Journal,* 1998: **7124:** 49–52.

Li FP, Fraumeni JF. Prospective study of a family cancer syndrome. *Journal of the American Medical Association,* 1982: **247:** 2692.

Morris-Jones PH, and Craft AW. Childhood cancer: cure at what cost? *Archives of Disease in Childhood,* 1990; **65:** 638–40.

Related topics of interest

Malignancy – leukaemia and lymphoma (p. 257)
Malignancy – solid tumours (p. 261)

MALIGNANCY – LEUKAEMIA AND LYMPHOMA

Leukaemia is the commonest childhood malignancy with 400–450 new cases per year in the UK. This gives a prevalence of 3.5 per 100 000 children under the age of 15 years. Acute lymphoblastic leukaemia (ALL) accounts for 75% of cases; the peak age is 2–6 years, and it is slightly more common in boys (1.2M:1F). Non-Hodgkin's lymphoma is the third most common childhood malignancy, and it can be thought of as 'lumpy leukaemia'. The peak age is 7–10 years and it is three times more common in boys than in girls. Hodgkin's lymphoma occurs in older children and is four times more common in boys.

Leukaemia

Presentation

Presenting features include fatigue, pallor, bruising, frequent or severe infections, lymphadenopathy or bone pain. Hepatosplenomegaly may be present. Cranial nerve palsies (particularly seventh nerve) are uncommon presenting features but indicate CNS involvement. There may be testicular enlargement in boys owing to leukaemic infiltration

Investigation

- FBC and film. Typically shows anaemia, thrombocytopenia, neutropenia and blasts, but the blood count may be normal. A high white count ($> 50 \times 10^9$/l) is a poor prognostic indicator.
- Bone marrow aspirate and trephine. Myeloperoxidase or Sudan black reaction distinguishes lymphoblasts from myeloblasts (negative or less than 3% positive blasts in ALL). Immunological markers determine the cell lineage of the blasts (T, B, null, common, pre-B, etc.).
- Cytogenetics. Numerical or structural chromosomal abnormalities in blood or bone marrow are of prognostic importance, e.g. hyperdiploidy has a good prognosis, while some translocations are associated with a worse prognosis.
- Lumbar puncture. Less than 5% of affected children have CNS disease at diagnosis. If there is any suggestion of CNS involvement or raised intracranial pressure, a CT scan should be performed before LP.
- Culture. Blood, urine, CSF, surface swabs.
- Chest radiography. Mediastinal widening is seen particularly in T-cell ALL.
- U&Es, creatinine, calcium, phosphate and urate. Baseline pretreatment. There may be a degree of renal failure at diagnosis, and the urate is often raised.

- Liver function tests (LFTs) are usually normal at diagnosis but enzymes may be elevated due to leukaemic infiltration. Many of the anti-leukaemic drugs can impair liver function.
- Viral antibodies (varicella, measles, CMV).

Adverse prognostic features

- High white blood cell count (WBC).
- Age < 2 years or >10 years (survival is only 20% if over 16 years).
- Boys have a slightly worse prognosis than girls.
- Massive mediastinal widening.
- CNS disease.
- T-cell ALL, acute or chronic myeloid leukaemia (AML, CML).
- Chromosomal abnormalities, e.g. translocations.
- Slow responders (not in remission after 4 weeks' induction).
- Relapse during treatment.

Treatment

Most children with ALL in the UK are treated according to national protocols as part of the UK Acute Lymphoblastic Leukaemia (UKALL) trial. The current protocol (UKALL XI) consists of a 4-week period of remission induction followed by consolidation with two or three blocks of intensification. Regular intrathecal methotrexate, with or without high-dose intravenous methotrexate, is given as prophylaxis against CNS relapse. Following consolidation, a further 18 months' maintenance treatment (mainly oral chemotherapy) is given to complete a total of 2 years' treatment. Cranial irradiation is now reserved for children with high-risk disease (high WBC, CNS disease). Bone marrow transplantation from a compatible sibling is considered in first remission in poor-prognosis patients. If there are no adverse prognostic features, 5-year survival is greater than 70%, but in high-risk patients it is only 40–50%.

Problems

1. Tumour lysis syndrome. Acute renal failure may occur when treatment starts, owing to acute lysis of blasts, with release of uric acid and phosphate (especially if high WBC or B-cell disease). Prehydration, alkalinization of the urine and allopurinol promote renal excretion and should be commenced at least 24 hours prior to treatment.

2. Immunosuppression. Children with leukaemia are relatively immunosuppressed for the duration of their treatment and for at least 6 months after. They are particularly at risk of infections (viral and fungal as well as bacterial) following intensification blocks when the child is neutropenic. Granulocyte colony-stimulating factors may be used to stimulate bone marrow recovery from intensive chemotherapy. Antibiotic prophylaxis against the opportunistic infection pneumocystis pneumonia is given routinely. Measles and chickenpox can be life-threatening and immunoglobulin should be given if exposed and non-immune. Immunizations should not be given during and for 6 months after treatment as antibody responses will be inadequate and live vaccines may be life-threatening.

3. Side effects of cytotoxic drugs. The introduction of antiemetics such as ondansetron has greatly improved the tolerability of treatment. Other side-effects include alopecia, mucosal ulceration (e.g. methotrexate), renal toxicity (e.g. methotrexate), cardiotoxicity (e.g. anthracyclines) and peripheral neuropathy (e.g. vincristine).

Non-Hodgkin's lymphoma (NHL)

Forty per cent of these lymphomas are abdominal (usually B-cell), and 30% are mediastinal (usually T-cell). Other sites include head and neck lymph nodes and the kidneys. There is an increased incidence in immunodeficiency syndromes, e.g. Wiskott–Aldrich, ataxia telangiectasia, AIDS, and post organ transplantation. NHL is treated using protocols similar to those for ALL. Staging and prognosis depends on the site and number of groups of lymph nodes involved. Five-year survival is 85–90% in localized disease, but only 30–40% in advanced disease.

Hodgkin's lymphoma (Hodgkin's disease, HD)

Epstein–Barr virus may have a role in the aetiology of HD. Histology of affected lymph nodes shows characteristic Reed–Sternberg cells. The disease itself causes relative immunosuppression and there is a high risk of second malignancies. Localized disease is treated with radiotherapy, and more widespread disease is treated with chemotherapy. Overall the 5-year survival is over 80%, but it tends to be a lifelong relapsing and remitting disorder.

Further reading

Chessells JM. Maintenance treatment and shared care in lymphoblastic leukaemia. *Archives of Disease in Childhood,* 1995; **73:** 368–73.

Plowman PN, Pinkerton CR (eds) *Paediatric Oncology: Clinical Practice and Controversies.* London: Chapman & Hall, 1992: Chapters 9–12.

Related topics of interest

Malignancy in childhood (p. 254)
Purpura and bruising (p. 330)

MALIGNANCY – SOLID TUMOURS

Brain and spinal cord tumours are the most common solid tumours, accounting for 25% of all childhood malignancy (~ 300 new cases per year in the UK). The two most common extracranial solid tumours are neuroblastoma and Wilms' tumour, each with about 70 new cases per year.

Brain and spinal cord tumours

The majority of CNS tumours arise from two histological cell types: glial cells (astrocytomas and ependymomas) and neuroectodermal cells (primitive neuroectodermal tumours and medulloblastomas). They have a high potential for local recurrence and neuroaxial dissemination but distant metastases are rare.

Presentation

- Headaches.
- Early morning vomiting.
- Focal neurological signs, e.g. cerebellar signs with posterior fossa tumour.
- Increasing head circumference (infants).
- Convulsions.
- Endocrine disturbance, e.g. precocious puberty, diencephalic syndrome.

Investigation

- *Radiology*. CT scan or MRI. Fifty per cent arise in the posterior fossa.
- *Histology*. Stereotactic biopsy if unresectable. Fifty per cent are astrocytomas. Biological markers such as p53 expression may help in predicting prognosis but are still research investigations at present.

Management

Acutely raised intracranial pressure is treated with mannitol and dexamethasone. A ventriculoperitoneal shunt is sometimes needed. Surgical resection and craniospinal radiotherapy are the mainstays of treatment. Chemotherapy has been shown to shrink some tumours, particularly those of neuroectodermal origin, and may delay progression in others. Radiotherapy is particularly damaging to the infant brain so chemotherapy is currently used in this age group.

Outcome

Overall there is only a 50% chance of 5-year survival. Low-grade astrocytomas which are completely resected carry the best prognosis and high-grade gliomas (glioblastoma multiforme) are associated with a very poor prognosis, with the majority of affected infants dying within months. Late effects of the treatment include the neuroendocrine and neuropsychological effects of radiotherapy.

Neuroblastoma

This is a malignant tumour derived from the sympathetic nervous system. The peak age of incidence is 2 years; it is rare over 5 years and is slightly more common in boys (1.4M:1F). In one-third the primary tumour arises from the adrenal, and the majority have metastases at presentation (bone, bone marrow, lymph nodes, less commonly liver, skin). Prognosis is inversely related to age at presentation. Under the age of 1 year the tumour behaves very differently and may even regress spontaneously. Despite even advanced disease, the prognosis in this age group is usually good.

Presentation

- Abdominal mass (> 50%).
- Bone marrow infiltration. Anaemia, thrombocytopenia, bone pain.
- Non-specific malaise.
- Local invasion and compression, e.g. proptosis in head and neck disease, venous compression in thoracic disease.
- Spinal cord compression. A 'dumb-bell' tumour grows through the intervertebral foramina and has retroperitoneal and intraspinal components.
- Metabolic effects. High levels of catecholamines and vasoactive intestinal peptides cause sweating, pallor and diarrhoea.
- Hepatomegaly.
- Bluish skin nodules.

Investigation

- Urinary catecholamine metabolites. Raised vanillyl-mandelic acid (VMA) and homovanillic acid (HVA) to creatinine ratios on a spot urine specimen.
- Radiology. Abdominal US, CT scan or MRI (chest, abdomen, ± head and neck). The tumour often contains flecks of calcification.
- Tumour histology and cytogenetics. More differentiated tumours have a better prognosis. Structural and numerical abnormalities of chromosome 1 and N-*myc* amplification (cellular oncogene) are associated with more advanced disease.
- Bone marrow examination.
- Radionucleotide bone scan.
- Meta-iodobenzylguanidine (MIBG) scan. An ^{131}I-labelled guanethine analogue which is taken up by > 90% of neuroblastomas.
- Serum ferritin. Raised ferritin associated with more advanced disease and worse prognosis.

Management

If the tumour is localized and completely resected no further treatment may be needed. However, the majority require adjuvant chemotherapy with or without radiotherapy. Very high-dose chemotherapy (megatherapy) with autologous bone marrow rescue and targeted radiotherapy using MIBG are used in some centres.

Outcome

Localized, completely resectable disease (stage 1) has a good prognosis, with more than 90% 5-year survival, but these children account for less than 5% of the total. More than 60% of children have disseminated disease at diagnosis (stage 4). Five-year survival is ~ 60% under the age of 1 year but is only ~ 20% over 1 year, prognosis worsening with increasing age. Stage 4S is a special group under the age of 1 year, who have a localized primary tumour with dissemination to liver, skin and bone marrow. This group has more than 80% 5-year survival. Mass screening of infants for raised urinary catecholamines, to detect early neuroblastomas, has not been widely accepted since many of the tumours detected have an intrinsically good prognosis and may even regress spontaneously.

Wilms' tumour (nephroblastoma)

This tumour arises from embryonal cells within the kidney (nephrogenic rests). The majority present under the age of 5 years, boys being affected slightly more commonly than girls. The left kidney is affected more often than the right and 5–10% of patients have bilateral tumours. Wilms' tumour is associated with aniridia, hemihypertrophy, Beckwith–Wiedemann syndrome and genitourinary abnormalities.

Abnormalities of chromosome 11 have been identified in some children. Staging depends on whether there is local extension beyond the renal capsule, involvement of local lymph nodes or distant lung metastases.

Presentation

- Asymptomatic renal mass (90%).
- Haematuria – rare.

Investigation

- Radiology. Abdominal US and CT scan. Chest radiography to identify lung metastases.
- Tumour histology. Unfavourable features include areas of anaplasia.

Management

Nephrectomy is performed either as a primary procedure or following shrinkage of the tumour by chemotherapy. The duration and intensity of post-operative chemotherapy depends on the tumour stage and histological features. Radiotherapy is used if the tumour is not limited to the kidney.

Outcome

Overall there is more than 85% 5-year survival. Age over 5 years, advanced stage and unfavourable histology are worse prognostic features, but even these children have a better than 60% chance of cure.

Further reading

Meller S. Targeted radiotherapy for neuroblastoma. *Archives of Disease in Childhood,* 1997; **77:** 389–91.

Murphy SB, Cohn SL, Craft AW *et al.* Do children benefit from mass screening for neuroblastoma? *Lancet,* 1991; **337:** 344–6.

Related topic of interest

Malignancy in childhood (p. 254)

MENINGITIS AND ENCEPHALITIS

Eighty per cent of all bacterial meningitis occurs in childhood, with a mortality of 10% (over 100 deaths per year in the UK). It is the commonest cause of acquired sensorineural deafness, and can lead to other neurological sequelae, including epilepsy. The organisms responsible vary with age, and the choice of antibiotics therefore depends on the age of the child as well as the local pattern of drug resistance. Meningitis may also follow infection with a wide variety of viruses, and the prognosis is usually good with no specific treatment. Encephalitis is usually viral or post-infectious and is characterized by fever, disturbed consciousness, convulsions and focal neurological signs. Tuberculous meningitis should be considered in every case of aseptic meningitis or encephalitis. The onset is usually insidious and these children often develop focal neurological signs before a diagnosis is made.

Problems

- Seizures.
- Inappropriate ADH secretion.
- Cerebral oedema.
- Subdural effusions.
- Septicaemic shock.
- Neurological sequelae.
- Prophylaxis for close contacts.

Meningitis

Aetiology

1. Bacterial

(a) Neonatal period

- *E. coli* and other Gram-negative organisms.
- Group B streptococcus.
- *Listeria monocytogenes.*

(b) Over 3 months

- *Neisseria meningitidis.*
- *Haemophilus influenzae* (usually under 6 years).
- *Streptococcus pneumoniae.*

(c) 1 to 3 months

- Any of the above.

2. *Viral.* Most commonly coxsackie, echovirus, mumps.

3. *Tuberculosis.*

4. *Fungal.* Rare unless immunocompromised.

Clinical features

The characteristic features are pyrexia, headache, neck stiffness and photophobia. In a neonate or infant the symptoms are less specific with fever, poor feeding, irritability, vomiting, a full fontanelle, apnoea or drowsiness. A convulsion may be the presenting feature, so a lumbar puncture (LP) should always be considered in a child under 1 year who has a convulsion with fever. Neonatal meningitis is uncommon but has a high mortality and morbidity; most have an associated bacteraemia and many are shocked at diagnosis. Meningococcal meningitis may be associated with septicaemia (characteristic rash ± shock). Haemophilus meningitis is much less common since the introduction of routine immunization. Symptoms of viral meningitis are usually less severe than bacterial meningitis and there may have been a preceding upper respiratory or gastrointestinal illness, but it is not always clear-cut.

Investigation

- FBC, clotting studies.
- Blood cultures.
- Serum viral titres – acute and convalescent.
- Blood glucose.
- CSF protein, glucose, bacteriology and virology. In bacterial meningitis there is a raised WBC (mainly polymorphs), raised protein and low glucose (< 50% of blood glucose). Organisms may be seen on Gram stain. In viral meningitis there is a raised WBC (mainly lymphocytes), protein is normal or raised and CSF glucose is normal. In tuberculous meningitis there is a raised WBC (mainly lymphocytes), raised protein and low glucose.
- U&E.
- Swabs (throat, nose, purpuric skin) for bacterial and viral culture.
- Urine culture.

Management

1. Lumbar puncture. If meningitis is suspected, an LP should be performed immediately unless the child's cardiovascular system is unstable or there is evidence of raised intracranial pressure (e.g. deep coma, protracted seizures, focal neurological signs, unequal pupils or abnormal pupillary reflexes plus gradual onset of symptoms/signs). If the LP is contraindicated, antibiotic treatment should not be delayed. Antibiotic guidelines should be reviewed regularly to take account of the continually changing pattern of antibiotic resistance. Treatment should be reviewed with culture and sensitivity results after 24–48 hours. In the presence of a meningococcal rash penicillin should be given immediately. If the CSF and clinical picture suggests viral meningitis it is usual to treat with 48 hours' antibiotics, awaiting negative CSF culture.

2. *General measures.* Cardiopulmonary support may be necessary. Restrict fluid to two-thirds of normal requirements and record strict fluid balance. Inappropriate ADH secretion is common. Monitor neurological status – any deterioration suggests worsening cerebral oedema or development of a subdural collection. Detect and treat seizures.

3. *Steroids.* Much of the cerebral damage in bacterial meningitis is due to activation of the host inflammatory responses rather than the direct effect of the invading organism. The role of steroids in reducing this inflammatory response is controversial, but the early use of dexamethasone in haemophilus meningitis may be of benefit, particularly in reducing the incidence of deafness. The role of steroids in meningococcal and pneumococcal meningitis is still unclear, and their routine use is not recommended.

4. *Prophylaxis.* The disease must be notified to P.H.L. Close contacts (household or kissing contacts) of a child with meningococcal disease should be treated with rifampicin. The patient should also be given rifampicin to clear carriage as soon as oral intake is tolerated. Children under 5 years who have been in close contact with a child with haemophilus meningitis and who are not immunized should be given rifampicin. Rifampicin causes orange–red discoloration of urine and tears (stains contact lenses). It interferes with other drugs (including the oral contraceptive pill) and is contraindicated in pregnancy. In the case of an outbreak of meningococcal disease where the serotype is A or C, vaccination of close contacts may be offered in addition to chemoprophylaxis. At present there is no vaccine available for type B.

Encephalitis

Aetiology

1. *Infectious*

- Herpes simplex.
- Enterovirus (coxsackie, echovirus).
- Mumps.

2. *Post-infectious*

- Measles.
- Varicella zoster.

- Live vaccines (e.g. measles – very rare).
- Subacute sclerosing panencephalitis (SSPE).

Clinical features

Herpes simplex is the most common cause of severe encephalitis. Mortality is high and neurological sequelae in the survivors are common. The CSF shows a raised white count, and the EEG and CT scan show characteristic changes in the temporal lobes. An acute self-limiting encephalitis may follow chickenpox, resulting in cerebellar ataxia. Encephalitis may also follow measles, with irritability and seizures a few days after the rash. There may be complete recovery or it can progress to severe neurological impairment or death. SSPE is a late complication of measles owing to persistence of the virus in the brain. Degeneration of the brain occurs several years after the initial infection.

Further reading

Mayon-White RT, Heath PT. Preventative strategies on meningococcal disease. *Archives of Disease in Childhood.* 1997; **76:** 178–81.

Report of the Meningitis Working Party of the British Paediatric Immunology and Infectious Diseases Group. Should we use dexamethasone in meningitis? *Archives of Disease in Childhood,* 1992; **67:** 1398–401.

Gandy G, Rennie J. Antibiotic treatment of suspected neonatal meningitis. *Archives of Disease in Childhood,* 1990; **65:** 1–2.

Related topics of interest

Coma (p. 89)
Immunization (p. 206)
Neonatal convulsions (p. 272)
Rashes and blisters (p. 337)
Shock (p. 344)

MUSCLE AND NEUROMUSCULAR DISORDERS

Disorders of muscle (myopathies) present with floppiness, delayed motor milestones, abnormal gait, clumsiness or progressive muscle weakness. The majority of myopathies are inherited, and all are uncommon. Dystrophies are characterized by degeneration of muscle fibres. Myotonia is the failure of muscle relaxation after contraction. Myotonia may occur as an abnormal response to muscle relaxant agents (e.g. scoline) during anaesthesia resulting in total opisthotonus. There is an increased risk of this reaction in children with muscle disease. Disorders of the neuromuscular junction include myasthenia gravis and botulism.

Myopathies

- Developmental, e.g. nemaline myopathy, central core disease.
- Degenerative, e.g. muscular dystrophy.
- Metabolic, e.g. glycogen storage disease (Pompe's), carnitine deficiency, periodic paralysis, mitochondrial abnormalities.
- Endocrine, e.g. hypothyroidism.
- Myotonic, e.g. myotonic dystrophy, abnormal response to scoline.
- Inflammatory, e.g. polymyositis, dermatomyositis.

Duchenne muscular dystrophy

Problems

- Progressive muscle wasting and weakness.
- Repeated respiratory infections.
- Psychological problems.
- Family disruption and modifications to the home.
- Genetic counselling. There is a 50% risk of recurrence in males.
- Future therapies. Gene replacement, myoblast transfer.

Clinical features

Duchenne muscular dystrophy is the most common muscular dystrophy with a prevalence of 1 in 3000 male births. It is inherited as a sex-linked recessive condition, although new mutations are responsible for up to one-third of cases. Female carriers are unaffected. Presentation is usually in the first 5 years of life with a waddling gait due to weakness of the pelvic girdle. Other early features include frequent falls, difficulty climbing stairs, climbing up the legs to get up from the floor (Gower's sign), pseudohypertrophy of the calf muscles and lordosis. The intellect is usually normal but there is an increased incidence of mild learning difficulties. Weakness and wasting is progressive with the majority unable to walk by 10 years. Cardiac muscle is also affected.

Late features include scoliosis, contractures and aspiration pneumonia. Death usually occurs between 15 and 25 years. Becker muscular dystrophy is less common and progresses more slowly, with death usually in middle age.

Investigation

- Creatine phosphokinase (CPK). Very high (normal up to 150), falls as disease progresses.
- Neurophysiology. Characteristic myopathic changes.
- Muscle biopsy. Degenerative changes, dystrophin immunofluorescence.
- Cytogenetics. A very large gene involved in Duchenne and Becker muscular dystrophy has been located on the short arm of the X chromosome (Xp21). It codes for the protein dystrophin, which forms part of the cytoskeleton of muscle cells. Mutations can be identified in about 60% of cases. The level of dystrophin seems to correlate with clinical severity, and therapeutic measures to correct dystrophin abnormalities are the subject of current research.
- Antenatal diagnosis. Identification of a known mutation, or dystrophin analysis.

Myotonic syndromes

Myotonic dystrophy is the most common of the myotonic syndromes. Inheritance is autosomal dominant and the gene has recently been identified on chromosome 19. Muscle weakness produces a myopathic facies, ptosis and a sagging jaw. Myotonia causes difficulty in relaxing the grasp. It is associated with mild learning difficulties, cataracts and frontal balding. Congenital dystrophia myotonica occurs in infants of an affected mother and many die of respiratory difficulties in the neonatal period as a result of severe hypotonia. Those who survive often have severe learning difficulties. Myotonia is detected by shaking hands with the mother.

Dermatomyositis

This is an inflammatory disorder characterized by generalized proximal muscle weakness and pain (polymyositis) associated with a violaceous skin rash (eyelids, cheeks, knees and bony prominences). There is an underlying vasculitis of small blood vessels of unknown aetiology. Treatment is with steroids. Severe disease may be associated with subcutaneous calcification.

Myasthenia gravis

This is an autoimmune disorder of the neuromuscular junction which can occur at any age. Antibodies are produced against the acetylcholine receptors. It is associated with other autoimmune diseases and is more common in girls. Clinical features include ptosis, squint, difficulty in chewing and swallowing, and dysarthria. Generalized weakness and hypotonia is an uncommon presentation. Weakness is exacerbated by repetitive or sustained contraction. Diagnosis is confirmed by reversal of weakness with edrophonium and treatment is with long-acting anticholinesterase inhibitors. Acute exacerbation of muscle weakness can be precipitated by exertion, infections or some drugs, such as aminoglycosides (myasthenic crisis), or by excessive anticholinesterase treatment (cholinergic crisis). Neonatal myasthenia gravis occurs in some infants of affected mothers owing to placental transfer of antiacetylcholine receptor antibodies, and resolves in 4–6 weeks. Congenital myasthenia gravis is an autosomal recessive condition which presents in the newborn period and is relatively resistant to treatment.

Further reading

Bushby KMD. Recent advances in understanding muscular dystrophy. *Archives of Disease in Childhood,* 1992; **67:** 1310–2.

Related topics of interest

Disability (p. 124)
Floppy infant (p. 150)

NEONATAL CONVULSIONS

Many disorders may cause fits in the neonatal period, the commonest being perinatal asphyxia, metabolic derangements and meningitis. Asphyxia due to disturbances in fetal circulation and lack of oxygen during labour may lead to hypoxic–ischaemic encephalopathy in the first few days of life, and this is a major cause of death and neurological disability.

Aetiology

- Hypoxia. Perinatal asphyxia.
- Metabolic disorders. Hypoglycaemia, hypocalcaemia, hyponatraemia, hypomagnesaemia.
- Infection. Meningitis, congenital viral infection, encephalitis
- Intracranial haemorrhage. Intraventricular, subdural, intracerebral.
- Drug withdrawal. Maternal drug abuse.
- Cerebral malformation.
- Inborn error of metabolism.

Clinical features

Convulsions in neonates are different from those in older children. They may be manifested by extension and stiffening of the body with upward deviation of the eyes. Other more subtle features include apnoea and bradycardia, sucking and chewing movements of the mouth or cycling movements of the limbs.

Investigation

- Blood sugar. BM Stix immediately.
- U&E.
- Serum calcium and magnesium.
- Acid–base status.
- Full septic screen including lumbar puncture.
- FBC.
- Other tests as indicated, e.g. metabolic screen, cerebral US, clotting screen, EEG.

Management

1. Correct underlying metabolic disorder, e.g. hypoglycaemia (i.v. dextrose infusion), hyponatraemia (fluid restriction). These may be the primary cause of the convulsion or may be secondary to other conditions such as birth asphyxia, meningitis or an inborn error of metabolism.

2. Anticonvulsants to control fits and prevent further convulsions. Phenobarbitone is the first-line drug. Other useful drugs include paraldehyde, phenytoin and clonazepam. If convulsions continue despite these, consider thiopentone.

3. Fluid balance. Cerebral insults (e.g. birth asphyxia, prolonged convulsions, meningitis) result in a degree of cerebral oedema. Fluids should be restricted by 20–40% in the first 24–48 hours to reduce the risk of fluid overload, which exacerbates cerebral oedema and may lead to hyponatraemia. Oliguria may result from ADH secretion or renal ischaemia. The use of diuretics (e.g. mannitol) and the place of intracranial pressure monitoring are controversial.

4. Respiratory support. Ventilation may be needed to maintain good oxygenation. Hyperventilation to maintain a low–normal $P\text{CO}_2$ may help reduce cerebral oedema.

5. Broad-spectrum i.v. antibiotics should be commenced once a full septic screen has been performed. The common causes of neonatal meningitis are group B streptococcus, *E. coli* and *Listeria.*

Birth asphyxia

Problems

- Hypoxic–ischaemic encephalopathy and neurological sequelae.
- Meconium aspiration.
- Cardiovascular complications – myocardial ischaemia, persistent fetal circulation.
- Renal ischaemia.
- Necrotizing enterocolitis.
- Inappropriate ADH.
- Disseminated intravascular coagulopathy (DIC).

Diagnosis and outcome

There is no accepted definition of birth asphyxia so the prevalence is difficult to ascertain, but in the UK it is in the region of 5 per 1000 full-term live births, with 1 in 1000 dying or being left severely disabled. Prompt cardiorespiratory resuscitation at birth and early supportive care (glucose, oxygen, management of cerebral oedema, treatment of seizures) are important in limiting the cerebral injury.

Hypoxic stress is an invariable consequence of labour, but the level of stress which an individual fetus can withstand is unclear. Meconium staining of the amniotic fluid and an abnormal cardiotocograph are currently used as indications of fetal distress during labour but are poorly predictive of long-term neurological problems. Fetal scalp blood sampling can be used to assess the degree of acidosis as a measure of fetal distress, and a pH < 7.2 is often taken as an indication for assisted delivery (forceps, Caesarean). The mean umbilical venous pH in uncompromised fetuses is reported to be 7.32, but there is poor correlation between cord blood acidosis and subsequent neurological impairment. The Apgar score is routinely recorded at 1 and 5 minutes after birth and assesses five variables: heart rate, respiratory effort, muscle tone, reflex irritability and colour. Severe depression of the Apgar score (0–3) is directly related to the risk of death, but it is otherwise poorly predictive of neurological outcome and there is a poor correlation with cord blood acidosis. Delay in establishing spontaneous respiration may indicate asphyxia but is influenced by gestational age and maternal drugs.

Three grades of hypoxic–ischaemic encephalopathy (HIE) following asphyxia are described: mild, moderate and severe. The duration and severity of neurological signs (level of consciousness, tone and posture, sucking reflex, seizures, autonomic function) together with EEG findings are the best predictors of neurological outcome. Mild encephalopathy carries a good prognosis, but moderate and severe encephalopathy result in a high risk of impairment. The severity of HIE, however, can only be diagnosed retrospectively after symptoms have developed. New therapeutic interventions such as allopurinol (a free radical scavenger) and inhibitors of the excitatory neurotransmitter glutamate may prove to be useful but need to be given early, so there remains a need for an early marker of asphyxia. Newer techniques such as magnetic resonance spectroscopy to evaluate the ATP energy state of the brain and Doppler measurement of cerebral blood flow may be useful in assessing the extent of asphyxia.

Ultrasound and CT scanning are used to identify treatable complications of asphyxia (e.g. subdural collection) and to predict outcome. Poor prognostic findings include injury to the basal ganglia and subcortical cysts due to infarction in the vascular watershed area, but these do not develop until after the first week of life.

Further reading

Evans D, Levene M. Neonatal seizures. *Archives of Disease in Childhood,* Fetal and Neonatal edn, 1998; **78:** F70–5.

Levene MI. Management of the asphyxiated full term infant. *Archives of Disease in Childhood,* 1993; **68:** 612–6.

Marlow N. Do we need an Apgar score? *Archives of Disease in Childhood,* 1992; **67:** 765–7.

Related topics of interest

Coma (p. 89)
Disability (p. 124)
Fits, faints and funny turns (p. 144)
Meningitis and encephalitis (p. 265)

NEONATAL JAUNDICE

Jaundice occurs in 60% of term and 80% of pre-term infants within the first week. Although it is usually physiological and benign, it may also signify serious underlying disease. Jaundice should always be investigated if there is a deviation from the normal pattern of physiological jaundice.

Jaundice requiring investigation

- Visible jaundice within 24 hours of birth.
- Baby unwell and jaundiced.
- High or fast-rising levels of bilirubin (level > 220 μmol/l in a term baby, or a rate of rise above 85 μmol/l/day).
- Jaundice persisting beyond 14 days.
- Conjugated hyperbilirubinaemia (associated with pale stools, dark urine) is always pathological.

History

The following points in the history are important:

- Parental history. Past obstetric history, ethnic origins, blood groups, consanguinity.
- Antenatal/perinatal history. Illnesses during pregnancy, gestational age and mode of delivery .
- Postnatal history. Feeding problems, failure to pass meconium, vomiting, fever and colour of the baby's stool and urine.

Examination

Weight, length and head circumference should be plotted, and any dysmorphic features noted. Examination may reveal pallor, bruising, purpura, or hepatosplenomegaly. Specimens of stool and urine should be inspected by the clinician. More specific diagnostic clues may be present, e.g. cataracts in galactosaemia, cystic mass if there is a choledochal cyst.

Presentation in first 24 hours of life

The commonest causes for early jaundice are:

- Haemolysis, e.g. rhesus disease or ABO incompatibility, red cell defects, e.g. spherocytosis, glucose-6-phosphate dehydrogenase deficiency.
- Extravascular blood, e.g. cephalhaematoma, swallowed blood.
- Polycythaemia, e.g. recipient of twin-to-twin transfusion, small for dates.
- Sepsis.

Investigation

- Haematology. FBC, film, reticulocyte count, blood group and save, Coombs' test, maternal haemolysins.

- Biochemistry. Serum bilirubin, conjugated and unconjugated, blood glucose.
- Septic screen. Blood and urine cultures, lumbar puncture.

Presentation >24 hours and <14 days

Physiological jaundice

This occurs in healthy newborn infants. Jaundice is noted after the age of 24 hours, reaches a peak on the third or fourth day of life (approximately 120 μmol/l), and fades by the seventh to tenth day of life. There is a later peak and trough in the pre-term infant. Aetiological factors include the shortened red cell survival in neonates, reduced bilirubin conjugation and increased enteric reabsorption of bilirubin.

Breast milk jaundice

Jaundice is more common in breast-fed babies. This is thought to be due to the presence of β-glucuronidase in the milk which deconjugates bilirubin in the bowel, causing increased enterohepatic circulation.

Pathological jaundice

This may be due to unconjugated or conjugated hyperbilirubinaemia. A high or rapidly rising bilirubin level should be investigated further. Any of the causes listed below under prolonged jaundice may present within the first 10 days.

Investigation

Apart from establishing the bilirubin level if the jaundice appears significant, no investigations are usually necessary if there are no findings to suggest pathology.

Prolonged jaundice

Although physiological jaundice may rarely continue beyond a couple of weeks, the cause should be assumed to be pathological at this stage until proven otherwise. The causes of prolonged jaundice or jaundice present in a baby more than 2 weeks old include:

Unconjugated hyperbilirubinaemia

- Haemolysis, e.g. rhesus disease or ABO incompatibility, red cell defects, e.g. spherocytosis, glucose-6-phosphate dehydrogenase deficiency.
- Extravascular blood, e.g. cephalhaematoma, swallowed blood.
- Sepsis.
- Increased enterohepatic circulation, e.g. meconium plug, pyloric stenosis.
- Metabolic, e.g. galactosaemia.

- Hypothyroidism.
- Decreased conjugation, e.g. Crigler–Najjar (rare).

Conjugated hyperbilirubinaemia

- Bile duct obstruction, e.g. biliary atresia, choledochal cyst.
- Biliary hypoplasia, e.g. Alagille's syndrome or non-syndromic.
- Neonatal hepatitis. In many conditions, cholestasis represents a final common pathway of hepatic injury:
    - Metabolic. Galactosaemia, α_1-antitrypsin deficiency, cystic fibrosis.
    - Infective. Bacterial infection, congenital viral infection, hepatitis B.
    - Endocrine. Hypothyroidism, hypopituitarism.
    - Miscellaneous, e.g. parenteral nutrition, lipid storage disorders.

Investigation

All babies will need baseline investigations of:

- FBC and film.
- Serum bilirubin, conjugated and unconjugated.
- Liver function.
- Thyroid function.
- Serum for antibodies to toxoplasmosis, rubella, etc (CMV on urine).
- Urine for culture.
- Urine for reducing sugars.

According to the clinical picture, further tests may include:

1. Unconjugated hyperbilirubinaemia

- Osmotic fragility studies and red cell enzyme measurements for congenital haemolyses.
- Blood culture if sepsis suspected.

2. Conjugated hyperbilirubinaemia (>15% conjugated). The cause of the cholestasis should be determined with urgency because biliary atresia requires urgent surgery before 60 days of age if irreversible liver damage is to be avoided.

- Coagulation screen.
- Urine for the presence of bile, organic and amino acids, and reducing sugars.

- Serum α_1-antitrypsin phenotype (total serum level is unreliable), galactose-1-phosphate uridyl transferase activity, amino acids.
- Plasma immunoreactive trypsin or DNA studies to exclude cystic fibrosis. Sweat test unreliable before 6 weeks of age.
- Imaging: hepatobiliary scintigraphy scan after pretreatment with phenobarbitone may determine bile duct patency. Cerebral and abdominal US, spinal X-rays (for Alagille's syndrome).
- Tissue diagnosis: liver biopsy. Occasionally bone marrow or skin biopsy is needed to exclude a storage disorder.

Management of neonatal jaundice

Unconjugated hyperbilirubinaemia

If a cause is identified it should be treated appropriately, e.g. septicaemia. Unconjugated bilirubin is lipid soluble and readily dissociates from albumin and diffuses into the CNS. It may cause kernicterus (acute: shrill cry, opisthotonus, fits; long-term: choreoathetosis, deafness, learning disability) in those with very high bilirubin levels, although this can occur at lower levels if the neonate is sick or pre-term.

1. Phototherapy. Unconjugated bilirubin is isomerized by exposure to light (ideal frequency 420–470 nm), and converted into a more water-soluble form, which can then be excreted in bile. Phototherapy is usually considered at bilirubin levels of 250 μmol/l and above in term babies, but at lower levels in the sick or pre-term infant. Additional fluids should be given and the eyes covered.

2. Exchange transfusion. This should be considered for Coombs' test positive haemolytic disease, or if the rate of rise of bilirubin is > 10 μmol/l/hour.

Conjugated hyperbilirubinaemia

Immediate priority should be given to the treatment of life-threatening complications, e.g. sepsis, coagulopathy, hypoglycaemia. The cause of the cholestasis should then be determined. In biliary atresia, the Kasai procedure achieves biliary drainage by the formation of a Roux-en-Y loop of jejunum sutured into the porta hepatis. Other causes of cholestasis may need specific treatment, e.g. surgical excision of a choledochal cyst, and supportive therapy such as coagulation factors, fat-soluble vitamins, added medium chain triglyceride in feeds.

Further reading

Kliegman RM. Jaundice and hyperbilirubinaemia in the newborn. In: Behrman RE, Kliegman RM, Arvin AM, eds. *Nelson Textbook of Paediatrics*, 15th edn. Philadelphia: WB Saunders, 1996; 493–9.

Related topics of interest

Congenital infection (p. 93)
Jaundice (p. 225)
Liver disease (p. 244)

NEONATAL RESPIRATORY DISTRESS

Respiratory distress is characterized by tachypnoea (respiratory rate > 60 per minute), expiratory grunting and recession. Cyanosis without oxygen is common. About 2% of all babies and 20% of those under 2500 g have breathing difficulties in the neonatal period. The commonest pulmonary causes of respiratory distress are respiratory distress syndrome (RDS), transient tachypnoea of the newborn, streptococcal pneumonia and meconium aspiration. RDS is due to surfactant deficiency and affects about 7000 UK babies each year. Improvements in neonatal intensive care, including the use of surfactant replacement therapy, have significantly reduced the mortality. The differential diagnosis of a cyanosed baby includes lung disease, cyanotic heart disease and persistent fetal circulation.

Problems

- Hypoxia.
- Acidosis.
- Pneumothorax.
- Chronic lung disease (CLD).
- Sequelae of prolonged ventilation, e.g. airway stenosis.

Differential diagnosis

- Respiratory distress syndrome (hyaline membrane disease).
- Pneumonia (particularly group B streptococcus).
- Transient tachypnoea of the newborn.
- Meconium aspiration.
- Pneumothorax.
- Congenital heart disease (cyanosis, heart failure).
- Diaphragmatic hernia.
- Increased intra-abdominal pressure, e.g. post-repair of gastroschisis.
- Upper airway obstruction, e.g. choanal atresia, Pierre Robin syndrome.
- Cystic lung malformations, e.g. cystic adenomatoid malformation.
- Pleural effusion, e.g. severe rhesus disease.
- Metabolic disorders.
- Myopathies, e.g. Werdnig–Hoffmann, myotonic dystrophy.

Respiratory distress syndrome (RDS)

Clinical features

Predisposing factors include prematurity, hypoxia, hypothermia and maternal diabetes. Boys are more severely affected than girls, and Afro-Caribbean babies are less severely affected than Caucasian babies. Respiratory distress develops within 4 hours of birth and progressively worsens over the next 24–48 hours. Symptoms begin to resolve after 36–48 hours as surfactant synthesis increases, and this is usually associated with a diuresis. Corticosteroids reduce the incidence and severity of RDS when given to mothers in preterm labour. Growth retardation, prolonged rupture of membranes and maternal pre-eclamptic toxaemia advance fetal maturation and may reduce the severity of RDS. The CXR in RDS typically shows granular opacity (ground-glass appearance) with air bronchograms.

Management

1. Supportive care. Management is aimed at supportive care with supplemental oxygen with or without ventilation until spontaneous recovery occurs. Worsening hypoxia, hypercarbia, acidosis and apnoea are indications for ventilation. In mild RDS nasogastric feeding may be possible, but most need intravenous fluids in the acute phase.

2. Ventilation. Most babies manage well on conventional intermittent positive pressure ventilation which may be time controlled or patient triggered. However very premature babies and those with severe disease may benefit from the newer forms of ventilation. High frequency oscillation (HFO) avoids some of the lung damage of conventional ventilation and may improve oxygenation and outcome. It may also benefit babies with pneumothorax or pulmonary haemorrhage who are requiring more than minimal ventilation. Severely ill babies with a high mortality risk who have been ventilated for less than 7 days, weigh >2 kg and have no neurological problems may be considered for extracorporeal membrane oxygenation (ECMO) at a specialist centre. Future possibilities include liquid ventilation using perfluorocarbon through which gases passively diffuse.

3. Surfactant. Pulmonary surfactant is a complex mixture of lipids, proteins and carbohydrate. It is synthesized and secreted by type II epithelial cells, and the quantity increases throughout gestation. It has surface tension-lowering properties in the alveoli and deficiency leads to atelectasis at end-expiration. Manufactured surfactant preparations can be given directly down the endotracheal tube. They may be animal derived (Survanta (bovine), Curosurf (porcine)) or synthetic (ALEC and Exosurf). The speed of action differs between the products but the outcome (improvement in oxygenation and reduction in ventilation pressures) appear to be similar. Large, randomized, multicentre trials in the last few years have shown a 40% reduction in mortality, and a significant reduction in the incidence of pneumothorax with surfactant therapy. It may also reduce the incidence of ischaemic and haemorrhagic cerebral lesions. Survival with severe CLD is reduced but the overall incidence of CLD seems unchanged.

Surfactant has been given prophylactically to babies at risk of RDS, but there is no clear evidence of the benefit of early administration. Adverse effects include problems with administration (e.g. hypoxia if too rapid, blocked endotracheal tube if not reconstituted properly) and a possible increase in the incidence of pulmonary haemorrhage in infants < 700 g.

Surfactant therapy in other pulmonary diseases may have a transient beneficial effect, e.g. meconium aspiration, pneumonia, congenital diaphragmatic hernia.

4. *Antibiotics.* It is often difficult to distinguish RDS from early streptococcal pneumonia so penicillin is usually given for the first 48 hours until blood cultures and surface swabs are negative.

Transient tachypnoea of the newborn

Delayed clearance of fetal lung fluid results in respiratory distress which is usually mild (rarely need > 40% oxygen) and settles in 24–48 hours. Predisposing factors include Caesarean or precipitate delivery. CXR shows diffuse streaky shadowing and fluid in the horizontal fissure.

Meconium aspiration

Acute or chronic intrauterine hypoxia causes 15–20% of babies to pass meconium before or during delivery. Aspiration occurs in 5% of these and results in airway obstruction, inhibition of surfactant synthesis and a chemical pneumonitis. CXR shows patchy atelectasis and hyperinflation due to airway obstruction. The risk of pneumothorax is high, and ventilation should be avoided if possible. Aspiration may be prevented by suctioning the oropharynx immediately after birth. If meconium is seen on the cords at direct laryngoscopy the infant should be intubated and the airway suctioned. The use of bronchial lavage is controversial as it may wash meconium further into small airways. If respiratory distress develops, management is supportive, with supplemental oxygen and i.v. fluids. Antibiotics should be given as there is an increased risk of secondary infection. Symptoms usually settle within 2–7 days but 30% may require ventilation. Mortality is 5–10%.

Chronic lung disease (CLD)

An infant who has a need for supplemental oxygen at 28 days and has an abnormal CXR has CLD (previously known as bronchopulmonary dysplasia, BPD). It occurs in ~ 5% of all admissions to neonatal units and is commonest in infants < 1500 g. The most common predisposing factor is ventilation for RDS, but it may occur as a result of other conditions, e.g. meconium aspiration, congenital heart disease. Lung fibrosis and cystic changes occur as a result of barotrauma and oxygen toxicity, and signs of right heart strain may develop. CXR shows coarse shadowing, cysts, hyperexpansion and variable cardiomegaly. Management aims to gradually wean the infant off respiratory support, maintain nutrition (increased calorie requirements) and treat infections promptly with antibiotics and physiotherapy. Diuretics may be of benefit, and steroids have been used to decrease oxygen requirements. The use of steroids is now being advocated earlier in the course of RDS to try to achieve earlier extubation and reduce the incidence and severity of CLD. The use of surfactant has reduced the incidence of severe CLD but there remain a few infants who have a long-term oxygen requirement and are managed with home oxygen. Rehospitalization in the first year of life is common due to respiratory infection, and mortality from respiratory failure or cor pulmonale is increased.

Further reading

Finer N. Inhaled nitric oxide in neonates. *Archives of Disease in Childhood,* 1997; **77:** F81–4.

Marlow N. High frequency ventilation and respiratory distress syndrome: do we have an answer? *Archives of Disease in Childhood,* Fetal and Neonatal edn. 1998; **78:** F1–2.

Morley CJ. Systematic review of prophylactic vs rescue surfactant. *Archives of Disease in Childhood,* 1997; **77:** F70–4.

Samuels MP, Southall DP. Home oxygen therapy. In: David TJ ed. *Recent Advances in Paediatrics,* Vol. 14. Edinburgh: Churchill Livingstone, 1995; 37–52.

Sinha SK, Donn SM. Advances in neonatal conventional ventilation. *Archives of Disease in Childhood,* 1997; **75:** F135–40.

Vyas J, Kotecha S. Effects of antenatal and postnatal corticosteroids on the preterm lung. *Archives of Disease in Childhood,* 1997; **77:** F147–50.

Wilkinson AR. Surfactant therapy. In: David TJ, ed. *Recent Advances in Paediatrics,* Vol. 11. Edinburgh: Churchill Livingstone, 1993; 53–66.

Related topics of interest

Cyanotic congenital heart disease (p. 104)
Prematurity (p. 323)

NEONATAL SURGERY

Disorders of the gastrointestinal tract are common causes of referral for neonatal surgery. Congenital abnormalities may be detected antenatally or present early in the neonatal period. Necrotizing enterocolitis (NEC) is usually managed medically, but surgery is indicated in some cases. Pyloric stenosis, inguinal hernias and intussusception may present in early infancy. Other congenital abnormalities which may require early surgical intervention include congenital heart defects, cleft lip and palate, choanal atresia, congenital lung malformations (e.g. congenital lobar emphysema), urological problems (e.g. posterior urethral valves), sacrococcygeal tumours and biliary atresia, and some of these are discussed elsewhere.

Presentation of gastrointestinal (GI) tract abnormalities in the neonatal period

- Antenatal diagnosis (gastroschisis, diaphragmatic hernia).
- Polyhydramnios (oesophageal atresia).
- Respiratory distress (diaphragmatic hernia).
- Vomiting (intestinal atresia, malrotation, pyloric stenosis, NEC).
- Constipation (meconium ileus, Hirschsprung's disease, anorectal abnormalities).
- Abdominal pain (intussusception, strangulated inguinal hernia).
- Abdominal distension and bloody stools (NEC).

Necrotizing enterocolitis (NEC)

NEC may affect any part of the GI tract, but the commonest sites are terminal ileum, caecum and ascending colon. Damage to the normally impermeable mucosal barrier (hypoxia, ischaemia, immature mucosa) allows organisms, endotoxins and gas to escape from the lumen into the gut wall. NEC is often associated with a septicaemia, but no one organism has been implicated. Nearly all affected infants have received oral feeds, which may act as a substrate for bacterial proliferation. There is an increased risk of NEC with hyperosmolar feeds and when the feed volume is rapidly increased. Breast milk has a protective effect. Coagulation necrosis of the mucosa with microthrombi leads to patchy ulceration, oedema and haemorrhage. This may progress to transmural necrosis and perforation.

Clinical features

NEC can affect term or preterm neonates but is particularly common in those <1500 g. Predisposing factors include hypoxia, hypotension, umbilical catheterization, intrauterine growth retardation, patent ductus arteriosus and exchange transfusion. It can occur at any stage during a baby's stay in a special care baby unit but is most common in the first week of life. Presentation may be non-specific, with lethargy, apnoeas, temperature instability or shock and DIC. More specific features include abdominal distension, bile-stained vomiting and bloody stools. Bowel sounds are absent, the abdomen is tender and there may be palpable distended bowel loops.

Investigation

- FBC and clotting studies.
- U&E.
- Full septic screen (blood, urine, CSF, stool cultures).
- Abdominal radiography. Dilated bowel loops, thickened gut wall, fluid levels, intramural gas (pneumatosis intestinalis), gas in the biliary tree, evidence of perforation.

Management

1. Medical. Most settle with broad-spectrum i.v. antibiotics (including metronidazole) and stopping feeds. Parenteral nutrition should be continued for at least 7 days before feeds are slowly reintroduced. Cardiorespiratory support may be needed and metabolic homeostasis should be maintained. Umbilical catheters should be removed.

2. Surgery. Indications for surgery are continued deterioration despite medical treatment, persistent bowel obstruction and perforation. Some perforations can be managed conservatively if the infant is too unstable for surgery.

Outcome

The majority recover fully, but recurrence occurs in ~ 10% of cases, usually within 1 month. Mortality is associated with DIC and septicaemia. Longer term sequelae include strictures, short gut syndrome and fistulae.

Diaphragmatic hernia

Congenital diaphragmatic hernia occurs in about 1 in 2500 live births and is more common on the left side. The infant presents with respiratory distress, usually on the first day of life. Examination reveals a scaphoid abdomen, displacement of the cardiac impulse, and reduced air entry with or without bowel sounds on the affected side of the chest. The degree of pulmonary hypoplasia ranges from mild to severe. Smaller defects, particularly on the right side, may present later and may be confused radiologically with cystic lung lesions (e.g. cystic adenomatoid malformation). Diagnosis is usually made on chest or abdominal radiographs, but can be confirmed by barium swallow. Antenatal diagnosis is becoming increasingly common. Resuscitation with bag and mask ventilation should be avoided as this will cause gastric distension and worsening of respiratory distress. Most affected children are now electively paralysed, ventilated and stabilized for at least 12 hours before surgery. The bowel is decompressed with a nasogastric tube. High ventilation pressures may be needed and there is a risk of pneumothorax. Pulmonary hypertension is treated with hyperventilation and pulmonary vasodilators (e.g. tolazoline). The optimum time for surgery is controversial, but survival is improved if hypoxia and acidosis have been corrected. Survival rates are now better than 50%. The outcome is dependent on the degree of pulmonary hypoplasia and the presence of associated abnormalities. The pulmonary reserve is reduced in the first 1–2 years of life, but the majority of surviving children achieve virtually normal lung function in later childhood.

Oesophageal atresia and tracheo-oesophageal fistula

The majority of cases (> 85%) of oesophageal atresia are associated with a tracheo-oesophageal fistula (TOF). The incidence is 1 in 3000 live births and it is associated with polyhydramnios, which may precipitate premature labour. Affected infants typically have frothy secretions and choke on the first feed. Oesophageal atresia should be excluded in all infants born to mothers with polyhydramnios, by passing a nasogastric tube into the stomach soon after birth. The catheter will not pass more than 8–10 cm from the lips in the presence of oesophageal atresia and the position of the tube can be confirmed radiologically. Air in the stomach confirms the presence of a TOF. The oesophageal pouch is drained with a Replogle tube and all fluids are given intravenously. If there is evidence of aspiration, antibiotics and physiotherapy should be commenced.

Surgery is carried out as soon as the baby is stable. Primary end-to-end anastomosis of the oesophagus is usually possible, with division of the fistula. Contrast studies are performed post-operatively to ensure integrity of the anastomosis before commencing oral feeds. Gastro-oesophageal reflux is common in these children and may require surgical treatment. The brassy TOF cough may persist for several years and is due to a degree of tracheomalacia. Anastomotic stricture may occur.

Gastroschisis and exomphalos

Exomphalos is persistence of the gut herniation which normally occurs between the sixth and 14th weeks of gestation. There may be a large abdominal wall defect covered by a sac of amnion and peritoneum (exomphalos major) or a herniation of abdominal contents into the umbilical cord (exomphalos minor). The incidence is about 1 in 10 000 live births. Exomphalos major has a high incidence (~ 40%) of associated abnormalities (e.g. chromosomal abnormalities, cardiac defects, anencephaly, Beckwith–Wiedemann syndrome). Gastroschisis is evisceration of small and large bowel through a defect of the anterior abdominal wall to the right of the umbilicus. The incidence is about 1 in 6000 live births. The aetiology is unknown. The bowel is often thickened, matted together, and may be shortened. Associated abnormalities are rare. The majority of cases of both gastroschisis and exomphalos are now diagnosed antenatally. Caesarean section does not improve the outcome and these infants can be delivered vaginally. The lesion should be covered with a plastic bag or cling-film to minimize fluid and heat loss, and the bowel decompressed with a nasogastric tube. It may be possible to return the gut to the abdominal cavity as a primary surgical procedure, but larger defects require staged reduction over several days or weeks using a silastic silo. Bowel resection for ischaemic damage is more common with gastroschisis.

Intravenous fluids and nutrition are continued until enteral feeding is established post-operatively, which may take weeks or months. Post-operative complications include sepsis, respiratory embarrassment, hypoproteinaemia, renal vein thrombosis and short gut syndrome.

Further reading

Davies CF, Young DG. Gastroenterology. Part IV: Congenital defects and surgical problems. In: Roberton NRC, ed. *Textbook of Neonatology*, 2nd edn. Edinburgh: Churchill Livingstone, 1992: 655–86.

Related topics of interest

Neonatal respiratory distress (p. 281)
Vomiting (p. 377)

NEPHROTIC SYNDROME

The nephrotic syndrome occurs when heavy proteinuria results in hypoproteinaemia and oedema. It is an uncommon condition with 2–4 new cases per 100 000 children per year. The peak age is 2– 6 years and boys are more commonly affected than girls (2.5 : 1). In most cases (>90%) the cause is unknown (idiopathic or minimal change nephrotic syndrome) and the proteinuria is steroid responsive. There is thought to be an immunological basis and there is an association with atopy. The prognosis is good with < 10% progressing to chronic renal failure. Genetic predisposition is associated with HLA-DRW7 and DR3 (six times increased risk) and there is an increased risk in siblings of an affected child. Less commonly the nephrotic syndrome occurs secondary to another disorder and is not steroid responsive. In these children the prognosis is generally poor, more than 30% progressing to renal failure.

Problems

- Hypovolaemia.
- Infection.
- Thrombosis.
- Acute renal failure.
- Hyperlipidaemia.
- Complications of prolonged steroid treatment, e.g. poor growth, obesity, hypertension.

Aetiology

(a) Idiopathic (minimal change nephrotic syndrome – MCNS).

(b) Secondary to:

- Henoch–Schönlein purpura.
- Glomerulonephritis.
- Malaria.
- Renal vein thrombosis.
- Toxins, e.g. lead, gold, snake venom.
- Allergy, e.g. bee sting, immunization.
- Miscellaneous conditions, e.g. amyloid, sickle cell anaemia, SLE, hepatitis B infection.

(c) Congenital (Finnish type nephrotic syndrome).

Pathology

The light microscopic findings in MCNS are unremarkable and electron microscopy shows fusion of the epithelial cell foot processes. In the steroid unresponsive group the underlying pathology is usually focal segmental glomerulosclerosis (less commonly membrano-proliferative glomerulonephritis).

Clinical features

Oedema is the usual presenting feature, typically facial and periorbital. There may be associated peripheral oedema (legs, scrotal, sacral), ascites and pleural effusions. The child is often irritable, with a poor appetite and may have diarrhoea and/or vomiting. It is vital to recognize symptoms and signs of hypovolaemia including cold peripheries, poor capillary refill, and abdominal pain (due to splanchnic underperfusion). Hypovolaemia and an increased clotting tendency can lead to peripheral ischaemia and infarction resulting in loss of digits and even limbs from gangrene. Hypertension may be a feature if the nephrotic syndrome is secondary to glomerulonephritis.

Congenital nephrotic syndrome is very rare, and presents at birth with placental oedema, or develops in the first few months of life. It is an autosomal recessive condition, more common in Scandinavia.

Investigations

- Urinalysis.

  Heavy proteinuria = proteinuria > 40 mg/m^2/hour or early morning protein:creatinine ratio >200 mg/mmol.

  Haematuria may be present (10–25% of patients) and may indicate an underlying glomerulonephritis.

Some centres determine the protein selectivity index, the proteinuria of MCNS being highly selective (i.e. small proteins only, e.g. albumin) and of focal segmental glomerulosclerosis being poorly selective. However steroid responsiveness is the best indicator of MCNS.

- FBC. The haematocrit is a useful guide to hypovolaemia.
- Plasma U&Es, creatinine, albumin. Hypoalbuminaemia = albumin < 25 g/l. The urea may be raised due to hypovolaemia but the creatinine is usually normal in MCNS. Hyponatraemia may occur.
- Urinary sodium. A very low urine sodium suggests critical hypovolaemia (maximal renal retention of salt and water in an attempt to compensate).
- Calcium and magnesium. Levels are reduced in parallel with albumin (ionized calcium normal).
- Hepatitis B surface antigen.
- ASO titre, complement screen and autoantibody screen. If there is a mixed nephritic/nephrotic picture.
- Immunoglobulins. IgG is reduced and IgE may be raised.
- Lipids. Hyperlipidaemia is common.

Management

1. Correct hypovolaemia. Plasma expansion with plasma or salt-poor (20%) albumin if critically hypovolaemic. Diuretics should be used with caution as they may induce hypovolaemia. Rapid infusion of fluids may precipitate pulmonary oedema. Consider monitoring central venous pressure in the acute phase. Acute renal failure may occur due to hypovolaemia or due to the underlying condition. Strict fluid input/output monitoring including daily weighing is essential. A low sodium diet, and bedrest may help to reduce oedema.

2. Steroids. Many different steroid regimens are used, e.g. prednisolone 2 mg/kg/day or 60 mg/m^2/day until in remission (protein free for 3 days) and then 40 mg/m^2 alternate days for 4 weeks. 80% will be in remission within 28 days and most of these will have MCNS. Those who are steroid resistant (no response in four weeks) should be referred to a paediatric nephrologist for further management. Relapses are common (> 75% have at least one relapse – proteinuria 2+ for three or more consecutive days) and are often associated with infections or exacerbations of asthma/eczema. These are treated with further courses of prednisolone. Frequent relapses (two or more relapses within 6 months of initial response, or four or more relapses within any 12 month period) may warrant the use of alternate day prednisolone for up to 6 months to prevent recurrences.

3. Other drugs. If relapses occur on prednisolone or the side effects of steroids become unacceptable levamisole, cyclophosphamide, or cyclosporin A may be considered. Renal biopsy is not performed routinely and is only indicated in those who fail to respond to steroids, or in those with poor prognostic features at diagnosis (haematuria, hypertension, raised creatinine, age <1year or > 10 years). Biopsy may also be indicated prior to starting cyclosporin treatment. Relapses eventually cease and active disease is rare beyond puberty.

4. Prevent infections. Nephrotic patients are immunocompromised because of low IgG levels, impaired lymphocyte function, protein malnutrition, and immunosuppressive drugs. Prophylactic penicillin should be given when oedematous to prevent pneumococcal peritonitis. Fever will be masked by steroid treatment and abdominal pain may be the only indication of peritonitis. Live vaccines should be avoided until the child has been off daily steroids for at least 3 months, but are permissable if the child is on low dose alternate day prednisolone (< 0.5 mg/kg alternate days).

5. *Prevent thrombosis.* The increased clotting tendency is due to elevated clotting factors and enhanced platelet aggregability. This may be exacerbated by hypovolaemia. Renal vein thrombosis may further complicate the nephrotic syndrome.

Further reading

Report of a Workshop by the British Association for Paediatric Nephrology and Research Unit, Royal College of Physicians. Consensus statement on management and audit potential for steroid responsive nephrotic syndrome. *Archives of Disease in Childhood,* 1994; **70:** 151–7.

Watson AR, Coleman JE. Dietary management in nephrotic syndrome. *Archives of Disease in Childhood,* 1993; **69:** 179–80.

Related topics of interest

Acute renal failure (p. 15)
Chronic renal failure (p. 82)
Glomerulonephritis (p. 164)

NEUROCUTANEOUS SYNDROMES

These disorders are syndromes of genetic or developmental anomalies which involve structures of ectodermal origin, i.e. peripheral and central nervous system, skin and eye. Only some of these conditions are discussed below.

Problems

- Neurological.
- Cosmetic.
- Visceral.
- Developmental delay.
- Visual disturbance.

Tuberous sclerosis (TS)

The classical features of this autosomal dominant condition are learning disability, seizures and facial angiofibromas. However, it has a wide range of clinical features, and a high mutation rate accounting for up to two-thirds of cases. Birth prevalence is thought to be as high as 1 in 6000. A gene locus has been found on the long arm of chromosome 9, but also on other sites, e.g. 11q, and this genetic heterogeneity means that antenatal diagnosis is not yet possible.

Skin lesions include hypomelanic 'ash leaf'-shaped macules which fluoresce under UV light (Wood's lamp) and may be present from birth. The fibrous forehead plaque may also appear early.

Adenoma sebaceum rarely appears before the age of 2–3 years and is a papular acneiform eruption in a butterfly distribution over the face, sparing the upper lip. Periungual fibromata of fingers or toes are rarely seen before puberty, but may be the sole sign of TS. Shagreen patches are raised, roughened areas of skin over the lumbosacral area. Neurological features include learning disability (50%) and seizures, commonly infantile spasms. Psychotic and autistic behaviour is common. Intracranial lesions occur, e.g. subependymal glial nodules, cortical tubers and giant cell astrocytomas (rare but can cause hydrocephalus by obstruction to the third ventricular outflow).

Cardiac rhabdomyoma may be an important prenatal marker, and may present with obstructive cardiac symptoms but then regress later. Renal involvement occurs in 80% of cases, as polycystic kidneys or angiolipomata.

Retinal phakomata may be a feature, normally symptomless, appearing as a fleshy, raised lesion, often around the optic disc.

Management of TS should involve effective control of seizures, and active surveillance for the recognized complications of the disease. Argon laser therapy has been successful in the treatment of facial angiofibromas.

Sturge–Weber syndrome

The main features of this rare and sporadically occurring syndrome are leptomeningeal angiomatosis (all cases), facial angiomatous naevus ('portwine stain') of the ophthalmic division of the trigeminal nerve (85% of cases) and choroidal angioma (40% of cases). The leptomeningeal angioma is common in the parieto-occipital area, and is bilateral in 15% of cases. The facial port-wine stain is usually ipsilateral to the leptomeningeal angioma.

Clinical features are seizures (often partial motor seizures in early infancy), learning disability, glaucoma and hemiplegia. Characteristic appearances on skull radiographs are of 'rail-road' track calcification after the first year of life, but MRI and CT scanning will reveal changes earlier.

Management involves the control of seizures, regular ophthalmological assessment and laser treatment of skin lesions. Neurosurgery may be suitable in selected cases.

Neurofibromatosis (NF)

This is the most common of the neurocutaneous syndromes, and can be separated into type 1 neurofibromatosis (classical, von Recklinghausen), assigned to chromosome 17, and type 2 (central) neurofibromatosis, assigned to chromosome 22. Both are autosomal dominant disorders.

1. Type 1 neurofibromatosis (NF1). Two or more of the following diagnostic criteria must be present for diagnosis:

- Six or more *café au lait* macules (over 5 mm diameter in prepubertal children and over 15 mm in post-pubertal children). These often appear in the first year of life, and are nearly always present by 6 years of age.
- Two or more neurofibromas of any type, or one plexiform neurofibroma.
- Axillary or inguinal freckling (tends to follow the appearance of *café au lait* lesions).
- Optic glioma.
- Two or more Lisch nodules.
- A distinctive osseous lesion such as sphenoid dysplasia or pseudoarthrosis.
- A first-degree relative with NF1.

Complications include malignant change in the skin lesions, especially the diffuse subcutaneous plexiform tumours. CNS malignancy (optic nerve pathway gliomas), phaeochromocytoma, renal artery stenosis, spinal (dumb-bell) tumours, gastrointestinal neurofibromas and epilepsy are all rare but serious complications.

2. *Type 2 neurofibromatosis (NF2).* It is unusual for NF2 to present in the paediatric age group (average age of onset is 20 years), and new mutations are common. Symptoms occur from bilateral acoustic neuromas, cranial meningiomas and spinal tumours. Skin signs may be minimal.

Incontinentia pigmenti

This is an X-linked dominant disorder, usually lethal in males. A triphasic rash (vesicular, verrucous, hyperpigmented) tends to fade altogether by adulthood. Seizures, mental retardation, spasticity and ocular abnormalities are associated features.

Klippel–Trenaunay–Weber syndrome

Complex angiomatous malformations occur over one or more limbs, associated with hypertrophy of soft tissue and bone. Cerebral angiomatous malformations may occur.

Further reading

Ruggieri M, Huson SM. What's new in neurofibromatosis? *Current Paediatrics,* 1997; **7:** 167–76.

Webb DW, Osborne JP. Tuberous sclerosis. *Archives of Disease in Childhood,* 1995; **72:** 471–73.

Related topics of interest

Developmental delay (p. 115)
Rashes and blisters (p. 337)

NEWBORN EXAMINATION

Every newborn baby should be fully examined within the first 2 to 3 days of life. This examination should include:

1. Review of the family history, pregnancy and birth, e.g.:

- Maternal history including blood group and any illnesses, e.g. diabetes.
- Gestation, mode of delivery (forceps, ventouse etc), condition at birth (Apgar scores), presence of meconium, prolonged rupture of the membranes.
- Abnormalities noted on antenatal ultrasound such as renal tract abnormalities.
- Previous baby with a congenital abnormality.
- Family history such as sensorineural hearing loss (consider audiology referral).
- Consider haemoglobinopathy screening, BCG or hepatitis B immunization according to local policies.

2. Enquiry about any parental concerns.

3. Physical examination.
(a) Document weight and head circumference.
(b) Note and discuss any birth marks.
(c) Check for:

- Jaundice (see related topic Neonatal jaundice, p. 276).
- Cyanosis and respiratory distress (see related topics Neonatal respiratory distress, p. 281 and Cyanotic congenital heart disease, p. 104).
- Congenital dislocation of the hips and talipes.
- Testicular descent.
- Red reflexes to exclude cataracts.
- Heart murmurs (remember – absence of a murmur in the early days of life does not exclude serious congenital heart disease – see related topic Heart murmurs, p. 194).

This chapter cannot possibly be comprehensive but the following are some common or important findings.

General examination

1. Caput succedaneum. A serosanguinous subcutaneous effusion over the presenting part of the head which subsides within 24 hours.

2. Chignon. The oedematous part of the scalp that is sucked into a Ventouse extractor. Occasionally there is haemorrhage into the chignon or necrosis of the skin, with secondary infection.

3. Cephalhaematoma. A subperiosteal haemorrhage which most frequently occurs over the parietal bones (sometimes bilateral). The extent of the haemorrhage is limited by the suture lines and it usually presents as a fluctuant swelling on the second day of life. It is associated with a hairline fracture of the underlying bone and is more common following instrumental deliveries. No treatment is required and it resolves over 2–12 weeks, with a hard calcified rim sometimes giving the impression of a depressed skull fracture.

4. Petechiae and subconjunctival haemorrhages. Facial petechiae and bruising are particularly common if the cord has been tight around the neck, and the face may appear cyanosed and bloated. Subconjunctival haemorrhages due to raised intrathoracic pressure are common following vaginal delivery.

5. Abrasions and skin punctures. From forceps, scalp electrodes, or fetal blood sampling occasionally become infected resulting in abscess formation. Accidental scalpel incisions during caesarian delivery may require suturing.

6. Polydactyly, syndactyly. Polydactyly may be sporadic or inherited as an isolated autosomal dominant condition. Extra digits may be attached to either the radial or ulnar side of the hand. Even if the digit has a narrow connecting pedicle, surgical removal is advised rather than simply tying it off with silk as there may be a cartilaginous connection and there is a risk of infection. Polydactyly is also associated with syndromes such as Patau's, Laurence Moon Biedl and infantile thoracic dystrophy. Syndactyly (fusion of the fingers) is associated with syndromes such as Apert's, Waardenberg's, and orofacial digital syndrome.

7. Preauricular skin tags (accessory auricles). These are common and of no significance. They can be surgically excised when the child is older if there are concerns about their cosmetic appearance. Preauricular pits are less common but may become infected.

8. Sacral dimple. A pit at the top of the natal cleft which is almost always blind ending with no connection with the underlying spine. No action is required if the base of the pit can be identified.

9. Meconium and urine. Meconium should be passed within the first 24 hours, although there may be some delay in preterm babies. If passage of meconium is delayed more than 48 hours ano-rectal anomalies, cystic fibrosis, and Hirschsprung's disease should be considered.

Urine should be passed in the first 24 hours. Apparent delay is often due to urine having been passed during delivery, but check for a palpable bladder (e.g. posterior urethral valves in boys). Poor urine output due to acute tubular necrosis may occur following birth asphyxia.

10. Umbilicus. The cord dries and drops off after 7–10 days. A sticky umbilicus can usually be managed with cleaning and antiseptic powders. However, as the umbilical vessels remain patent for the first few weeks, periumbilical inflammation may have serious consequences (e.g. septicaemia, portal vein thrombosis). Antibiotics are required. Umbilical herniation is common. Strangulation or rupture are virtually unknown and even large hernias usually resolve spontaneously by school age. Umbilical granulomas usually resolve with the application of silver nitrate. A patent urachus or vitello-intestinal fistula should be considered if there is a persistent umbilical discharge. Delayed separation of the cord is associated with some types of immunodeficiency.

Rashes and naevi

1. Erythema toxicum. This is a very common, benign, self-limiting rash of unknown aetiology. The erythematous maculopapular rash usually appears in the first few days of life. It can occur anywhere on the body and tends to come and go over several days. Small pustules may be present which contain eosinophils. No treatment is required but it must be distinguished from staphylococcal skin infection.

2. Milia (milk spots). These are pearly white retention cysts of the pilosebaceous follicles on the nose. They are very common and usually disappear after the first month.

3. Stork mark. A dull pink, non-raised capillary naevus commonly found in the nape of the neck and over the eyelids, forehead, and bridge of the nose. Fading of the facial naevus is usual over the first year, but it may persist in the nape of the neck.

4. Superficial cavernous haemangiomas (strawberry marks). These are not present at birth but appear as red spots in the first few weeks. They are usually superficial, and may be single or multiple. They often grow rapidly during the first year of life into raised, well-demarcated, bright red masses. Complications include bleeding and infection. They are particularly common on the face and may interfere with vision or feeding. Although they may be cosmetically unsightly, treatment is usually avoided as spontaneous regression occurs within 4–5 years leaving little or no mark. If very large or encroaching on vital structures, surgical debulking or steroid therapy may be considered.

5. Deeper cavernous haemangiomas may be present at birth and can enlarge with time. The overlying skin is normal or bluish in colour. These naevi usually persist, although partial resolution may occur.

6. Port wine stain. A dark capillary naevus which does not fade. This can occur on any part of the body, but if the area of the ophthalmic division of the trigeminal nerve is affected, there may be an associated intracranial haemangioma (Sturge–Weber syndrome). Laser therapy may be helpful.

7. Mongolian blue spot. Blue-black discoloration commonly seen over the buttocks and lumbo-sacral region in babies of Asian or Afro-Caribbean origin. Usually fades over the first few years and should not be mistaken for bruising.

8. Pigmented naevi. These vary from small brown moles to giant hairy, pigmented naevi. There is a small risk of malignant change particularly with very large naevi, which can be treated by excision and skin grafting.

Peripheral nerve injuries

1. Facial nerve palsy is usually unilateral and is associated with pressure from forceps or the maternal pelvis. The weakness generally resolves within days or weeks. Congenital defects of the 7th nerve are usually bilateral.

2. Erb's palsy. Lateral flexion of the neck or traction on the arms during delivery may result in injury to the upper roots of the brachial plexus (C5, C6). The arm is held in the waiter's tip position and an associated fracture of the clavicle or humerus should also be considered. The weakness usually resolves in a few weeks but may take several months. A small number are left with residual weakness which may be improved with surgery.

3. Klumpke's palsy. Damage to the lower brachial roots (C8, T1) is less common but can occur when the arms are extended up beside the head.

Genitalia

1. Undescended testes. The testes of boys born at term should be in the scrotum. Those that are not in the scrotum may be retractile, incompletely descended (e.g. in the inguinal canal) or intra-abdominal (cryptorchidism). Orchidopexy to bring down the testis is recommended before school age as there is an increased risk of infertility, torsion, and malignancy in undescended testes.

2. Hypospadias. The urethral meatus opens more proximally than normal. The degree of hypospadias is described as glandular, coronal, penile or perineal. Operative repair is usually performed in the first 2 to 3 years of life. The foreskin may be used in reconstructive surgery so the infant should not be circumcised. Renal tract ultrasound is usually performed as there is an association with other renal tract abnormalities.

3. Epispadias. A rare anomaly where the urethral opening is situated on the dorsal aspect of the penis. In its extreme form it is associated with bladder exstrophy.

Congenital dislocation of the hip (CDH)

CDH occurs in 1.5 per 1000 live births and is six times more common in girls than boys. There is an increased incidence in first degree relatives of an affected individual. Dislocation occurs secondary to abnormal laxity of the joint capsule with elongation of the ligamentum teres. There may be a shallow acetabulum and hypoplasia of the femoral head. Unilateral defects are twice as common as bilateral defects. Predisposing factors include breech delivery, spina bifida, and hypotonia. There is an association between talipes and CDH.

Diagnosis

It is essential to detect CDH early as the treatment is then relatively simple. Ortolani's and Barlow's tests are used in the newborn period and throughout early infancy to detect dislocated or dislocatable hips. With the hips and knees flexed the thighs are abducted and a dislocated femoral head will 'clunk' back into the acetabulum. Application of backward pressure as abduction is commenced will detect a dislocatable hip. By 2–3 months of age instability of the joint is lost and important signs are asymmetrical skin folds and limitation of abduction. Late signs include shortening and external rotation of the limb, and a waddling gait with a positive Trendelenburg test.

X-rays are not useful in the early detection of CDH as before the hips are ossified interpretation is difficult. Ultrasound is used in some centres as a screening procedure, particularly for those at higher risk of CDH, e.g. family history, breech delivery.

Management

Treatment of an unstable or dislocated hip should be commenced immediately with an abduction splint (e.g .Von Rosen). This maintains the femoral head in the correct position until the acetabulum has developed sufficiently to prevent dislocation (usually 6–12 weeks). Occasionally dislocated hips cannot be reduced in a splint and these require surgical intervention. CDH which is detected late is difficult to treat because of the relatively fixed displacement of the femoral head with limitation of abduction and adductor contracture. Surgical correction with a period of traction may be successful.

Talipes

Talipes occurs in 1 in 1000 live births and is three times more common in boys than girls. 50% are bilateral and predisposing factors include oligohydramnios, spina bifida, and a family history of talipes. The most common deformity consists of fixed plantar flexion with inversion of the foot and adduction of the forefoot (talipes equinovarus). A less common deformity consists of dorsiflexion and eversion of the foot (talipes calcaneovalgus). All cases must be carefully examined for associated hip and spine problems. Gradual manipulative correction with adhesive strapping over a period of 6 to 8 weeks will correct the majority of the less rigid deformities. Surgical correction with soft tissue release and tendon transplantation to correct the inversion of the hindfoot, followed by splinting with Denis Browne boots, may be necessary for more rigid deformities. Corrective bone surgery is sometimes necessary in later childhood.

Further reading

Dezateux C, Godward S. Screening for congenital dislocation of the hip in the newborn and young infants. In: David TJ, ed. *Recent Advances in Paediatrics.* Edinburgh: Churchill Livingstone, 1997.

Johnston PGB. *The Newborn Child,* 8th edn. New York: Churchill Livingstone, 1998.

Related topics of interest

Cyanotic congenital heart disease (p. 104)
Heart murmurs (p. 194)
Neonatal jaundice (p. 276)
Neonatal respiratory distress (p. 281)

NUTRITION

Good nutrition is vitally important for growth and development, particularly during early childhood. For the seriously ill child or the child with a chronic illness, nutritional support should be considered as a priority. Oral feeds may be supplemented with enteral feeds via a nasogastric tube or gastrostomy, but if the gut cannot be used (e.g. severe inflammatory bowel disease, necrotizing enterocolitis) total parenteral nutrition should be considered.

There is increasing evidence that early nutrition may have influences on health in later life. Barker and co-workers (see Further reading) suggest that undernutrition *in utero* may be a risk factor for the development of hypertension, diabetes or cardiovascular disease.

Iron deficiency is common in the UK and may have adverse effects on immunological, neuromuscular and cognitive function (see related topic Anaemia, p. 31). Vitamin deficiencies are less common but may occur in association with malabsorption syndromes, chronic liver disease and chronic renal failure. Malnutrition remains a major health issue in the developing world.

Infant feeding

1. Breast-feeding. Breast-feeding should be promoted by all health care workers. The composition of breast milk is ideal for human growth and development. The fat is particularly well absorbed. Breast milk also provides appropriate amounts of the essential fatty acids linoleic and alpha linoleic acid, as well as long chain polyunsaturated fatty acids, which are particularly important for brain and retinal development. The protein content is lower than other milks, with a casein:whey ratio of 40:60. The salt content is low. Iron concentrations are relatively low but absorption is good, possibly promoted by the iron being bound to lactoferrin. Breast-feeding reduces the risk of gastrointestinal and respiratory infections as the milk contains IgA and immunologically active proteins, e.g. lactoferrin, which inhibit growth of microorganisms. It has a trophic effect on the gut, enhances mother–infant bonding and suckling promotes oromotor function. There is debate as to whether there is a beneficial protective effect against atopy in infants with a strong family history. Colostrum is the milk produced in the first few days after birth. It has a higher concentration of protein (mainly immunoglobulins), vitamins A and B_{12}, and a lower fat content.

2. Formula milk feeds. For mothers who are unable to breast-feed or do not wish to, modified cow's milk formulas are available. There are numerous brands with little variation between them. Unmodified cow's or goat's milk is unsuitable for infants due to the high solute load (protein and salt). The casein:whey ratio and the salt content of cow's milk is modified to be closer to that of breast milk and the formulas are fortified with iron and vitamins. The amino acid composition of whey-dominant milks is closest to breast milk, but casein-dominant milks are available. These claim to provide greater satisfaction for a hungry baby but there is little evidence for this. All have approximately the same calorie content (67 kcal per 100 ml).

Soya based milks are available for infants who are cow's milk protein intolerant, but there is also an increased risk of soya allergy in these infants. Soya formulas also have a high content of phytoestrogens. The long-term effects of these, particularly on sperm production and fertility, have been debated recently. Special formulas and semi-elemental diets using 'high degree' hydrosylates may be indicated for infants with severe milk protein intolerance or inborn errors of metabolism, e.g. PKU, galactosaemia.

3. Preterm formula milks. These provide a greater density of nutrients, aiming to achieve intrauterine growth rates without feeding large volumes. Studies have shown that infants fed these formula milks achieve better growth and development (motor and mental performance) than those fed standard formula milks. However, expressed breast milk (EBM) provides protection against necrotizing enterocolitis and may have advantages in terms of improved IQ. EBM can be enriched with human milk fortifiers for very low birth weight babies.

4. Weaning. Introduction of solids is usually considered at around 4–5 months of age. Delayed weaning is associated with iron deficiency anaemia particularly in breast-fed infants.

5. Cow's milk. The introduction of 'doorstep' cow's milk should be deferred until the age of 1 year, as the protein and sodium contents are too high and the iron and vitamin content is too low. There is also some evidence that unmodified cow's milk can cause microscopic gastrointestinal bleeding in infancy and subclinical iron deficiency may occur. 'Follow-on' milks are now available which are similar in composition to cow's milk but have added iron and vitamins. These are suitable for infants over 6 months of age. Skimmed and semi-skimmed milk is not recommended for children because of their reduced energy contents.

Table 1. Human breast milk vs 'doorstep' cow's milk (composition per 100 ml)

Milk	kcal	KJ	Protein (g)	Fat (g)	CHO (g)	Na (mg)
Human	65–75	270–315	1.2–1.4 (whey:casein = 60:40)	3.7–4.8	7.1–7.8	15
Cow's	68	284	3.3 (whey:casein = 20:80)	4.0	4.9	56

Normal requirements

The recommended volume of feed for a young infant is approximately 150 ml/kg/day (105 kcal/kg/day) but there is enormous variation in requirements and good growth is evidence of sufficient intake. (*Note* 1oz = 30 ml). Daily energy requirements are approximately 80–120 kcal/kg during the first year and decrease by ~10 kcal/kg per year over the subsequent 3 years. Energy requirements are increased during periods of rapid growth and development (e.g. puberty) and during fever (raises basal metabolic rate by 10% for each degree of fever).

Assessment of nutritional status

- Anthropometry – height, weight, head circumference, skin fold thickness, mid-upper arm circumference.
- Clinical evidence of iron or vitamin deficiency, e.g. rickets, anaemia.
- Body mass index = wt (kg)/ht^2 (m).
- Body composition analysis, bone mineral density
- Blood tests, e.g. haematological indices (iron deficiency), albumin, calcium group, vitamin levels.

Vitamin deficiencies

Vitamin deficiencies are rare in the UK. Supplemention is not needed routinely but should be considered for children at high risk of deficiency, e.g. prematurity, vegan mother, poor diet, malabsorption, chronic renal or liver failure.

- vitamin A (retinol) deficiency causes xerophthalmia, the major preventable cause of childhood blindness worldwide.
- vitamin B_1 (thiamine) deficiency causes infantile beri beri.
- vitamin B_2 (riboflavin) deficiency causes angular stomatitis, fissuring of lips.
- nicotinic acid deficiency causes pellagra.
- vitamin B_{12} deficiency causes megaloblastic anaemia, glossitis, neurological complications.

- vitamin C (ascorbic acid) deficiency causes scurvy. Results in impaired collagen synthesis. Perifollicular haemorrhage is an early feature.
- vitamin D deficiency causes nutritional rickets (see related topic Calcium metabolism, p. 56).

Nutritional support for the ill child

1. Enteral nutrition. This is the method of choice if the small bowel is intact. Specialized formula feeds may be given via nasogastric tube or gastrostomy.

Situations in which enteral feeds might be useful include:

- Prematurity
- Neurological disorders leading to poor feeding, e.g. cerebral palsy.
- Anatomical problems of the oropharynx, e.g. severe cleft lip and palate.
- Chronic cardiorespiratory disease, e.g. heart failure secondary to a moderate VSD (to improve weight gain prior to surgery), cystic fibrosis (improved nutrition may reduce severity and frequency of chest infections).
- To maintain hydration during an acute illness, e.g. bronchiolitis, gastroenteritis.
- Chronic renal failure.
- Chronic liver disease.
- Severe anorexia nervosa.
- Crohn's disease – elemental formula feed may be indicated for the induction of remission.

2. Total parenteral nutrition (TPN). When the gut cannot be used, TPN provides a balanced preparation of amino acids, lipids, carbohydrates, vitamins, electrolytes and trace elements. Ideally, a catheter should be placed in a central vein but TPN can be given via peripheral veins for short periods. Complications of TPN administration include burns and scarring secondary to extravascation, central line infection or occlusion, bacterial endocarditis, electrolyte imbalance, cholestatic jaundice, hyperglycaemia, hyperlipidaemia, and trace metal deficiency. Electrolytes, liver function tests, and blood levels of vitamins and trace elements should be monitored regularly. Long-term bowel rest may lead to small intestinal and pancreatic atrophy so enteral feeds should be introduced as soon as possible.

Further reading

Aihie Sayer A, Cooper C, Barker DJP. Is lifespan determined *in utero*? *Archives of Disease in Childhood,* 1997; **77:** F162–4.

Barker DJP. *Mothers, Babies, and Disease in Later Life.* London: BMJ Publishing Group, 1994.

Barker DJP, Gluckman PD, Godfrey KM *et al.* Fetal nutrition and cardiovascular disease in adult life. *Lancet,* 1993; **341:** 938–41.

Dalzell AM, Dodge JA. Enteral nutrition. *Current Paediatrics,* 1992; **2** (3): 168–71.

Department of Health. *Weaning and the Weaning Diet.* HMSO, 1994.

Howie PW, Forsyth JS, Ogston SA, Clark A, Florey C du V. Protective effect of breastfeeding against infection. *British Medical Journal,* 1990; **300:** 11–16.

Lucas A, Morley R, Cole TJ *et al.* Early diet in preterm babies and developmental status at 18 months. *Lancet,* 1990; **335:** 1477–81.

Wilson AC, Forsyth JS, Greene SA *et al.* Relation of infant diet to childhood health: seven year follow up of cohort children in Dundee infant feeding study. *British Medical Journal,* 1998; **7124:** 21–5.

Related topics of interest

Anaemia (p. 31)
Calcium metabolism (p. 56)
Chronic diarrhoea (p. 77)
Failure to thrive (p. 138)

ORTHOPAEDIC PROBLEMS IN CHILDHOOD

There is a wide range in normality for limb shape and the development of gait. Even where it is outside the normal range, a problem may be a cosmetic rather than functional one.

The spine

1. Congenital abnormalities may be isolated or associated with other abnormalities. They may lead to obvious deformity (such as hemi vertebrae) or may be picked up incidentally on imaging (such as 'butterfly' vertebrae in Alagille syndrome). Syndromes which include spinal abnormalities include Klippel-Feil, the mucopolysaccharridoses and VATER anomaly.

2. Back pain should always be taken seriously in childhood and malignancy and infection excluded. Scheuerman's epiphysitis presents as a painful thoracic kyphosis. The aetiology is unknown and diagnosis is radiological.

3. Scoliosis may be postural (due to pelvic tilt) or fixed. Idiopathic scoliosis is commonest in adolescent girls. Scoliosis may be secondary to muscle imbalance (e.g. in cerebral palsy or muscular dystrophy) or bony abnormality (e.g. vertebral collapse or hemi vertebra). It is also more common in certain conditions such as neurofibromatosis. Problems are cosmetic, pain, and if severe, respiratory difficulties. A transient scoliosis may occur with pneumonia.

Lower limbs

Examination should include observing the gait with the child barefoot and examining the lower limb joints and neurology and the shoes for wear pattern.

1. In-toeing is very common in small children. Spontaneous resolution is the norm. Causes include:

- Metatarsus adductus. The commonest cause in toddlers. The forefoot is adducted and supinated.
- Medial tibial torsion. Presents at around 3–6 years with internal rotation of the trans-malleolar axis. There may be associated tibial bowing.
- Persistent femoral anteversion. Occurs more commonly in girls and the entire lower leg is internally rotated. The child commonly sits in the 'W' position which should be discouraged to promote resolution.

2. *Out-toeing* is less common unless associated with slipped upper femoral epiphysis when it is usually unilateral. Causes are external tibial torsion or femoral retroversion.

3. *Genu valgus* or knock knees are common between 3 and 5 years and may represent a physiological correction of genu varum. Resolution usually occurs by age 8. Operation may be necessary in adolescence for persistent deformity. Pathological causes include renal osteodystrophy, congenital dislocation of the patella and neuromuscular problems such as cerebral palsy.

4. *Genu varum* or bow-legs, are usually physiological and may be associated with medial tibial torsion. Unilateral deformity is more likely to pathological. Causes include Blount's disease, epiphyseal injury, rickets or bone dysplasia such as achondroplasia.

5. *Flat feet* may be painful or painless. All toddlers have painless flat feet until they develop medial arches at the age of 2–3 years. Older children may have flat feet due to lax ligaments, but when they go onto tip toe the arch should form. If it does not the foot is abnormal and a neurological cause should be suspected. Painful flat feet are usually due to a talo-navicular bar which may need surgical excision.

6. *Osgood-Schlatter disease* affects boys more than girls and is thought to be due to recurrent trauma to the tibial tubercle, where it attaches to the patella tendon, during rapid growth in active children. It presents with swelling, tenderness and prominence of the tibial tubercle. Resolution takes 12–24 months and requires rest and restriction of activities.

Upper limbs

1. *Sprengel's shoulder.* This is caused by failure of the scapula to descend during fetal development and so the shoulder on the affected side is abnormally high.

2. *Radial abnormalities.* The radius may be absent or abnormal in a number of rare syndromes such as thrombocytopenia and absent radius syndrome (TAR), Holt–Oram syndrome and Fanconi's anaemia.

3. *Hand abnormalities.* Trigger finger is caused by a thickening in the flexor tendon which may need surgical release if it becomes fixed in flexion. Polydactyly may be

simple or complex depending on whether there is bone in the extra digit. Surgery may be required for removal of the extra digit which will otherwise interfere with hand function and be cosmetically undesirable.

Further reading

Behrman RE, ed. Torsional and angular deformities. In: *Nelson Textbook of Paediatrics*, 15th edn. Philadelphia: WB Saunders, 1996; 1925–34.

England SP, ed. Common orthopedic problems I and II. In: *Paediatric Clinics of North America*, 1996; **42:** 4.

Related topics of interest

Juvenile chronic arthritis (p. 229)
Limping (p. 239)
Newborn examination (p. 296)

PERIPHERAL NEUROPATHY

Peripheral nerve disorders may affect sensory and/or motor nerves, involving one nerve (mononeuropathy) or causing a more generalized neuropathy (polyneuropathy). A neuropathy can present acutely (e.g. foot drop, facial palsy) or more chronically with muscle wasting and weakness. Sensory nerve involvement results in paraesthesia or anaesthesia, typically of the hands and feet. Neurophysiology shows slowed nerve conduction velocity and muscle biopsy may show denervation.

Aetiology

- Trauma. Birth injuries, fractures.
- Hereditary degenerative. Motor and sensory neuropathies, peroneal muscular atrophy (Charcot–Marie–Tooth).
- Metabolic. Diabetic (rare in childhood), Refsum's disease, metachromatic leucodystrophy.
- Toxins. Vincristine, lead, solvent abuse.
- Deficiencies. B_{12}, thiamine (rarely cause neuropathy in childhood).
- Parainfectious. Guillain–Barré syndrome.
- Idiopathic.

Guillain–Barré syndrome

This is an uncommon condition which mainly affects older children and adults but has been reported in infants as young as 6 months. A mild preceding febrile illness is common. Typically, there is sudden onset of symmetrical flaccid paralysis affecting the legs first and then ascending to involve the trunk and arms. Sensory loss is often a prominent early feature in children, with paraesthesiae causing severe limb pain and ataxia. Limb weakness and hyporeflexia may be unimpressive initially, leading to difficulties with diagnosis. Meningism and papilloedema are present in about one-third of cases and may cause further diagnostic confusion. Progression of muscle weakness may continue for several days and even weeks. Involvement of respiratory muscles necessitates mechanical ventilation in 10–20% of cases. In severe cases bilateral facial palsy and bulbar palsy occur. Autonomic involvement may cause hypertension and arrhythmias, excessive sweating, disturbed gut function and urinary retention.

The condition is usually self-limiting, with more than 80% making a full recovery, but the convalescent period may be very prolonged.

The underlying pathophysiology is demyelination of the peripheral nerves, which is thought to occur as a result of an autoimmune reaction. Suggested aetiological agents include mycoplasma and viruses, such as coxsackie B and Epstein–Barr virus.

Investigation

- CSF. Raised protein (may be normal early in illness). Normal white cell count.
- Viral cultures and serology, Paul Bunnell test.
- Neurophysiology (may be normal early in illness).

- Urine for porphyrin screen. Exclude acute intermittent porphyria.
- U&E. Exclude hypokalaemic periodic paralysis.
- Radiology. Exclude spinal cause of flaccid paralysis.
- Toxicology screen, e.g. exclude lead poisoning.

Management

1. *Supportive care.* If Guillain–Barré syndrome is suspected, the child should be admitted. A peak flow rate is measured 4-hourly in older children. Transcutaneous oxygen monitoring is useful in children unable to do a peak flow, and arterial blood gas measurements may be necessary. A falling peak flow rate, hypoxia, hypercarbia and exhaustion are indications for ventilation. The blood pressure should be monitored for evidence of autonomic involvement and the child may require catheterization for urinary retention. Regular turning and passive exercises help prevent the development of pressure sores and contractures. Pain relief may be needed for severe muscle pain. Nutrition is important and fluids should be given intravenously because of the risk of aspiration. Paralysis without impairment of awareness can be terrifying and requires reassurance and good communication. Sedation may be indicated.

2. *Specific treatments.* Steroids have not been shown to improve the outcome. Plasmapheresis may produce a clinical improvement and speed recovery if used early in the acute phase, but should be reserved for the most severely affected patients. Intravenous gammaglobulin has been reported to be helpful but has only been used in small studies.

Outcome

3. *Rehabilitative physiotherapy.* Acute mortality from respiratory failure and arrhythmias (including cardiac arrest) is now less than 5%. Over 80% make a complete recovery, but this may take several years. Severity of initial weakness does not correlate with long-term prognosis, but evidence of early improvement (before 3 weeks) is a good prognostic indicator.

Facial palsy

Aetiology

- Idiopathic (Bell's palsy).
- Infections, e.g. Ramsay Hunt (herpes zoster), infectious mononucleosis, mastoiditis, Lyme disease (characteristic rash, polyarthritis).
- Trauma, e.g. forceps delivery.

- CNS leukaemia.
- CNS tumour, e.g. pontine glioma.
- Hypertension.
- Guillain–Barré syndrome – usually bilateral.
- Myasthenia gravis.
- Post-ictal (Todd's paralysis).
- Drugs, e.g. vincristine.

Clinical features

Facial palsy in childhood is usually idiopathic, but may be associated with viral infections or Lyme disease. There is sudden onset of lower motor neurone weakness of one side of the face. Problems include conjunctivitis and corneal abrasion (owing to inability to close the eye), dribbling and slurring of speech. There may be facial pain either at the onset or during recovery. More than 80% will recover spontaneously with some improvement seen within 3 weeks.

Management

1. Careful history and clinical examination. Exclude hypertension and features of an intracranial tumour (headache, vomiting, other neurological signs), CNS leukaemia (bruising, anaemia) and middle ear disease. The majority of cases will be idiopathic and require symptomatic treatment and observation only. Investigations such as FBC, viral titres, Lyme disease serology or brain imaging may be indicated on the basis of clinical findings.

2. Pain relief and prevention of conjunctival irritation. Taping eye closed, artificial tears.

3. Steroids. May be beneficial if given within the first 48 hours, but the evidence to support their use is mixed. FBC to exclude leukaemia is essential before giving steroids.

4. Surgery. A few cases do not resolve and these patients may require plastic surgery to restore facial symmetry and protect the eye.

Lead poisoning

Chronic lead poisoning is a rare cause of peripheral neuropathy. Other features include anorexia, vomiting, abdominal pain, constipation, behavioural problems and failure to thrive. More severe poisoning may cause an encephalopathy with seizures, drowsiness and coma. Sources of lead include paint, old water pipes, batteries, surma eye make-up used by Asians and pollution. Symptoms are unlikely if the blood lead level is $< 80\ \mu g/100$ ml.

Investigations show a microcytic hypochromic anaemia, basophilic stippling, raised plasma δ-aminolaevulinic acid and free erythrocyte porphyrin, and raised urinary coproporphyrin. Radiographs may show lead lines at the end of long bones. Management consists of identifying and removing the source of lead and the use of chelating agents (e.g. D-penicillamine, EDTA).

Further reading

Korintherberg R, Mönting JS. Natural history and treatment effects in Guillain–Barré syndrome: a multicentre study. *Archives of Disease in Childhood,* 1996; **74:** 281–7.

The Guillain–Barré Study Group. Plasmapheresis and acute Guillain–Barré syndrome. *Neurology,* 1985; **35:** 1096–104.

Related topic of interest

Floppy infant (p. 150)

POISONING

Accidental poisoning is very common, resulting in over 40 000 attendances at casualty each year. It is most common in young children, particularly 1–3 year olds. A wide variety of medicines, household products and plants are ingested. Fewer than 30 children a year die as a result of poisoning, but large numbers of children are seen and observed in an attempt to prevent these occasional deaths. Education of parents about the dangers of poisoning and the use of lockable cupboards, childproof containers and blister packaging have all helped to reduce the incidence of serious poisoning.

Intentional self-poisoning (suicide, parasuicide) is most common in young people in their teens. Full psychiatric and social assessment is essential during hospital admission. Poisoning may also result from alcohol or solvent abuse. There may be no history of poisoning, but if a previously well child presents with unexplained symptoms (e.g. drowsiness, coma, convulsions, respiratory depression) then a diagnosis of poisoning should be considered, and blood and urine should be saved for toxicology.

Management

Establish exactly what and how much has been ingested, and how long ago. Advice can be sought from regional poisons units on the possible toxic effects of various substances, and the availabilty of antidotes or specific removal methods (e.g. alkaline diuresis). The majority of children do not have serious symptoms, but occasionally a child presents with respiratory depression, hypotension or reduced consciousness and requires cardiorespiratory resuscitation and support.

1. Activated charcoal is now widely used because it binds most poisonous substances, preventing systemic absorption. Repeated doses are recommended after ingestion of aspirin, barbiturates or theophylline. It is not recommended for iron or alcohol.

2. Emesis. Traditionally ipecachauna syrup was given to induce vomiting after ingestion. Evidence now suggests that emesis is only useful within 1 hour after ingestion. It remains the treatment of choice for substances that do not bind to charcoal.

3. Gastric lavage is indicated when significant amounts of poison, at high lethality, have been ingested. Intubation may be necessary for children with a reduced conscious level to protect the airway.

Salicylates

Problems

- Hyperventilation. Deep sighing respirations due to metabolic acidosis.
- Hyperglycaemia.
- Tinnitus.
- Hyperpyrexia, vasodilatation, sweating.
- Vomiting and abdominal pain.
- Dehydration.

Management

1. Gastric lavage can be undertaken up to 4 hours after ingestion as aspirin slows stomach emptying.

2. Repeated charcoal doses are recommended for ingestion of sustained preparations.

3. Measure blood salicylate level at 2 hours post- ingestion and repeat regularly as levels will increase over the first 6 hours. A level of <40 mg/100 ml requires no treatment. Admit the child if the level is > 40 mg/100 ml, or if the child is symptomatic. If the level is mildly raised (40–65 mg/100 ml) encourage a high fluid intake and commence i.v. fluids if the patient is not drinking well. If the level is high (> 65 mg/100 ml) alkalinization can be achieved by giving sodium bicarbonate by slow infusion. Forced diuresis is no longer recommended.

4. Supportive management of severe poisoning. Monitor acid–base status (metabolic acidosis, respiratory alkalosis), blood glucose (mild to moderate hyperglycaemia), U&E and prothrombin time. Tepid sponging may be necessary for hyperpyrexia. Strict fluid balance is essential with the risk of fluid overload from alkalinization, and the risk of dehydration from vomiting, hyperpyrexia and hyperglycaemia.

Paracetamol

Problems

- Nausea and vomiting. Lack of early symptoms other than some nausea and vomiting may be deceptive.
- Acute hepatic failure. Damage due to hepatocellular necrosis is maximal at 3–4 days post ingestion and leads to confusion, drowsiness, coagulopathy and jaundice.
- Acute tubular necrosis.

Management

1. *Activated charcoal* is currently recommended to reduce absorption.

2. *Measure blood paracetamol level* at least 4 hours post-ingestion and compare with a nomogram of level against time since ingestion. A level of < 200 μg/ml at 4 hours requires no treatment. Levels above a line joining 200 μg/ml at 4 hours and 30 μg/ml at 15 hours on a semilogarithmic graph require treatment. Patients on liver enzyme-inducing drugs (e.g. carbamazepine) may develop toxicity at lower paracetamol levels.

3. *Methionine or acetylcysteine.* These protect the liver if given within 12 hours of ingestion. Methionine is given orally as four doses over the first 12 hours. Acetylcysteine is given as an i.v. infusion over 20 hours.

4. *Monitor prothrombin time and liver function tests* for 3–4 days for evidence of hepatocellular damage if the paracetamol level was high.

5. *Supportive management of acute liver failure.*

Iron

Problems

- Phase 1 (6–12 hours), gastric irritation. Nausea, vomiting, abdominal pain, gastrointestinal haemorrhage.
- Phase 2 (12–24 hours), quiescent phase. Asymptomatic. Deposition of iron in the liver.
- Phase 3 (onset 16–24 hours), cardiovascular collapse, acute encephalopathy and hepatic failure.
- Phase 4, pyloric scarring and stenosis. If phase 3 is survived.

Management

1. *Initial resuscitation* of shocked child, may require intubation and ventilation.

2. *Gastric lavage* is recommended once airway is secured. Charcoal is not helpful.

3. *Desferrioxamine* can be left in the stomach following lavage to chelate the iron. Desferrioxamine by i.v. infusion is indicated if the serum iron level is > 5 mg/l.

4. Supportive management.

Tricyclic antidepressants

Problems

- Anticholinergic effects. Tachycardia, dilated pupils, convulsions.
- Cardiac effects. Arrhythmias and conduction delay.

Management

1. Convulsions should be treated with regular medication.

2. Arrhythmias are treated with phenytoin, which enhances conduction, or lignocaine.

3. Alkalinization (arterial pH 7.5), using sodium bicarbonate and hyperventilation, can reduce the toxic effects on the heart.

Opiates (including methadone)

Problems

- Bradycardia.
- Hypotension.
- Small pupils.

Management

1. Stabilize the airway, breathing and circulation.

2. Give Naloxone (antidote). Initial bolus may need repeating or start a continuous infusion.

Further reading

Poisoning. In: Advanced life support group. *Advanced Paediatric Life Support – the Practical Approach,* 2nd edn. London: BMJ Publications, 1997; 129–34.

Related topics of interest

Accidents (p. 7)
Adolescent health (p. 19)
Cardiac arrest (p. 61)
Jaundice (p. 225)
Liver disease (p. 244)
Shock (p. 344)

POLYURIA AND RENAL TUBULAR DISORDERS

Polyuria is the passing of excessive amounts of urine. It is a frequent presenting symptom which may indicate renal, metabolic or endocrine disease.

Aetiology

(a) Excessive fluid intake
(b) Renal disease
- Renal tubular disorders.
- Acute tubular necrosis – recovery phase.
- Chronic renal failure.
- Nephrogenic diabetes insipidus.

(c) Metabolic/endocrine disorders
- Diabetes mellitus.
- Diabetes insipidus.
- Hypercalcaemia.
- Adrenogenital syndrome.
- Conn's syndrome.

(d) Drugs, e.g. antihistamines

Diabetes insipidus

Diabetes insipidus (DI) is the inability to concentrate urine because of total or partial vasopressin (antidiuretic hormone, ADH) deficiency. Large amounts of dilute urine are passed and polydipsia maintains the plasma osmolality in the normal range. If oral intake is inadequate, hypernatraemic dehydration results. ADH is synthesized in the supraoptic hypothalamic neurones and then stored in the posterior pituitary. Secretion is controlled by plasma osmolality. Central DI may result from hypothalamic disease (e.g. craniopharyngioma, Langerhans cell histiocytosis) but is often idiopathic. It may be associated with other pituitary hormone deficiencies. Treatment is with synthetic ADH (DDAVP) given by nasal spray (occasionally orally). Unresponsiveness of the distal tubules and collecting ducts of the kidney to ADH may also cause polyuria and polydipsia (nephrogenic DI). It is present at birth and occurs mainly in boys. No specific treatment is available other than adequate fluid replacement and reduction of dietary solute load.

Investigation of polyuria

1. *History and examination.* Including age, duration of symptoms, family history, any evidence of failure to thrive, muscle weakness, headaches and visual disturbance, rickets or bone pain.

2. *Urinalysis.* For glucose, amino acids, pH – excludes diabetes mellitus and most renal tubular disorders if normal.

3. Paired urine and plasma osmolalities and a water deprivation test to distinguish between central and nephrogenic DI and psychogenic polydipsia. (*Note*: Water deprivation is potentially dangerous in DI and the test should be carefully monitored. The child should be weighed 2-hourly and the test must be discontinued if the weight falls below 97.5% of the starting weight.) Plasma osmolality will be normal or raised in both types of DI, and normal or low in psychogenic polydipsia (normal = 275–295 mosmol/l). The urine osmolality is inappropriately low (50–200 mosmol/l) in DI with failure to concentrate >300 mosmol/l following water deprivation (normally concentrate to >750 mosmol/l). DDAVP raises the urine osmolality in central DI but not in nephrogenic DI. In psychogenic polydipsia urine osmolality is appropriately low and, although concentrating ability may be impaired, it should still rise to >500 mosmol/l on water deprivation.

Renal tubular disorders

Eighty per cent of the glomerular filtrate is reabsorbed in the proximal tubules of the kidney (mainly sodium, chloride, phosphate, glucose, amino acids and water). Bicarbonate is regenerated by carbonic anhydrase and reabsorbed in exchange for hydrogen ions. Further sodium and water are reabsorbed in exchange for potassium or hydrogen ions in the distal tubules under the control of the renin–angiotensin system. Defects in this process of absorption and secretion may be confined to a specific transport system or cause a generalized transport defect. Many of these defects are genetically determined.

Problems

- Electrolyte imbalance.
- Polyuria, polydipsia.
- Failure to thrive.
- Muscle weakness.
- Rickets.

1. Proximal tubule defects

(a) Generalized transport defects

- Fanconi's syndrome
  - Primary
    - Cystinosis.
    - Adult-type.
  - Secondary
    - Heavy metals (e.g. lead, cadmium).
    - Wilson's disease.
    - Hereditary fructose intolerance.
    - Galactosaemia.

Tetracycline which has deteriorated.
Tyrosinosis.

- Lowe's (oculo-cerebro-renal) syndrome.

(b) Specific transport defects

- Cystinuria. This is a disorder of intestinal absorption and renal tubular reabsorption of dibasic amino acids (cystine, lysine, arginine, ornithine). There is a risk of multiple calculi formation. It occurs in 1 in 600 of the population, but calculi form in only 3%.
- Hartnup disease. Failure of renal and intestinal absorption of tryptophan results in a deficiency of its metabolite nicotinamide. This causes a pellagra-type rash.
- Familial hypophosphataemic rickets (vitamin D-resistant rickets). This is an X-linked dominant condition. The rickets is due to the impaired renal reabsorption of phosphate.
- Renal tubular acidosis type 2 (proximal RTA).

2. *Distal tubule defects*

- Nephrogenic diabetes insipidus.
- Renal tubular acidosis type 1 (distal RTA).

Renal tubular acidosis (RTA)

1. *Distal RTA.* This is much more common than proximal RTA. It is due to failure of the distal tubules to excrete hydrogen ions. It is usually primary but may be secondary, e.g. following vitamin D intoxication, amphotericin toxicity or renal transplantation. Features include:

- Hyperchloraemic acidosis.
- Nephrocalcinosis.
- Rickets secondary to bone resorption to buffer the acidosis.
- Failure to thrive and weakness.
- Hyponatraemia and hypokalaemia due to increased urinary loss.
- Polyuria.
- Inappropriately alkaline urine and inability to acidify urine (ammonium chloride test).

2. *Proximal RTA.* This is due to increased bicarbonate loss secondary to a defect in bicarbonate reabsorption. It may be primary but often occurs as part of Fanconi's syndrome. It is usually sporadic but may be inherited. Primary proximal RTA with no associated glycosuria or aminoaciduria is more common in boys, and usually presents in infancy with failure

to thrive, muscle weakness and persistent vomiting. There is a hyperchloraemic acidosis with appropriately acidic urine. Nephrocalcinosis is very rare.

Fanconi's syndrome

This is a generalized defect of proximal tubular function resulting in excess glucose, amino acids, uric acid, phosphate, sodium, potassium, bicarbonate and protein in the urine. The defect may be primary or secondary to tubular damage in other conditions (see above). Presenting features include failure to thrive, anorexia, vomiting, polyuria, polydipsia, rickets, muscle weakness, hypotonia, paralytic ileus and acute dehydration with metabolic acidosis. The primary defect is divided into two forms which affect both sexes equally:

1. Cystinosis (Lignac–Fanconi syndrome). This is a severe autosomal recessive condition in which cystine is deposited in many tissues. Renal tubular deposition and progressive glomerular damage lead to renal failure in early life. Cystine crystals can be identified in bone marrow, on renal biopsy or by slit-lamp examination of the cornea.

2. Adult-type Fanconi's syndrome. The inheritance of this condition is less clear. It is not associated with cystinosis, and progression to renal failure is slow.

Further reading

Perheentura J. The neurohypophysis and water regulation. In: Brook CGD, ed. *Clinical Paediatric Endocrinology*, 3rd edn. Oxford: Blackwell Science, 1995; 580–615.

Related topics of interest

Adrenal disorders (p. 23)
Chronic renal failure (p. 82)
Diabetes mellitus (p. 119)

PREMATURITY

Prematurity is defined as delivery before 37 completed weeks of gestation and is the second most common cause of neonatal death after malformation. Survival rates have improved with advances in perinatal and neonatal intensive care over the last 20 years. The majority of infants over 32 weeks' gestation who weigh over 1500 g are now expected to survive. Some infants delivered as early as 22 weeks have survived with intensive care, but those of less than 500 g or 22 weeks are considered unviable in most centres. Low birth weight (LBW < 2500 g) infants account for about 6% of the total births, and very low birth weight infants (VLBW < 1500 g) make up less than 1% of the total. An infant may be both small for gestational age and preterm. Premature delivery is due to either preterm labour or obstetric intervention when the risks to the mother or the fetus of continuing the pregnancy are very high, e.g. pre-eclamptic toxaemia (PET), severe IUGR. Prematurity is more common in young mothers, smokers, those with poor socioeconomic backgrounds and those with a previous history of a preterm delivery.

Problems

- Hypothermia.
- Hypoglycaemia.
- Respiratory distress.
- Nutrition.
- Jaundice.
- Susceptibility to infections.
- Necrotizing enterocolitis.
- Patent ductus arteriosus.
- Haemorrhagic and ischaemic cerebral lesions.
- Retinopathy of prematurity.
- Neurodevelopmental outcome.
- Parent–child bonding.

Aetiology of preterm labour

- Idiopathic (~ 50%).
- Multiple pregnancy.
- Antepartum haemorrhage.
- Premature rupture of membranes.
- Polyhydramnios.
- Cervical incompetence, e.g. previous surgery, congenital.
- Uterine malformations, e.g. bicornuate uterus.
- Maternal illness, e.g. diabetes mellitus, PET, intercurrent viral infection, UTI.
- Infection, e.g. *Listeria*. Other organisms (e.g. *Mycoplasma hominis, Ureaplasma urealyticum*) may have a role in the aetiology of premature rupture of membranes.

Survival

For infants born after 32 weeks' gestation without congenital abnormality there is over 95% survival. Those of between 30 and 32 weeks have a survival rate of 90–95%, and this falls to 75–80% for those of between 28 and 30 weeks. Infants of 28 weeks' gestation or less show improved survival when treated in recognized neonatal intensive care units. At 26 weeks ~ 45% survive, at 24 weeks only ~ 30% survive and at 23 weeks less than 10% survive.

Intraventricular haemorrhage (IVH) and hypoxic-ischaemic encephalopathy (HIE)

Impaired autoregulation of cerebral blood flow, cardiopulmonary instability, sepsis and metabolic derangements predispose the preterm infant to cerebral haemorrhage and ischaemia. Haemorrhage arises from friable capillaries of the germinal layer and may be limited to this layer, or extend into the ventricular space or the surrounding parenchyma. In 25–30% of infants < 1500 g an IVH will develop, and 90% occur by the third day of life. Many are small, clinically silent and have no sequelae. A fall in the haematocrit may be the only clue. Large haemorrhages may result in death or neurological sequelae as a result of periventricular cerebral injury or progressive hydrocephalus. Thirty per cent of IVHs increase in size in the first week of life, and post-haemorrhagic hydrocephalus is common following moderate and large IVHs. Hydrocephalus becomes static or resolves spontaneously in >50% of cases but, if progressive, serial lumbar punctures or ventricular shunts may be needed. There is no evidence that Caesarean delivery reduces the incidence of IVH, and the role of prophylactic treatments (e.g. ethamsylate, vitamin E) is unclear.

HIE is associated with perinatal and post-natal asphyxia. Cerebral ischaemia may result from a period of hypotension and occurs particularly in arterial watershed areas (e.g. periventricular leucomalacia, PVL).

Retinopathy of prematurity (ROP)

ROP is a vasoproliferative retinopathy which can result in retinal detachment and blindness. The underlying mechanism by which damage to the immature retina occurs is still poorly understood. The association with hyperoxia has been well documented, but there is no absolute level of arterial oxygen tension above which ROP will occur, and it is occasionally seen in infants who have never received supplemental oxygen. Risk factors include low gestation, low birth weight (particularly < 1000 g), and multiple birth. It is associated with ischaemic and haemorrhagic cerebral lesions and almost all cases have neurological impairment at follow-up. All infants under 31 weeks gestation and < 1500 g should be screened with indirect ophthalmology at 7–9 weeks of age. Acute changes are seen in 70–80% of infants < 1000 g but many regress. Severe ROP has a 50% risk of causing blindness if not treated. Treatment is with cryotherapy. Results of surgery once the retina has become detached are poor.

Neurodevelopmental outcome

About 15–20% of surviving infants of < 1000 g and about 10% of those of 1000–1500 g have a moderately serious disability. Between 8 and 10% of surviving infants of 24–25 weeks' gestation have a major impairment (e.g. cerebral palsy, blindness). Prematurity is particularly associated with spastic diplegia and relative sparing of intellect. There is no conclusive evidence about the cause of neurological sequelae, but the sickest infants are at the greatest risk. Ischaemic and moderate to severe haemorrhagic cerebral lesions detected on US scan are predictive of a worse neurological outcome. Magnetic resonance studies have shown an association between deranged cerebral energy metabolism in the first week and neurodevelopmental impairment at 1 year of age. The effects of early diet on long-term neurodevelopment and intellect are controversial.

Further reading

Campbell AGM. Follow-up studies. In: Roberton NRC, ed. *Textbook of Neonatology,* 2nd edn. Edinburgh: Churchill Livingstone, 1992: 43–74.

Rennie JM. Perinatal management at the lower margin of viability. *Archives of Disease in Childhood,* 1996; **74:** F214–8.

Report of Joint Working Party of The Royal College of Ophthalmologists and British Association of Perinatal Medicine. *Retinopathy of Prematurity: Guidelines for Screening and Treatment.* London: Royal College of Ophthalmologists, 1995.

Ventriculomegaly trial group. Randomised trial of early tapping in neonatal posthaemorrhagic ventricular dilatation. *Archives of Disease in Childhood*, 1990: **65:** 3–10.

Related topics of interest

Neonatal jaundice (p. 276)
Neonatal respiratory distress (p. 281)

PUBERTY – PRECOCIOUS AND DELAYED

Puberty is a period of changing patterns of hormone secretion resulting in physical and physiological changes which culminate in sexual maturation and fertility. There is great variability in the onset of these changes, but 95% of girls will have commenced puberty by the age of 13 years and 95% of boys will have commenced before the age of 14 years. Precocious puberty may be central (true) resulting from activation of the hypothalamic–pituitary–gonadal axis, or peripheral (false), involving an abnormal pathway and usually resulting in incomplete maturity. Precocious puberty is more common in girls (10:1) but is usually idiopathic. In boys, the majority will have a pathological cause and they therefore require more careful investigation. Delayed puberty is more common in boys and is usually constitutional.

Normal puberty

Normal puberty requires the secretion of both growth hormone and sex steroids. Pulsatile release of gonadotrophin-releasing hormone (GnRH) from the hypothalamus is initially nocturnal, and stimulates release of luteinizing hormone (LH) and follicle-stimulating hormone (FSH) from the pituitary. Spikes of hormone release are detected before clinical signs of puberty, and these increase in amplitude and frequency as puberty progresses. By late puberty, pulsatile LH and FSH secretion occurs throughout the 24 hours. The average duration of puberty is 2–3 years.

Girls

LH stimulates ovulation and FSH stimulates release of oestradiol from the ovaries. Breast development is the first sign of puberty. The growth spurt occurs early in puberty with the attainment of breast stage B2, and continues to menarche and breast stage B4.

Boys

LH stimulates release of testosterone from the testes. FSH stimulates spermatogenesis and thus determines testicular volume. Puberty starts approximately 0.6 years later than in girls, the first indication being increase of testicular volume to 4 ml. The growth spurt occurs later in puberty than in girls, when the testicular volume has reached 10–12 ml.

Children requiring investigation

- Girls commencing puberty < 8 years.
- Boys commencing puberty < 9 years.
- Lack of any pubertal development in a girl > 13 years or a boy > 14 years.
- Puberty which pursues an abnormal sequence or stops before completion.

Precocious puberty

Aetiology

1. Central/true

- Idiopathic.
- Intracranial tumours.
- Hydrocephalus.
- Radiotherapy (e.g. CNS prophylaxis in the treatment of leukaemia).
- Post-infection, e.g. meningitis
- Neurofibromatosis.
- McCune–Albright syndrome (*café au lait* patches, polyostotic fibrous dysplasia, precocious puberty. Commoner in girls. GnRH independent).
- Ectopic gonadotrophin release, e.g. hepatoblastoma.

2. Peripheral/false

- Ovarian, testicular or adrenal tumours.
- Virilizing congenital adrenal hyperplasia.
- Exogenous sex steroids.

Clinical features

If a child shows signs of early pubertal development it is important to decide if the normal sequence of physical development (consonant with puberty) has occurred. This suggests stimulation of the hypothalamic–pituitary–gonadal axis (true precocious puberty) usually by premature activation of GnRH pulsatility. In the majority of girls this is idiopathic, but in boys a central precipitating cause should be suspected. If there is lack of consonance (e.g. pubic hair and acne without breast development) peripheral causes should be considered (false precocious puberty). Signs of virilization associated with hypertension suggest an adrenal cause. Early breast development (premature thelarche) with no other signs of puberty (i.e. normal growth rate, no pubic hair, appropriate bone age) is a benign condition due to isolated pulsatile FSH secretion which requires no treatment. Gynaecomastia in boys of pubertal age is extremely common and usually subsides as puberty progresses. Isolated vaginal bleeding may be due to a foreign body.

Investigation

- Growth assessment and pubertal staging.
- LH, FSH profiles. Pulsatile release is seen in true precocious puberty, low levels in false precocious puberty (research investigations).
- GnRH stimulation test. Elevated basal FSH and LH levels with exaggerated response to LHRH in true precocious puberty.

- Pelvic US. Multicystic appearance of pubertal ovaries.
- Bone age. Often advanced.
- CNS imaging. Always in boys, only if neurological signs in girls.
- Plasma 17-hydroxyprogesterone, plasma and urinary androgens, if virilized.
- Thyroid function. Thyroid-releasing hormone stimulates prolactin and FSH release as well as thyroid-stimulating hormone (TSH), so breast development in girls or testicular enlargement in boys may be seen in hypothyroidism.

Management

If a cause is identified it may be removed, although the endocrine abnormality may not resolve. GnRH analogues are used to arrest puberty by blocking pulsatile release of FSH and LH from the pituitary. They can be given intranasally, subcutaneously or by depot injection. Growth hormone may be given to accelerate growth in an attempt to compensate for advanced skeletal maturity.

Delayed puberty

Aetiology

- Constitutional in the majority.
- Primary gonadal failure (e.g. Turner's syndrome (XO), irradiation, chemotherapy).
- Secondary gonadal failure (e.g. hypogonadotrophic hypogonadism, pituitary or hypothalamic tumours).
- Chronic illness, anorexia nervosa.

Clinical features

If there are no signs of puberty, general history and examination may identify the presence of chronic illness. Constitutional pubertal delay is usually associated with short stature, whereas normal stature is usual in hypogonadotrophic hypogonadism. Features of Turner's syndrome may be present (see related topic Chromosomal abnormalities, p. 73). Incomplete or abnormal puberty (lack of consonance) is uncommon and causes include disorders of steroidogenesis and ACTH deficiency.

Investigation

- LH, FSH. Low in hypothalamo-pituitary problems (secondary gonadal failure due to decreased gonadotrophin release) and also in constitutional delay. Elevated in primary gonadal failure, e.g. Turner's syndrome. The GnRH stimulation test is unreliable in distinguishing hypogonadotrophic hypogonadism from simple pubertal delay.

- Bone age. Often delayed.
- Thyroid function tests.
- Chromosomes – particularly in girls to exclude Turner's syndrome.

Management

If constitutional delay is causing psychological distress, puberty may be induced with sex steroids in low doses. Hormone replacement treatment is indicated in Turner's syndrome.

Further reading

Brook CGD. Puberty. In: *A Guide to the Practice of Paediatric Endocrinology.* Cambridge University Press, 1993; 55–82.

Merke DP, Cutler GB. Evaluation and management of precocious puberty. *Archives of Disease in Childhood,* 1996; **75:** 269–71.

Related topics of interest

Chromosomal abnormalities (p. 73)
Growth assessment (p. 167)
Growth – short stature, tall stature (p. 171)

PURPURA AND BRUISING

Purpura and bruising may be due to thrombocytopenia, platelet dysfunction, a vascular problem or a coagulation factor deficiency. The commonest causes in childhood are trauma, Henoch–Schönlein purpura (HSP), idiopathic thrombocytopenic purpura (ITP) and leukaemia. Less common but important causes are meningococcal septicaemia and inherited coagulopathies, which are discussed elsewhere. Conjunctival haemorrhages and facial petechiae are common following raised intrathoracic pressure (e.g. whooping cough, vomiting, newborn following vaginal delivery) but may occur spontaneously in leukaemia and other bleeding disorders.

Aetiology

(a) Vascular

- Trauma (accidental, non-accidental).
- HSP.
- Infection, e.g. meningococcal sepsis.
- Rare, e.g. hereditary haemorrhagic telangiectasia.

(b) Thrombocytopenia ($< 150 \times 10^9$/l)

- ITP.
- Hypersplenism, e.g. haematological (spherocytosis), malignancy (lymphoma), infections (infectious mononucleosis), metabolic (Gaucher's disease).
- Consumption, e.g. DIC, giant haemangioma.
- Decreased production, e.g. bone marrow infiltration (leukaemia, neuroblastoma), drugs (chloramphenicol).
- Immune, e.g. drugs (quinine), autoimmune (SLE).

(c) Platelet dysfunction

- Drugs, e.g. aspirin.
- Metabolic, e.g. uraemia.
- Inherited, e.g. von Willebrand's, thrombasthenia.

(d) Coagulopathy

- Inherited (haemophilia, Christmas disease, von Willebrand's disease).
- Acquired (DIC, haemorrhagic disease of the newborn, liver disease).

Investigation

- FBC. The two most likely causes of thrombocytopenia are ITP and leukaemia. The platelet count is usually $< 30 \times 10^9$/l before abnormal bruising and petechiae occur.
- Partial thromboplastin test (PTT). This is a test of the intrinsic clotting factors (VIII, IX, XI, XII). It is abnormal in haemophilia, Christmas disease and von Willebrand's disease.
- Prothrombin time (PT). This is a test of the extrinsic clotting factors (II, V, VII, X). It is normal in haemophilia

and Christmas disease, prolonged in liver disease and vitamin K deficiency.

- Bleeding time. A prolonged bleeding time in the presence of a normal platelet count suggests platelet dysfunction, e.g. von Willebrand's disease, thrombasthenia.

Henoch–Schönlein purpura (HSP)

Problems

- Rash.
- Joint pains.
- Glomerulonephritis.
- Abdominal pain.

Clinical features

HSP is a diffuse, self-limiting allergic vasculitis of unknown aetiology (also known as anaphylactoid purpura). It occurs particularly in pre-school children, and is twice as common in boys. Peak incidence is in the winter. The first symptom in most (>50%) is the appearance of a purpuric rash in a relatively well child. The characteristic distribution is over the extensor surfaces of the limbs and buttocks, but it may involve the trunk and occasionally the face. It begins as a raised urticarial rash, rapidly progressing to purpura. Pain and swelling of one or more joints (particularly ankles and knees) occurs in two-thirds of cases and is the presenting symptom in 25%. Gastrointestinal involvement is common with colicky abdominal pain due to haemorrhage into the gut wall. Less common problems include melaena, bloody diarrhoea and intussusception.

Renal involvement is common, occurring in 25–50% of patients. Most have asymptomatic microscopic haematuria, but features of acute glomerulonephritis (microscopic haematuria, oliguria, hypertension) or nephrotic syndrome (oedema, proteinuria) may develop. Rare cases progress to end-stage renal failure. CNS symptoms (fits, behaviour disturbance) are uncommon. Scrotal involvement may present as a testicular torsion.

Investigation

There are no specific laboratory findings and diagnosis is made on the clinical presentation. The platelet count and clotting studies are normal.

Management

Treatment is symptomatic with analgesics for joint and abdominal pain, plus bed rest if joint pain is marked. A short course of steroids can be used for severe abdominal pain. Urinalysis for blood and protein, and regular blood pressure monitoring are important. The benefits of specific therapies for severe renal involvement (aspirin, pulsed methylprednisolone, plasma exchange, cyclophosphamide) are unclear.

Outcome

HSP runs a variable course with the majority settling within 2–6 weeks. Relapses can occur but rarely beyond 1 year. Microscopic haematuria may persist for several months or even years. The renal function of those with acute nephritis or nephrosis may continue to deteriorate even after 5 years so long-term surveillance is essential.

Idiopathic (immune) thrombocytopenic purpura (ITP)

Problems

- Chronic blood loss.
- Intracranial haemorrhage (risk < 1%).
- Side-effects of treatment.

Clinical features

ITP presents with acute onset of bruising, purpura and petechiae. Less commonly mucosal bleeding occurs. Eighty per cent report a preceding viral illness, but the child is usually well at presentation and associated symptoms, e.g. pallor, lethargy, bone pain, should suggest leukaemia. In 75% the platelet count returns to normal within 3 months, but in 10–20% thrombocytopenia persists beyond 6 months (chronic ITP). Mortality is low and is usually due to intracranial haemorrhage.

Investigation

- FBC. Thrombocytopenia often $< 10 \times 10^9$/l.
- Immunoglobulins. IgG, IgA. Platelet-associated IgG is almost always present but difficult to detect with very low platelet counts. Platelet antibody tests are usually unhelpful.
- Viral titres, e.g. Epstein–Barr virus, rubella, CMV (if under 1 year).
- Bone marrow aspirate. Probably not necessary if the platelet count is $> 30 \times 10^9$/l, but the child should be observed and one performed if spontaneous remission does not occur within 2–3 weeks. A bone marrow aspirate is *essential* if any features suggestive of marrow infiltration or aplasia are present, or if treatment (particularly steroids) is planned. In ITP there are normal or increased numbers of megakaryocytes.
- Anti-nuclear factor, anti-DNA antibodies. Exclude SLE if ITP becomes chronic.

Management

Children are usually admitted to hospital to make the diagnosis. There is no need to keep them in hospital or restrict activities other than to try to prevent fights and vigorous knockabouts, particularly when the platelet count is $< 10 \times 10^9/l$. No treatment is necessary if there is no mucosal bleeding or serious haemorrhage, but a short course of low-dose steroids may lead to slightly faster recovery of the platelet count. Bone marrow aspiration to exclude leukaemia must be performed before starting treatment. Chronic ITP has been treated with pulses of high-dose methylprednisolone, immunoglobulin infusions and splenectomy, but in view of the side-effects of these treatments they are best reserved for serious haemorrhagic emergencies, together with massive allogeneic platelet transfusion. ITP may remit at any time even after years, and serious haemorrhage is rare. Treatment is symptomatic, not curative, so the child should be treated on the basis of symptoms and not the platelet count.

Further reading

Eden OB, Lilleyman JS on behalf of the British Paediatric Haematology Group. Guidelines for management of idiopathic thrombocytopenic purpura. *Archives of Disease in Childhood,* 1992; **67:** 1056–8.

Reid MM. Chronic ITP, incidence, treatment and outcome. *Archives of Disease in Childhood,* 1995; **72:** 125–8.

Related topics of interest

Bleeding disorders (p. 53)
Child protection (p. 65)
Glomerulonephritis (p. 164)
Haemolytic uraemic syndrome (p. 179)
Malignancy – leukaemia and lymphoma (p. 257)

PYREXIA OF UNKNOWN ORIGIN

Pyrexia of unknown origin (PUO) may be defined as a fever of over one week's duration which remains unexplained despite investigation. Most children admitted to hospital with fever have a viral upper respiratory tract infection and the fever settles in less than one week. Symptoms or signs of common bacterial infections (e.g. dysuria, cough, tachypnoea, meningism) should be excluded. Fever is a normal part of the body's response to infection but complications of fever in childhood include febrile convulsions and dehydration.

In a child who has a persistent or recurrent fever, other conditions need to be considered and extensive investigations are sometimes required to identify the cause. A careful history and examination will help direct investigations. New symptoms or signs may develop with time, giving further clues to the underlying cause, so repeated clinical assessment is vital. In general, antibiotic treatment should be withheld until the diagnosis has been established, but this is clearly inappropriate in a sick or deteriorating child.

Causes to consider in a child with a persistent or recurrent fever

- Infection is the underlying cause in the majority of cases.
  Bacterial infections particularly cerebral abscess, subphrenic abscess, osteomyelitis, tuberculosis, infective endocarditis, brucellosis.
  Viral infections, e.g. Epstein–Barr virus, CMV.
  Tropical infections, e.g. malaria, typhoid, amoebic liver abscess.
  Other, e.g. toxoplasmosis, psittacosis.
- Kawasaki disease (see related topic, p. 233).
- Malignancy – fever is rarely the only presenting feature, e.g. Hodgkin's lymphoma, neuroblastoma.
- Connective tissue disorder, e.g. Still's disease, SLE, polyarteritis nodosa.
- Drug-induced pyrexia, e.g. salicylates.
- Other rare causes, e.g.
  Riley–Day syndrome (familial dysautonomia) – absent tear production and corneal reflex.
  Familial Mediterranean fever.
  Inflammatory bowel disease – rarely presents with fever alone.
  Diabetes insipidus.
  Ectodermal dysplasia – overheating due to absence of sweat glands.
- Münchausen syndrome by proxy.

Clinical assessment of a child with a PUO

1. *History. Noting particularly:*

- Any associated symptoms (e.g. rash, joint pains, night sweats).

- Underlying heart defect.
- Exposure to unpasteurized milk (tuberculosis, brucellosis).
- Contact with animals.
- Insect bites.
- Recent travel abroad.
- Family history.
- Any recent medication (previous antibiotics may have modified the illness).

2. *Examination.* The pattern of fever may be helpful (e.g. spiking fever in malaria or infective endocarditis, persistent low-grade fever with a cerebral abscess or osteomyelitis). Careful examination of the chest and abdomen (including rectal examination) may provide localizing signs. All joints should be examined and local bony tenderness excluded. A swinging fever may precede any joint manifestations in Still's disease by several weeks. Signs of raised intracranial pressure (e.g. headache, papilloedema) may occur in the presence of a cerebral abscess, but there may be no localizing neurological signs. The diagnosis should be considered in all children with a PUO, particularly if there has been a recent ear or scalp infection or if there is underlying congenital heart disease. Splenomegaly may be found in glandular fever, typhoid, and malignancy. Infective endocarditis should be considered in any child with a heart defect, but it can occur in a structurally normal heart. Predisposing factors include dental or surgical procedures. The onset is often insidious (subacute bacterial endocarditis, SBE) with fever, malaise and weight loss but it may follow a fulminant course. Features of infective endocarditis include a new or altered murmur and microscopic haematuria. Splenomegaly, Osler nodes, petechiae (especially oral mucosa, eyelids and optic fundi), and splinter haemorrhages are less common in childhood than in adults.

Investigations

- FBC and film. Thick and thin films are needed if malaria is suspected. The platelet count may be raised in Kawasaki disease.
- ESR, CRP. Raised in active inflammation or infection.
- Blood cultures. Repeated frequently particularly with spikes of fever, especially if infective endocarditis is suspected (majority of cases of SBE are due to *Streptococcus viridans*).
- Monospot or Paul Bunnell test, for Epstein–Barr virus.

- Serum for viral serology.
- Urine and stool cultures. Bacterial, viral.
- Gastric aspirate, early morning urines, sputum culture for acid-fast bacilli (tuberculosis).
- Mantoux test.
- Imaging, e.g. CXR, abdominal US, CT brain, isotope bone scan, white cell scans (labelled with gallium or technetium) – may reveal occult sites of infection.
- CSF culture/serology. Bacterial and viral. But consider deferring the LP until a cerebral abscess has been excluded by CT brain.
- Bone marrow examination. To exclude infiltration with malignancy (lymphoma, leukaemia, neuroblastoma) or tuberculosis.
- Autoimmune profile.
- Urinary catecholamines. To exclude neuroblastoma.

Related topics of interest

Juvenile chronic arthritis (p. 229)
Kawasaki disease (p. 233)
Malignancy – leukaemia and lymphoma (p. 257)

RASHES AND BLISTERS

Viral illnesses in childhood are often accompanied by widespread erythematous macular or maculopapular rashes. It is important to distinguish these from petechial or purpuric rashes which do not blanch when compressed (see related topic Purpura and bruising, p. 330). Other common causes of skin rashes in childhood include impetigo, molluscum contagiosum, atopic eczema and allergic reactions (food allergy, drug reactions). Rashes in the nappy area are usually due to ammoniacal dermatitis, candidal infection or seborrheic dermatitis.

Blisters or vesicular skin lesions are associated with staphylococcal infection and certain viral infections (e.g. varicella zoster, herpes simplex, coxsackie virus). Blistering may also result from physical trauma to the skin (e.g. tight shoes, scalds, sunburn). Genetically inherited blistering conditions are very rare (epidermolysis bullosa) and usually present at birth or in early childhood. Other rare causes of vesicular skin lesions include chronic bullous disease of childhood and dermatitis herpetiformis.

Insect bites, stings and infestations (e.g. scabies) are typically itchy and may cause erythema and vesicular lesions. Desquamation (skin peeling) is a typical feature of scarlet fever and Kawasaki disease.

Some systemic disorders are associated with typical rashes which are described elsewhere, e.g. Henoch–Schönlein purpura, Kawasaki disease, dermatomyositis, Langerhan's cell histiocytosis. Mumps does not cause a rash but is included in this chapter along with other childhood viral infections (measles, chickenpox, etc.).

Viral infections

1. Measles

- Cause: RNA virus.
- Transmission: Respiratory droplet.
- Incubation period: 10 days.
- Clinical features: Prodomal illness for 3–4 days before the appearance of the rash – fever, malaise, irritability, conjunctivitis, coryza, dry cough, lymphadenopathy, Koplik's spots (tiny white spots on bright red buccal mucosa). A florid maculopapular rash starts behind the ears and spreads from the head and neck to cover the whole body. The spots become confluent and then fade over 3–4 days.
- Infectious period: Start of prodrome to 4 days after the appearance of the rash.
- Complications: Otitis media, pneumonia, encephalitis (rare), subacute sclerosing panencephalitis (SSPE) (late, rare). High mortality in immuno-suppressed patients and in children in developing countries especially if malnourished.
- Prevention: Measles vaccine available since 1968. Combined measles, mumps and rubella (MMR) vaccine

given at 12–18 months in the UK since 1988. Pre-school booster now being introduced. Human normal immunoglobulin should be given to immuno-suppressed children within 72 hours of contact with measles.

2. *Rubella (German measles)*
- Cause: RNA virus.
- Transmission: Respiratory droplet.
- Incubation period: 14–21 days.
- Clinical features: Usually mild fever and malaise. Transient pink macular rash lasts 2–3 days. Lymphadenopathy typically sub-occipital. Differentiation from other mild viral illnesses difficult clinically.
- Infectious period: One week before appearance of rash to 4 days after.
- Complications: Rare in childhood. Arthritis is common in adolescents and adults. Maternal infection particularly in the first trimester may result in congenital infection (deafness, cardiac defects, cataracts, microcephaly).
- Prevention: MMR at 12–18 months, pre-school MMR booster.

3. *Chickenpox*
- Cause: DNA virus *Varicella zoster.*
- Transmission: Respiratory droplet or direct contact.
- Incubation period: 14 days.
- Clinical features: No prodromal illness. Low grade fever. Vesicles appear in crops all over the body. May also occur in the mouth. Often intensely itchy. Vesicles may rupture to produce shallow ulcers which then dry and crust over.
- Infectious period: 2 days before rash until all lesions have crusted.
- Complications: Secondary bacterial infection of vesicles. Encephalitis with ataxia typically 7–10 days after the illness. Usually mild and resolves in 1–2 weeks. Pneumonitis (rare). Adults, immunosuppressed patients and neonates are at risk of severe disseminated disease which can be fatal. The virus can remain latent and recur years later as shingles (herpes zoster). Non-immune individuals may develop chickenpox when exposed to shingles, but not vice versa.
- Prevention: Vaccine available but not given routinely in the UK at present. Zoster immune globulin or acyclovir recommended for those at risk of severe disease.

4. Mumps

- Cause: RNA virus paramyxovirus.
- Transmission: Respiratory droplet.
- Incubation period: 14–21 days.
- Clinical features: Subclinical infection common. Fever, and malaise, with enlargement of one or both parotids. Settles in 7–10 days. No rash.
- Complications: Common cause of aseptic meningitis prior to routine immunization. Epididymo-orchitis and pancreatitis rare.
- Prevention: MMR at 12–18 months, pre-school MMR booster.

5. Fifth disease (slapped cheek disease)

- Cause: Human parvovirus B19.
- Transmission: Respiratory droplet.
- Clinical features: Mild febrile illness with bright red cheeks bilaterally. Maculopapular rash develops on trunk and limbs 1–4 days later. Becomes reticular as it fades over the next 1–3 weeks. Arthralgia and arthritis occur in about 10% of cases. Outbreaks classically in winter and spring.
- Complications: Intrauterine infection with this virus may result in spontaneous abortion or fetal hydrops. Parvovirus infection may precipitate an aplastic crisis in those with an underlying haemolytic disorder, e.g. hereditary spherocytosis.

6. Roseola infantum

- Cause: Human herpes virus type 6.
- Clinical features: Short febrile illness (2–4 days). Erythematous, macular rash appears as the fever settles.
- Complications: Febrile convulsions common during the febrile phase.

7. Herpes simplex virus (HSV)

- Clinical features: HSV type 1 is spread by infected saliva or direct contact and is often asymptomatic. Children with acute gingivostomatitis (fever, extensive ulceration of the buccal mucosa, cervical lymphadenopathy) may become dehydrated due to difficulty eating and drinking. Treatment is supportive (pain relief, fluids) and acyclovir (i.v., oral or topical) may be considered.

  Neonatal transmission of HSV type 2 from a mother who has active genital herpes at the time of delivery can result in severe disseminated disease with a high mortality. Elective caesarean section should be considered.

- Complications: Recurrent cold sores, encephalitis, congenital infection, kerato-conjunctivitis, eczema herpeticum.

8. *Hand, foot and mouth disease*

- Cause: Coxsackie virus type A16.
- Clinical features: Mild self-limiting illness occurring in epidemics. Papular–vesicular eruption of hands, feet, mouth and buttocks.

9. *Molluscum contagiosum*

- Cause: A pox virus.
- Transmission: Direct contact.
- Clinical features: Common self-limiting infection. Clusters of skin coloured papules which cause little or no discomfort. Found on the trunk (especially axillae), limbs and occasionally the face. Papules are 2–5 mm across and typically have a central dimple ('umbilication'). Spontaneous resolution within 6–9 months is usual, although freezing or cautery may be used.

Other infections and infestations

1. *Impetigo*. Highly contagious superficial infection, usually starting as a vesicle on the face which rapidly progresses to typical golden crusted lesions particularly around the mouth. The causative organisms are usually *Staphylococcus aureus* and/or a streptococcus. Treatment is with topical antibiotic preparations. Systemic antibiotics are rarely indicated.

2. *Scabies*. Very contagious infestation caused by *Sarcoptes scabiei* which burrows into the skin and lays its eggs. It produces intense itching and there may be a secondary erythematous rash. Burrows may be visible particularly between the fingers, and on the wrists, feet and genitalia. Treatment must be for the whole family with malathion or permethrin. Bedclothes should be thoroughly washed.

3. *Erysipelas*. Superficial, well demarcated skin infection caused by a group A beta-haemolytic streptococcus which can occur on any part of the body. It may be difficult to distinguish from more deep-seated cellulitis. Facial erysipelas must be differentiated from slapped cheek disease

and the violaceous cellulitis caused by *Haemophilus influenzae*. Treatment is with penicillin or erythromycin.

4. Scarlet fever. A widespread erythematous rash develops 2–3 days following tonsillitis due to an erythrogenic toxin-producing group A beta-haemolytic streptococcus. Typically there is circumoral pallor, and a thick white exudate may develop on the tongue which peels off leaving a 'strawberry tongue'. The rash fades and desquamates. Late complications include post-streptococcal glomerulonephritis and rheumatic fever. Treatment is with penicillin.

5. Staphylococcal scalded skin syndrome. A widespread tender erythematous rash progresses to bullae formation and then exfoliation which may involve the entire body surface. Caused by an epidermolytic toxin produced by certain strains of *Staphylococcus aureus* especially phage type 71. Mucous membranes are not involved (cf. toxic shock syndrome). Management includes pain relief, fluids and flucloxacillin.

6. Lyme disease. Caused by a tick-borne spirochaete *Borrelia burgdorferi*. First recognized in 1975 after an outbreak in Lyme, Connecticut. Particularly prevalent in areas where there are deer which act as hosts for the ticks (e.g. the New Forest). A small red macule or papule at the site of the tick bite spreads circumferentially to a maximum diameter of ~15 cm, with central fading of the erythema (erythema chronicum migrans). Associated symptoms include fluctuating fever, malaise, lymphadenopathy, myalgia and arthralgia. In about 15% of patients frank neurological symptoms (e.g. facial palsy, lymphocytic meningitis, encephalitis) occur weeks to months after the initial infection, which may have been asymptomatic. Other late complications include arthritis and myopericarditis. Diagnosis can be confirmed serologically. Treatment is with penicillin, erythromycin or a cephalosporin.

Nappy rash

1. Ammoniacal. Irritant or contact dermatitis associated with prolonged contact with a wet nappy. The rash is erythematous and there may be areas of ulceration. It is limited by the margins of the nappy and spares the flexures. Management is with frequent nappy changing or exposure, careful washing and drying at each change, and simple barrier creams, e.g. zinc and castor oil.

2. Candidiasis. Infection spreads from the perianal area causing an erythematous rash commonly with satellite lesions, and involving the flexures. Treatment is with topical and oral antifungals, e.g. nystatin.

3. Seborrheic dermatitis. Greasy, erythematous patches with scaling and crusting are seen particularly over the scalp ('cradle cap') or nappy area. It may spread to involve much of the body. Very common in the first 18 months of life. Aetiology unknown. Preparations containing salicylic acid may be used but can cause irritation. Mild topical steroids are sometimes used.

Other rashes in childhood

1. Atopic eczema (see also related topic Eczema, p. 132). Typical features include erythema, vesicles, ichthyosis and itching. Affected areas of skin are prone to secondary bacterial infection (staphylococcal, streptococcal) and there is a risk of severe widespread infection with herpes simplex virus.

2. Psoriasis. Typical erythematous plaques with silvery scales especially on the scalp and extensor surfaces of the limbs. Uncommon in childhood but there is often a family history of psoriasis. Treatments include coal tar preparations, dithranol, and UV light.

More common is guttate psoriasis, which is an acute eruption of small red scaling lesions following an intercurrent illness, particularly a streptococcal sore throat.

3. Epidermolysis bullosa. Inherited disorders in which there is an increased susceptibility to blister formation at the site of mechanical trauma. Many different types, of varying severity, classified on the basis of inheritance, clinical features and electron microscopic identification of the cleavage plane of the blister, e.g. junctional, dystrophic, simplex.

4. Chronic bullous disease of childhood. Persistent or recurrent bullae particularly around the neck and genitalia. Spontaneously resolves in a few months to years. Aetiology is unknown but may be autoimmune.

5. Erythema nodosum. Red tender nodular lesions usually present on the shins. Associated with streptococcal infection, and primary tuberculosis. Rarer causes in childhood include sarcoidosis, ulcerative colitis, Crohn's disease and drugs (e.g. sulphonamides).

6. Erythema multiforme. Typical target lesions associated with herpes simplex, mycoplasma infection, certain drugs (e.g. cotrimoxazole). When associated with severe mucosal ulceration, it is known as Stevens–Johnson syndrome.

7. Dermatitis herpetiformis. Recurrent extremely itchy papules and vesicles over the extensor surfaces of the elbows, buttocks, and knees. Associated with gluten-sensitive enteropathy in many cases.

8. Acrodermatitis enteropathica. Autosomal recessive condition in which there is defective absorption of zinc. Features include mucocutaneous ulceration (particularly around the mouth and ano-genital region), diarrhoea, alopecia and failure to thrive. Treatment is with high dose oral zinc.

9. Incontinentia pigmentosa. Very rare X-linked dominant condition. Lethal in males. Linear vesicles develop in the neonate. Associated with neurological, ocular and dental abnormalities.

Further reading

Verbov J, Morley N. *Colour Atlas of Paediatric Dermatology.* Lancaster: MTP Press, 1983.
Williams REA, Morley WN. Diagnosis of systemic disorders from skin signs. *Current Paediatrics,* 1992; **2:** 90–2.

Related topics of interest

Allergy and anaphylaxis (p. 27)
Congenital infection (p. 93)
Eczema (p. 132)
Immunization (p. 206)
Neurocutaneous syndromes (p. 293)
Newborn examination (p. 296)
Purpura and bruising (p. 330)

SHOCK

Shock is inadequate tissue perfusion due to impaired cardiovascular function, which may be the end result of many disease processes. Impaired delivery of nutrients and oxygen to the tissues leads to anaerobic metabolism, acidosis, impaired cellular function and subsequent organ failure. Prompt recognition and resuscitation is vital to reverse this process and reduce both mortality and morbidity.

Problems

- Hypotension.
- Metabolic acidosis.
- Multisystem failure – hypoventilation, acute tubular necrosis, cerebral anoxia.

Aetiology

(a) Hypovolaemic shock

- Fluid and electrolyte loss
  External, e.g. gastroenteritis, burns.
  Internal, e.g. nephrotic syndrome.
- Blood loss, e.g. trauma, gastrointestinal bleed

(b) Cardiogenic shock

- Severe heart failure.

(c) Septicaemic shock

- Gram-negative sepsis, e.g. meningococcal septicaemia.
- Toxic shock syndrome.

(d) Drugs

- Overdose, e.g. barbiturates.
- Anaphylaxis.

Pathogenesis of septic shock

The clinical features of Gram-negative shock result from disruption of the normal homeostatic mechanisms of the vascular endothelium following activation of the host inflammatory responses by bacterial endotoxin. The normal endothelium maintains vascular permeability and inhibits thrombosis. Release of inflammatory mediators, including neutrophil-derived enzymes and cytokines (e.g. interleukin 2 and tumour necrosis factor) leads to three major processes:

- Increased vascular permeability resulting in hypovolaemia and oedema.
- Vasoconstriction of some vascular beds and dilatation of others leading to impaired organ function.
- Intravascular thrombosis with platelet and clotting factor consumption (DIC) resulting in further tissue hypoxia.

Prostacyclin (PGI_2) is an inhibitor of platelet aggregation and a potent vasodilator which is actively produced by the endothelium together with other important inhibitors of thrombosis such as nitric oxide. It has been suggested that a deficiency of PGI_2 may have a role in the pathogenesis of Gram-negative shock, but the role of exogenous PGI_2 as a therapeutic intervention has yet to be proven.

Clinical features

Shock may occur at any age but is most commonly seen in children under 5 years. The child lies quietly and is poorly responsive, or can be restless and confused. The peripheries are grey, mottled, cold and clammy with sluggish capillary filling. There may be central cyanosis and the breathing is often laboured with grunting. The pulse is thready, rapid and is difficult to feel peripherally. Hypotension is not a feature of early shock due to compensatory vasoconstriction but will eventually occur. Oliguria is usual. There may be decerebrate posturing if cerebral anoxia is marked or if septicaemia is associated with meningitis. The characteristic rash of meningococcal septicaemia should be readily recognized.

Toxic shock syndrome is an acute illness characterized by fever, mucous membrane hyperaemia, oedema, desquamating erythroderma and rapidly progressive hypotension with multisystem failure. It was originally associated with *Staphylococcus aureus* and became more widely recognized as an illness of young women who used tampons. However, a significant proportion of cases are not associated with menstruation, but with focal staphylococcal infection, and many of these cases occur in children. A toxic shock-like syndrome can also be caused by group A haemolytic streptococcus.

Investigation

- FBC. Hb is usually normal in acute blood loss. The packed cell volume (PCV) will be raised if the shock follows fluid loss. The WBC is often raised. Thrombocytopenia occurs with DIC.
- Blood glucose. Often low.
- U&E, creatinine. The degree of renal failure and electrolyte imbalance depends on the aetiology. Hyperkalaemia will be aggravated by acidosis.
- Acid–base status. Metabolic acidosis due to tissue hypoxia.
- Blood cultures.
- Liver function tests. Hepatic ischaemia leads to a rise in transaminases and ammonia.
- Clotting. DIC is invariably present in severe shock with consumption of clotting factors and elevation of FDPs. It

is also associated with septicaemia, burns and major trauma.

- Calcium, phosphate, magnesium. Commonly deranged.
- CXR. Cardiomegaly suggests cardiogenic shock. Pneumonia may be the primary illness or an aspiration pneumonia secondary to impaired consciousness level. In late shock pulmonary oedema and shock lung may develop.
- Urine culture. UTI may cause Gram-negative septicaemia and shock, particularly in infants.
- Lumbar puncture. Resuscitate and stabilize first.
- Group and save serum.

Management

1. *Airway*. Clear and maintain.

2. *Breathing*. Give oxygen, and if the patient is requiring sodium bicarbonate to correct acidosis, hypoventilating, or requiring large volumes of fluid for resuscitation, intubate and ventilate.

3. *Circulation*. Insert an i.v. line (peripheral, central, intraosseous), take bloods for investigations (including BM Stix) and give 20 ml/kg plasma or normal saline bolus over 5–10 minutes. This may need to be repeated. Commence i.v. infusion – the type of fluid will depend on the underlying cause of shock.

4. *Obtain a brief history* of the illness from an accompanying adult (parent, paramedic), including any relevant past medical history, drugs, etc.

5. *Examine the child* noting level of consciousness (AVPU system), evidence of sepsis (rash, neck stiffness), dehydration (reduced skin turgor, sunken fontanelle), trauma, etc.

6. *Arterial blood gas*. Consider giving i.v. sodium bicarbonate to reduce the degree of metabolic acidosis.

7. *Admit to the intensive care area once stable.*

8. *Obtain a full history from the parents.*

9. *Further management* will depend on the underlying cause of the circulatory failure. General measures to improve myocardial contractility include volume replacement and correction of acidosis, hypoxia, anaemia and electrolyte imbalance. In hypovolaemic shock the child will rapidly improve with plasma expansion, whereas in cardiogenic shock inotropes may be needed to improve myocardial function. If sepsis is suspected commence broad-spectrum antibiotics. The roles of prostacyclin and monoclonal antibodies to endotoxin in the treatment of septicaemic shock remain unproven.

Further reading

Levin M. Shock. In: Black D, ed. *Paediatric Emergencies,* 2nd edn. London: Butterworths, 1987: 87–116.

Lloyd-Thomas AR. Paediatric trauma. In: *ABC of Major Trauma*. London: BMJ Publications, 1991; 73–83.

Shock. In: Advanced Life Support Group. *Advanced Paediatric Life Support – the Practical Approach*, 2nd edn. London: BMJ Publications, 1997; 85–98.

Related topics of interest

Accidents (p. 7)
Acute renal failure (p. 15)
Cardiac arrest (p. 61)
Heart failure (p. 190)
Meningitis and encephalitis (p. 265)

SICKLE CELL ANAEMIA AND THALASSAEMIA SYNDROMES

Each molecule of haemoglobin normally contains four globin chains. At birth, 50–80% of haemoglobin is fetal haemoglobin (HbF = $\alpha_2\gamma_2$) and 15–40% is adult haemoglobin (HbA = $\alpha_2\beta_2$). A small proportion is $HbA_2 = \alpha_2\delta_2$. By 6 months of age HbF represents less than 5% of the total. By 3 years HbA represents 98–99% with one α-chain and one β-chain inherited from each parent. Sickle cell anaemia (HbSS) is a disorder of haemoglobin synthesis due to a single amino acid substitution (valine for glutamine) in the β-globin chain. Other β-chain variants include haemoglobin C (HbC). The thalassaemia syndromes result from impaired globin chain synthesis which may affect either the α- or β-chains. Each haemoglobinopathy can exist in the heterozygous or homozygous state. Mixed haemoglobinopathies, e.g. HbS/HbC or HbS/β-thalassaemia, occur and tend to be milder than HbSS.

Sickle cell anaemia

Problems

- Microcytic, hypochromic anaemia.
- Crises (painful, anaemic).
- Infections (*Pneumococcus, Salmonella*).
- Impaired renal concentrating ability.
- Family and social disruption.

Incidence

Sickle cell anaemia occurs mainly in those of African origin, with up to 1 in 4 West Africans and 1 in 10 Afro-Caribbeans being carriers. The carrier state has reached high levels in these populations as it protects against malaria. In the UK it is a common inner city problem with approximately 7000 people who are homozygous (sickle cell anaemia) and many more who are heterozygous (sickle cell trait).

Clinical features

High concentrations of HbS within red cells leads to aggregation of the HbS molecules when deoxygenated, resulting in distortion of the red cells (sickling), with subsequent increased blood viscosity and capillary obstruction. Dehydration, infection, acidosis and hypoxia exacerbate sickling.

Sickle cell anaemia usually presents after the age of 6 months (when levels of HbF have fallen) with painful swelling of the hands or feet (dactylitis), anaemia, icterus and hepatosplenomegaly. There is an increased risk of infections with encapsulated organisms because of splenic dysfunction (pneumococcal septicaemia, salmonella osteomyelitis), and these are a significant cause of mortality. Repeated splenic infarction results in less prominent splenomegaly in older children. Life is punctuated by painful and anaemic crises.

Painful crises are due to vaso-occlusion, causing severe pain in any part of the body (particularly bones, muscle, abdomen). Severe abdominal pain may be mistaken for an 'acute abdomen'. Anaemic crises result from bone marrow aplasia (parvovirus associated with infection), megaloblastic crisis (folate deficiency), visceral sequestration of red cells (e.g. hepatic, splenic) or haemolysis. Stroke occurs in ~ 5% of patients. Other complications include enuresis (impaired renal concentrating ability following repeated renal infarcts), leg ulcers, priapism, chest syndrome (chest pain, fever, leucocytosis, thrombocytopenia, high mortality) and aseptic necrosis of the hip. Delayed puberty is common. Heterozygotes rarely have problems but it is important to keep them well oxygenated during general anaesthesia.

Investigation

- FBC. Chronic haemolytic anaemia (microcytic, hypochromic). The Hb is usually 6–9 g/dl, and the reticulocyte count is raised. Sickle cells, target cells, and Howell–Jolly bodies may be seen on film. Blood can be deoxygenated as a screening test for sickling.
- Haemoglobin electrophoresis
  Homozygote: HbS 90–95%, HbF 5–10%.
  Heterozygote: HbS < 40%, HbA > 60%.

Management

1. *Painful crises.* Pain relief and adequate fluid intake. Blood, urine and a throat swab should be taken for culture and broad-spectrum antibiotics started. Non-steroidal anti-inflammatories may be adequate but opiates are frequently needed.

2. *Anaemic crises.* Urgent blood transfusion. In babies, splenic sequestration results in a sudden drop in Hb associated with a rapidly enlarging spleen. It can be life-threatening.

3. *Prophylaxis.* Penicillin and vaccination against pneumococcal infection. Increased folic acid requirements due to haemolysis.

4. *Blood transfusion* is not used routinely to treat anaemia as it may exacerbate hyperviscosity. Acute exchange transfusion may be of benefit in patients with acute stroke or severe sickle chest syndrome. Repeated transfusions to reduce the percentage of HbS may be useful before surgery, following a stroke (recurrence risk high within 3 years), or if painful crises are frequent.

5. Bone marrow transplantation. Sickle cell anaemia has a high morbidity and mortality (median life expectancy approximately 45 years). Bone marrow transplantation from an HLA-compatible sibling offers the chance of cure and is now considered in children who have already suffered significant complications (see Further reading).

Screening and antenatal diagnosis

Screening of cord blood is now routine in some areas of the UK and is recommended in all high-risk groups. Screening of parents will identify carriers. Sickle cell anaemia can now be detected by chorionic villus biopsy or amniocentesis.

Thalassaemia

Problems

- Anaemia.
- Growth failure.
- Bone marrow hyperplasia (skull bossing, maxillary overgrowth, brittle long bones).
- Hepatosplenomegaly (extramedullary erythropoiesis).
- Iron overload from repeated transfusions (cardiomyopathy, cirrhosis, haemosiderosis, skin pigmentation, endocrine failure).

Clinical features

Thalassaemia is most common amongst Mediterranean and Asian races. β-Thalassaemia is more common than α-thalassaemia and homozygotes (β-thalassaemia major) usually present in the first year of life with pallor and failure to thrive. Impaired β-chain synthesis leads to excessive production of α-chains, which are deposited in the red cells, causing haemolysis. Repeated blood transfusions are required to avoid the severe bone problems associated with compensatory bone marrow hyperplasia, but chronic iron overload results in significant morbidity and mortality in adolescence and early adult life. Heterozygotes (β-thalassaemia minor) have only mild anaemia which may be confused with iron deficiency anaemia.

In α-thalassaemia there are two pairs of genes involved. Lack of all four genes is incompatible with life (Bart's hydrops). Three-gene deficiency (HbH) is of varying severity and may result in transfusion dependency. Deficiency of one or two genes (α-thalassaemia trait) results in mild anaemia.

Investigation

- FBC. Hypochromic microcytic anaemia. Severe anaemia (Hb 4–8 g/dl) with reticulocytosis, target cells, and basophilic stippling is seen in β-thalassaemia major.

- Haemoglobin electrophoresis.

  β-Thalassaemia major: HbF 15–100%.

  β-Thalassaemia minor: HbA_2 > 4%.
  HbF > 2%.

  α-Thalassaemia: HbH detected in the three-gene defect, but normal electrophoresis in the one- or two-gene defect.
- Radiology. Typical 'hair on end' appearance of the skull in β-thalassaemia major.

Management

Patients with β-thalassaemia are transfused regularly to maintain their haemoglobin > 11 g/dl to try to suppress erythropoiesis. Desferrioxamine and other iron-chelating agents may help reduce iron overload and delay the onset of complications. Hypersplenism often necessitates splenectomy. Iron supplements are contraindicated in thalassaemia. Bone marrow transplantation may offer a cure.

Further reading

Davies SC, Oni L. Management of patients with sickle cell disease. *British Medical Journal,* 1997; **315:** 656–60.

Davies SC, Roberts IAG. Bone marrow transplant for sickle cell disease – an update. *Archives of Disease in Childhood,* 1996; **75:** 3–5.

Grundy R, Howard R, Evans J. Practical management of pain in sickling disorders. *Archives of Disease in Childhood,* 1993; **69:** 256–9.

Vermylen Ch, Cornu G, Philippe M, Ninane J, Borja A, Latinne D, Ferrant A, Michaux JL, Sokal G. Bone marrow transplantation in sickle cell anaemia. *Archives of Disease in Childhood,* 1991; **66:** 1195–98.

Weatherall DJ. The thalassaemias. *British Medical Journal,* 1997; **314:** 1675–8.

Related topic of interest

Anaemia (p. 31)

SMALL FOR DATES, LARGE FOR DATES

A baby who is below the 10th centile for gestation is small for dates, and one who is above the 90th centile for gestation is large for dates. By definition, these groups will include normal small and large babies. Mortality and morbidity in these infants, particularly as a result of hypoglycaemia, has fallen dramatically as a result of better recognition both antenatally and postnatally.

Small for dates (SFD)

Problems

- Hypoglycaemia.
- Hypothermia.
- Polycythaemia.
- Jaundice.
- Birth asphyxia.
- Increased incidence of congenital abnormalities.

Aetiology

Babies who are SFD may be proportionately growth retarded with low weight, length and head circumference suggesting early onset of intrauterine growth retardation (IUGR) or there may be relative sparing of head circumference suggesting onset of growth retardation in the last few weeks of pregnancy.

1. *Proportionate IUGR*

(a) Fetal causes

- Congenital infection (CMV, toxoplasmosis, rubella).
- Chromosomal abnormalities.

(b) Maternal causes

- Severe placental insufficiency (e.g. pre-eclamptic toxaemia).
- Severe maternal disease (e.g. renal disease, SLE).
- Early toxins (e.g. alcohol).

2. *Disproportionate IUGR*

- Placental insufficiency (pre-eclampsia, twin-to-twin transfusion).
- Maternal smoking.
- Less severe maternal disease.

Management

1. *Hypoglycaemia* is common because of decreased glycogen stores. There may also be transient hyperinsulinism. It is often asymptomatic but clinical features include jitteriness, apnoea, irritability, floppiness

and convulsions. There is controversy over the definition of neonatal hypoglycaemia with values ranging from <1 mmol/l to <2.5 mmol/l given in various textbooks. The risk of neurological damage after repeated or prolonged episodes of hypoglycaemia is well recognized, so careful monitoring and management with early feeding, and i.v. dextrose if needed, are vital.

2. *Hypothermia* is common owing to the large surface area to volume ratio and poor fat stores. Hypothermia may exacerbate hypoglycaemia so it is important to dry the baby quickly after birth and ensure adequate wrapping. Overhead heaters and incubators are sometimes necessary.

3. *Polycythaemia* results from poor placental oxygen transfer (placental insufficiency). Blood viscosity increases exponentially when the venous haematocrit is > 65%, and this can exacerbate respiratory problems and hypoglycaemia, and may lead to long-term neurological sequelae. The precise level of haematocrit which warrants treatment is controversial, but if the baby is symptomatic (e.g. respiratory distress, irrritability, hypoglycaemia) or if the haematocrit rises to 70%, dilutional exchange should be performed. There may be an associated thrombocytopenia.

4. *Jaundice.* Increased red cell breakdown due to polycythaemia results in increased bilirubin levels. Phototherapy with or without exchange transfusion is frequently needed.

5. *Birth asphyxia.* SFD babies are at increased risk of intrapartum asphyxia because of the poor glycogen and fat stores resulting in poor ability to maintain anaerobic metabolism. There is also an increased risk of meconium aspiration.

Large for dates (LFD)

Problems

- Obstructed labour – shoulder dystocia.
- Birth trauma and nerve palsies.
- Birth asphyxia,
- Hypoglycaemia.

Aetiology

- Constitutionally large.
- Maternal insulin-dependent diabetes (IDDM including gestational diabetes).

- Severe rhesus disease.
- Beckwith–Wiedemann syndrome.
- Sotos' syndrome.

Infant of a diabetic mother

Problems

- LFD.
- Hypoglycaemia.
- Increased incidence of congenital abnormalities, particularly congenital heart disease, vertebral anomalies, caudal regression syndrome (e.g. sacral agenesis).
- Respiratory distress.
- Polycythaemia and jaundice.
- Hypocalcaemia.
- Cardiomyopathy.

IDDM in pregnancy increases the risk of early miscarriage, pre-eclampsia, polyhydramnios, intrauterine death and preterm labour. It is the commonest cause of a large baby (macrosomia). Congenital abnormalities are more frequent, occurring in 5–10% of infants of IDDM mothers.

Hypoglycaemia is common owing to transient hyperinsulinism (hyperglycaemia *in utero* stimulates hyperplasia of the islets of Langerhans) and reduced glucagon response to hypoglycaemia. Early feeding with regular blood sugar monitoring is essential, and an i.v. dextrose infusion may be needed.

Respiratory distress may occur even in term babies as a result of inhibition of surfactant production by hyperglycaemia *in utero*. Hypertrophic cardiomyopathy may be detected by echocardiography, with thickening of the interventricular septum, which resolves over the first year of life and only rarely causes symptoms. Other problems which are seen more frequently in these infants include polycythaemia, jaundice and hypocalcaemia.

Good diabetic control during pregnancy reduces the risk of many of these problems, but the evidence that it reduces the risk of congenital abnormalities remains to be proven. Perinatal mortality in this group is about 4%, and half of these deaths are due to major congenital abnormalities.

Beckwith–Wiedemann syndrome

This uncommon syndrome is of unknown aetiology. Features include gigantism, macroglossia, visceromegaly, hyperinsulinaemic hypoglycaemia, transverse creases on the ear lobes, and umbilical hernia or exomphalos. Symptomatic hypoglycaemia occurs in 50% of cases and may be transient, or occasionally prolonged and severe. The learning disability which has been a recognized part of the syndrome is probably secondary to repeated hypoglycaemia, so prompt recognition and treatment is essential. There is an increased risk of hemihypertrophy and of tumours such as Wilms' tumour and hepatoblastoma.

Further reading

Chiswick ML. Intrauterine growth retardation. *British Medical Journal,* 1985; **291:** 845–8.

Related topics of interest

Hypoglycaemia (p. 202)
Neonatal jaundice (p. 276)
Neonatal respiratory distress (p. 281)

STRIDOR

Stridor is a harsh noise produced by obstruction to breathing in the larynx or trachea. Inspiratory stridor usually predominates, but obstruction in the subglottic area or trachea may also produce a soft expiratory stridor. Stridor may arise from an acute condition, or from a chronic persistent cause with recurrent symptoms. The site of the obstruction may be supraglottic, glottic or subglottic (tracheal).

Problems

- Hypoxia – acute or chronic.
- Acute upper airways obstruction.
- Respiratory distress.
- Failure to thrive.
- Feeding problems.

Acute stridor

Hypoxia results from the obstruction, leading to bronchospasm, pooling of secretions and patchy lung consolidation. Intense respiratory muscle effort maintains tidal volume until the point of exhaustion. Increasing tachycardia, tachypnoea, restlessness or drowsiness indicates the need for urgent intervention to maintain the airway. Pulse oximetry may be of value but clinical signs are the most important indicators of impending obstruction.

Acute laryngotracheobronchitis ('croup')

This is the most common cause of acute stridor, commonly occurring during the second year of life, and is usually caused by influenza, parainfluenza and respiratory syncytial viruses.

Mild coryzal symptoms are followed by a barking cough, hoarse voice and inspiratory stridor. Symptoms are often worse at night and the majority can be managed at home. Children with moderate or severe croup may benefit from steroid treatment. Single doses or short courses of inhaled or oral steroids may reduce time spent in hospital. Nebulized adrenaline can give temporary relief in severe cases (5 ml of 1 in 1000 diluted with saline). Full monitoring and resuscitation equipment should be available. Intubation is occasionally needed.

Acute epiglottitis

The usual pathogen is *Haemophilus influenzae* type B, occasionally the cause is streptococcal or viral. There is gross swelling of the epiglottis and aryepiglottic folds, causing a rapid onset of drooling, fever, muffled voice and quiet inspiratory stridor. Cough is not prominent. Typically the child sits forward to relieve the obstruction. Throat examination and unnecessary upset to the child should be avoided – complete respiratory obstruction may result. Expert anaesthetic and ENT assistance should be sought immediately, and laryngoscopy and intubation performed. Intravenous antibiotics may be given once the airway is secure – cefotaxime is appropriate. If *Haemophilus influenzae* is the cause, rifampicin prophylaxis should be given to the index case and to household contacts. The reported incidence of epiglottitis has dramatically reduced since the introduction of Hib vaccine.

Foreign body

There may be a history of choking or aspiration. Stridor has a variable quality, depending on site and mobility of the object. Urgent rigid bronchoscopy under general anaesthetic is required.

Retropharyngeal abscess (less common)

This is often caused by anaerobic or Gram-negative organisms and may follow bacterial pharyngitis or pharyngeal trauma in the young child. Soft stridor, neck extension, cervical lymphadenopathy and dysphagia are features. Treatment should include expert airway management, surgical drainage and broad-spectrum intravenous antibiotics.

Other causes

Other causes of acute stridor are less common and include bacterial tracheitis, tonsillar obstruction (quinsy, severe infectious mononucleosis), angioneurotic oedema, diphtheria and thermal, chemical or mechanical trauma to the upper airway.

Chronic stridor

Chronic stridor may date from birth or the early neonatal period. Its quality and phase (inspiratory ± expiratory), the nature of the cry and the presence of associated symptoms such as feeding difficulties or dyspnoea may give diagnostic clues. There may be persistent sternal retraction, or a Harrison's sulcus if obstruction is chronic, and failure to thrive may reflect chronically increased respiratory effort.

Congenital laryngeal stridor (laryngomalacia)

There is an elongated epiglottis, a relatively small larynx and redundant epiglottic folds. There may be associated micrognathia. Inspiratory stridor presents within 4 weeks of birth, worsening by 3–6 months. Twenty per cent also have an expiratory stridor. Stridor is worse in the supine position, the cry and cough are normal and the child is usually thriving. A presumptive diagnosis is often made, but floppy aryepiglottic folds are seen on flexible bronchoscopy. Spontaneous improvement by 2–4 years is the rule.

Subglottic stenosis

There may be a congenital thickening of subglottic tissues or true cords, congenital malformation of the cricoid cartilage or acquired stenosis from prolonged endotracheal intubation. There is both inspiratory and expiratory stridor, worsened by intercurrent infection. Stridor usually improves with time as the child grows.

Subglottic haemangioma

From 1 to 3 months of age, there is variable inspiratory and expiratory stridor which worsens with crying. Fifty per cent have cutaneous haemangiomas. Tracheostomy is often required; cautery, sclerosants, steroids and laser therapy may all have a role in treatment.

Vocal cord palsy

This is often associated with severe CNS deformity or major cardiac lesions. Inspiratory stridor, respiratory distress and feeding difficulties are common features.

Other causes

Laryngeal webs, cysts, clefts and papillomas are infrequent causes of stridor. Tracheal compression, e.g. a vascular ring, is also uncommon. A double aortic arch or abnormally placed major artery may cause soft inspiratory stridor with expiratory wheeze. There may be associated dysphagia and regurgitation.

Investigation of chronic stridor

- Chest radiography and lateral neck radiography of soft tissue.
- Barium swallow.
- Angiography.
- CT scan and MRI scan.
- Direct laryngoscopy and bronchoscopy.

Management

The approach to management will depend on the causative lesion, e.g surgical relief of extrinsic compression from a vascular ring, awaiting spontaneous resolution in laryngomalacia. Tracheostomy itself carries risks of scarring, stenosis and obstruction, but may be necessary for temporary or permanent relief of airway obstruction.

Further reading

Couriel JM. Management of croup. *Archives of Disease in Childhood,* 1988; **63:** 1305–8.

Godden C, Campbell M, Hussey M, Cogswell J. Double blind placebo controlled trial of budesonide for croup. *Archives of Disease in Childhood,* 1997; **76:** 155–8.

Inhaled budesonide and adrenaline for croup. *Drug and Therapeutics Bulletin,* 1996; **34:** 23–4.

Kilham HA, McEniery JA. Acute upper airway obstruction. *Current Paediatrics,* 1991; **1** (1): 17–25.
MacFadyen U. Chronic upper airways obstruction. *Current Paediatrics,* 1991; **1** (1): 26–9.

Related topics of interest

Cough and wheeze (p. 100)
Immunization (p. 206)
Upper respiratory tract infection (p. 367)

SUDDEN INFANT DEATH SYNDROME

Sudden infant death syndrome (SIDS) is defined as the sudden death of an infant or young child which is unexpected by history, and in which a thorough post-mortem examination fails to demonstrate an adequate cause of death. SIDS is the most common cause of death in infants between 1 week and 1 year of age. SIDS is a diagnosis of exclusion. Investigation of sudden unexpected death in infancy (SUDI) or 'cot death' may, in a small minority of cases, identify a less common cause of death, such as infection, trauma or a metabolic disorder (e.g. MCAD).

Epidemiology

SIDS became a registerable cause of death in 1971. Throughout the 1980s, a stable incidence of 2 per 1000 live births was reported in England and Wales. In 1991 a national 'Back to Sleep' campaign, advising avoidance of the prone sleeping position, was introduced which coincided with a decline in the reported incidence to 0.6 per 1000 live births. Despite this, SIDS remains the most common cause of death in the post neonatal period.

Aetiology

The cause of death in SIDS is likely to be multifactorial, with an interaction between physiological and environmental factors. Consistently recognizable associations include:

- Male sex.
- Peak age at 2-3 months (between 1– 6 months).
- Low birth weight (IUGR) and pre-term infants.
- Multiple birth.
- Sibling of SIDS victim.
- Poor socioeconomic status.
- Young maternal age.
- Short inter-pregnancy interval.

However the prevalence of these factors changes little from year to year. Certain environmental factors are more variable and have now been highlighted as risk factors for SIDS.

Risk factors

1. Sleeping position. The mechanism is not fully understood; however placing babies prone to sleep increases the risk of SIDS. The side sleeping position also carries an increased risk, therefore it is recommended for all babies to be placed supine for sleep, 'Back to Sleep'.

2. Over-wrapping. Avoidance of over heating is important, many babies who died were found to be overwrapped by clothing. Arrangement of bed clothes also holds a risk, as a significant number of babies were found with covers over their head. Babies are best placed 'Feet to Foot', feet reaching the bottom of the bed, with no excess bed clothes.

3. Parental smoking. Exposure to cigarette smoke both during pregnancy and after birth has been identified as a main contributing factor in SIDS. The risk from smoking in pregnancy increases with the number of cigarettes smoked. The risk is higher if both parents smoke; however the risk remains if only the father or even household visitors smoke.

4. Bed sharing. Several studies reveal an increased risk of SIDS if babies sleep in the same bed as their parents, especially if the mother smokes. Recommendations are bed sharing only for comfort and feeding, not for sleep.

5. Infections. Many SIDS victims have visited a health professional with minor symptoms or signs of illness in the week prior to their death. However despite intensive investigation no clear association between SIDS and the presence of viral or bacterial pathogens has been found.

The suggestion that breast feeding and the use of dummies may be protective is still being formally assessed by CESDI (Confidential Enquiry into Stillbirths and Deaths). Research into the cause of SIDS is ongoing and messages from research must be noted if the incidence is to be reduced further.

Management

Many babies will be brought directly to the accident and emergency department for attempted resuscitation. When resuscitation is unsuccessful the coroner must be informed and an autopsy performed by an experienced pathologist to produce a comprehensive report. A senior paediatrician should lead the resuscitation and should see the parents as soon as possible, explaining the necessary early involvement of the coroner and police and the need for post-mortem. Ample time should be allowed for the parents to cuddle and hold their baby. Continued follow-up appointments should be offered, including the discussion of post-mortem findings. Counselling is particularly important and the Foundation for the Study of Infant Death run local support groups.The care of the next infant scheme (CONI) provides important support for mothers in their next pregnancy and after delivery. If there is a subsequent sibling, parents may seek the reassurance of an apnoea monitor. There is no evidence that they prevent SIDS; however they should be accompanied by practical and written training in cardiopulmonary resuscitation.

Primary prevention

Parent craft groups and early child surveillance programmes should include key messages:

- Back to Sleep.
- Feet to Foot/head uncovered.
- Smoke-free zone.
- Not too hot.
- Prompt medical attention.
- Bed sharing for comfort, not for sleep.

It is important for this advice to reach all those who care for children.

Further reading

Bacon C. Cot Death after CESDI. *Archives of Disease in Childhood*, 1997; **76:** 171–3.

Fleming PJ, Blair PS, Bacon C *et al.* Environment of infants during sleep and risk of the sudden infant death syndrome: results of 1993–5 case-control study for confidential enquiry into stillbirths and deaths in infancy. *British Medical Journal*, 1996; **313:** 191–5.

Related topics of interest

Cardiac arrest (p. 61)
Inborn errors of metabolism (p. 215)

THYROID DISORDERS

Thyroid-stimulating hormone (TSH) controls the synthesis and release of thyroxine (T_4) by the thyroid gland. TSH secretion by the pituitary is under the control of hypothalamic thyrotrophin-releasing hormone (TRH), and is inhibited by somatostatin and dopamine. Triiodothyronine (T_3) is more metabolically active than T_4. Some T_3 is synthesized by the thyroid gland, but most is produced by conversion of T_4 to T_3 in peripheral tissues. T_4 is bound in plasma to thyroid-binding globulin (TBG), and T_3 is bound to TBG and albumin. The metabolically active free (unbound) T_4 and T_3 concentrations can now be measured directly by radioimmunoassay and account for only a small percentage of the total plasma concentrations. T_3 and T_4 modulate many physiological processes including thermogenesis and growth factor production. They also potentiate the actions of catecholamines and have widespread functions in the development of the CNS.

Hypothyroidism

Aetiology

1. *Primary hypothyroidism (T_4 low, TSH high).*

(a) Congenital

- Thyroid gland dysgenesis (agenesis, hypoplasia, or ectopic gland).
- Rare, inherited disorders of hormone synthesis (dyshormonogenesis).

(b) Acquired

- Iodine deficiency.
- Goitrogens.
- Autoimmune thyroiditis.
- Post-irradiation or chemotherapy.

2. *Secondary hypothyroidism (T_4 low, TSH normal or low) – pituitary hypothyroidism.*

- TSH deficiency (congenital or acquired).

3. *Tertiary hypothyroidism (T_4 low, TSH normal or low) – hypothalamic hypothyroidism.*

- TRH deficiency (congenital or acquired)

4. *TBG deficiency*

- Total T_4 low but free T_4 normal – clinically euthyroid.

Clinical features

1. *Congenital hypothyroidism* occurs in 1 in 4000 live births. Neonatal screening was introduced in the UK in 1978. TSH with or without T_4 concentrations are measured on the blood spot cards collected for the Guthrie test (for PKU) in the first week of life. A raised TSH indicates primary hypothyroidism, but secondary and tertiary

hypothyroidism (accounting for less than 10% of cases) will not be detected by this screening method as the TSH is normal or low. Infants are usually asymptomatic at birth, with features such as umbilical hernia, prolonged jaundice, large tongue, feeding difficulties, constipation and lethargy developing over 6–12 weeks if the baby is untreated. Growth failure will become increasingly obvious over the first year. Congenital TRH or TSH deficiency may occur as a component of panhypopituitarism (hypoglycaemia, micropenis, midline cranial defects).

2. *Acquired hypothyroidism* can occur at any age, and the onset of clinical features, such as weight gain, short stature, constipation, dry skin, lethargy and mental slowness, is usually insidious. A goitre may develop, tendon jerks are slow-relaxing and the bone age is delayed. Other presenting features include isolated breast development or large testes, without other signs of puberty, since TRH also stimulates FSH and prolactin secretion. Autoimmune thyroiditis may present with hypothyroidism, thyrotoxicosis or compensated hypothyroidism (raised TSH, normal T_4 – clinically euthyroid). It is more common in girls, may be familial and is associated with other autoimmune conditions. Thyroid disease is more common in Down's, Turner's and Noonan's syndromes.

Investigation

- Total or free T_4 and T_3.
- TSH. May be physiologically elevated in the first 3 days of life.
- Radioisotope thyroid scan (e.g. technetium-99m) can be performed in congenital hypothyroidism before treatment is commenced, but if not readily available is not essential and treatment should not be delayed. Absent or reduced uptake of isotope in the neck (agenesis or hypoplasia of the gland) or ectopic thyroid tissue (e.g. lingual thyroid) may be identified. A normally sited/sized gland may suggest a rare inherited enzyme defect (e.g. Pendred's syndrome – goitre with sensorineural deafness). The perchlorate discharge test is used to identify enzyme defects.
- Radiology. Delayed bone maturation, epiphyseal dysgenesis (e.g. femoral heads). No longer routinely performed in congenital hypothyroidism.
- Thyroid antibodies. e.g. antithyroglobulin, antimicrosomal antibodies. Useful in the investigation of acquired hypothyroidism.

- TRH stimulation test. There is a negligible TSH response to TRH in secondary hypothyroidism ('pituitary' response) and a late, exaggerated rise in TSH in tertiary hypothyroidism ('hypothalamic' response). The basal level of TSH is high in primary hypothyroidism and does not rise much higher with TRH stimulation.

Management

1. Congenital hypothyroidism. If a raised TSH is detected on neonatal screening the diagnosis should be confirmed urgently by taking venous blood for TSH and thyroxine (total or free T_4). Treatment with oral thyroxine should be commenced as soon as possible, usually whilst awaiting the blood test results, and certainly within the first 28 days of life. Crushed tablets are used as no suitable suspension is available. The dose of thyroxine is adjusted to maintain a high normal T_4, a near normal TSH and a satisfactory growth velocity. A persistently raised TSH despite a reasonable dose of thyroxine should prompt enquiry about compliance. Early treatment of congenital hypothyroidism has led to a marked reduction in mental handicap, but mild learning and coordination difficulties may persist, particularly if the degree of pre-treatment hypothyroidism is marked (total $T_4 < 42$ nmol/l). The recurrence risk of congenital hypothyroidism in future pregnancies is low unless it is due to an inborn error of thyroid hormone synthesis – in these disorders there is a 1 in 4 recurrence risk.

2. Acquired hypothyroidism should be treated with oral thyroxine and parents should be warned that the behaviour of older children often deteriorates when they start treatment, as they emerge from hypothyroid docility.

For the majority of cases (congenital and acquired) treatment is life-long. A persistently raised TSH is a risk factor for thyroid carcinoma so should be treated with thyroxine even if the child is euthyroid. Hypothyroidism is a common late effect of cancer treatment and these children are particularly at risk of second tumours. Congenital hypothyroidism is sometimes transient but all babies with a raised TSH need treatment for at least the first year of life. Reassessment of the diagnosis with a trial off treatment should be considered at around 18–24 months. This is not necessary if repeatedly high levels of TSH have been obtained on treatment after the age of 6 months, an ectopic gland has been identified, or there were clinical signs of hypothyroidism with very low T_4 concentrations at birth.

Hyperthyroidism

Hyperthyroidism in childhood is usually autoimmune. It is more common in adolescent girls and may be familial. Presenting features include behavioural problems, poor school performance, accelerated growth and weight loss in spite of an increased appetite. Clinical signs include exophthalmos, tachycardia, tremor and lid-lag. There may be a thyroid bruit or a goitre. Investigations show a high T_4 and T_3, a low or occasionally normal TSH and no response to TRH stimulation. Thyroid autoantibodies are usually positive. Treatment is with carbimazole or propylthiouracil, and propanolol is used acutely to control the β-adrenergic symptoms. Approximately half of childhood cases will remit spontaneously within 2–4 years, and many will become hypothyroid. Partial thyroidectomy or treatment with radio-iodine are options if hyperthyroidism persists. Neonatal thyrotoxicosis is a transient condition resulting from placental transfer of thyroid-stimulating antibodies from a thyrotoxic mother. Symptoms are often severe but can usually be controlled with propanolol. Potassium iodide or carbimazole is used to suppress thyroid activity in severely affected babies. Treatment can be withdrawn slowly after 2–3 months.

Further reading

Brook CGD. The thyroid gland. In: *A Guide to the Practice of Paediatric Endocrinology*. Cambridge University Press, 1993: 83–96.

ESPE Working Group on Congenital Hypothyroidism. Guidelines for neonatal screening programs for congenital hypothyroidism. *Hormone Research,* 1994; **41:** 1–2.

Grant DB. Congenital hypothyroidism: optimal management in the light of 15 years' experience of screening. *Archives of Disease in Childhood,* 1995; **72:** 85–9.

Related topics of interest

Developmental delay (p. 115)
Growth – short stature, tall stature (p. 171)

UPPER RESPIRATORY TRACT INFECTION

Acute infection of the upper respiratory tract affects the average child approximately four times per year. The ears, nose, tonsils, pharynx or sinuses may be affected, or any combination of these. Viruses are most commonly responsible, although serious bacterial infection may also occur. Certain epidemiological factors, such as parental smoking and overcrowding, may increase the rate or severity of infection.

Problems

- Fever, febrile convulsions.
- Malaise.
- Poor feeding.
- Poor sleeping.
- Upper airway obstruction.

Common cold (coryza, nasopharyngitis)

Rhinovirus, adenovirus, respiratory syncytial virus, influenza and parainfluenza are commonly responsible. Sneezing, sore throat, nasal obstruction and discharge occurs after a 2- to 3-day incubation period and may persist for up to 2 weeks. Nasal obstruction may cause feeding difficulties in the younger infant; saline nose drops may help clear mucus. Complications include direct viral invasion of the middle ear, sinuses or lower respiratory tract and secondary bacterial infection. Symptomatic treatment should be given with attention to fluid balance and paracetamol if necessary. There is little evidence to suggest that decongestants or antihistamines are of benefit.

Pharyngitis and tonsillitis

Adenovirus, parainfluenza and influenza virus, Epstein–Barr virus, coxsackie- and echoviruses are responsible in the majority of cases. Group A β-haemolytic streptococcus and other bacteria are causative in a significant number of cases. Sore throat, fever and malaise is accompanied by a red throat or tonsils, with exudate and cervical lymphadenopathy. Clinically it is difficult to distinguish between viral and streptococcal aetiology, and since the streptococcus may lead to sequelae of rheumatic fever or acute glomerulonephritis the decision to withold treatment may be difficult. Treatment with oral penicillin for 10–14 days should eradicate streptococcus. Confirmation of a bacterial cause may be obtained by a throat swab if practical circumstances permit. Patients with a past history of rheumatic fever or nephritis should always be treated with antibiotics.

Acute otitis media

The aetiology is viral in many cases, e.g. respiratory syncytial virus, adenovirus, influenza, but a number of bacterial pathogens may also be responsible, including *Streptococcus pneumoniae, Haemophilus influenzae*, group A β-haemolytic streptococcus. Severe otalgia is accompanied by fever, irritability and a bulging tympanic membrane with loss of its light reflex. Purulent discharge may appear if the drum ruptures. Complications include chronic suppurative infection and secretory otitis media with effusion. Meningitis, mastoiditis and cerebral abcess may rarely complicate an acute bacterial episode. Treatment with antibiotics (penicillin, amoxycillin, erythromycin or trimethoprim) is appropriate, since clinical distinction between viral and bacterial otitis media is difficult. Paracetamol may be given for fever and pain.

Sinusitis

Infection of paranasal sinuses may arise from spread of a viral infection during an acute coryzal infection, or by secondary bacterial infection. Facial pain, fever, headache and a purulent nasal discharge may be seen, with localized tenderness over the affected sinus. Complications include periorbital cellulitis, cavernous sinus thrombosis and cerebral abscess. Antibiotics should be given if bacterial infection is suspected, with symptomatic treatment of pain and fever. Surgical drainage is rarely required. If sinusitis is chronic, conditions such as allergy, cystic fibrosis, ciliary dyskinesia and immunodeficiency should be considered.

Acute laryngotracheo-bronchitis, acute epiglottitis

See related topic Stridor (p. 356).

Adenotonsillectomy

This surgery is widely performed, although there has been little objective evidence in the past to show a definite beneficial effect for many children, and controversy continues. For children with recurrent tonsillitis in particular, it is important to apply careful selection criteria, which include an assessment of the frequency of documented tonsillitis episodes and the amount of education missed. However, indications for adenotonsillectomy may be considered as:

- Obstructive sleep apnoea. Tonsillar and adenoidal hypertrophy may contribute to chronic upper airway obstruction, with the development of right ventricular hypertrophy and, eventually, cor pulmonale.

- Peritonsillar abscess. Tonsillectomy is usually advised because of the risks of rupture with aspiration, upper airway obstruction, or involvement of the retropharyngeal tissues.
- Recurrent tonsillitis. If significant numbers of school days are missed during two successive years because of well-documented episodes of tonsillitis, tonsillectomy may be of benefit. Adeno-tonsillectomy may also be recommended for recurrent otitis media which is associated with tonsillitis.

Further reading

Del Mar CB, Glasziou PP, Hayem M. Are antibiotics indicated as initial treatment for children with acute otitis media? A meta-analysis. *British Medical Journal,* 1997; **314:** 1526–9.

Maw AR. Developments in ear, nose and throat surgery. In: David TJ, ed. *Recent Advances in Paediatrics,* Vol. 9. Edinburgh: Churchill Livingstone, 1991: 93–108.

Related topics of interest

Cough and wheeze (p. 100)
Stridor (p. 356)

URINARY TRACT INFECTION

Urinary tract infection (UTI) is common in infants and children. Infection in the presence of vesicoureteric reflux of urine is associated with renal cortical scarring (reflux nephropathy), particularly in the first year of life. This can have significant long-term implications, underlying up to 20% of cases of chronic renal failure in children and being a significant cause of end-stage renal failure in young adults. It is important that a UTI is proven on urine culture and not just treated on the basis of symptoms, as the diagnosis should initiate thorough radiological investigation of the renal tract.

Problems

- Enuresis.
- Failure to thrive.
- Septicaemia.
- Reflux nephrophathy (renal scarring also called chronic pyelonephritis).
  Hypertension.The long-term risk is approximately 10–20% in those with renal scarring. There is also an increased incidence of pre-eclamptic toxaemia in pregnancy.
  Chronic and end-stage renal failure (ESRF).

Aetiology

Most cases are caused by normal bowel commensal organisms which ascend the urethra (> 90% of first infections are due to *E. coli*). In the neonatal period, infection may be haematogenously acquired and bacteraemia is present in > 60%.

Predisposing factors include incomplete emptying of the bladder (neuropathic bladder, mechanical outflow obstruction, e.g. ureterocele), constipation and poor fluid intake.

Clinical features

In the neonatal period UTI is more common in males (2M:1F). Presenting features include irritability, refusal to feed, vomiting, failure to thrive and exacerbation of jaundice. If bacteraemic, the baby will be toxic and extremely unwell. In older children UTIs are more common in girls (prevalence 1–2% of schoolgirls, 0.2% of boys). The pre-school child may present with non-specific diarrhoea and vomiting, poor weight gain, fever or malaise. More specific symptoms include frequency, dysuria, enuresis, fever with or without haematuria, loin pain.

Frequency and dysuria may also be caused by irritation from nylon underwear, bubble baths or perineal *Candida* in the absence of a UTI.

Examination should include blood pressure, palpation of the kidneys, lower limb reflexes and examination of the lumbosacral spine.

Investigation

- Urine microscopy, culture and sensitivity. Reliability depends on the care of collection. Collection methods:
  older child, mid-stream urine (MSU) sample;
  in a young child/infant, bag urine, clean catch, urine collection pads or suprapubic aspirate (SPA).

  Pyuria suggests infection but is not diagnostic. Organisms may be seen on microscopy. Significant bacteriuria is defined as a pure growth of more than 10^5 organisms per ml of clean, freshly passed urine, or any growth from an SPA. Two urine specimens should be collected unless an SPA is performed.
- Blood cultures.
- FBC.
- U&E, creatinine.

Management

If a UTI is suspected appropriate antibacterial therapy should be commenced once the urine specimens have been collected. Antibiotics should be given intravenously if the child is vomiting or is toxic and unwell. High fluid intake should be encouraged. After a short course of antibiotics the urine should be re-examined to ensure that the infection has cleared. Low-dose prophylactic antibiotics should be continued at least until further investigation of the urinary tract has been completed

Further investigation

It is essential that all young children with a proven UTI are investigated radiologically to detect obstructive uropathy, scars and vesico-ureteric reflux (VUR) so that prophylaxis against further infections can be given in an attempt to prevent reflux nephropathy. VUR is found in 30–40% of children presenting with a UTI, and the prevalence of VUR is as high as 1 in 250 children with a high familial incidence. More than 80% will resolve spontaneously with age, but there is a high incidence of cortical scarring associated with VUR, particularly in children < 1 year, suggesting that susceptibility to scarring is greatest in infants. Renal scarring is found in approximately 10% of children investigated following a UTI. There is no consensus as to what investigations should be performed, but one suggested approach following a first proven UTI is:

1. Infants under 1 year. Ultrasound (US) to assess renal size and detect hydronephrosis, dimercaptosuccinic acid (DMSA) isotope scan to detect renal scars and measure differential function, and micturating cystourethrogram (MCUG) to detect VUR or urethral valves. DMSA should not be performed within 4 weeks of a UTI as it may detect transient areas of abnormality which do not develop into scars on long-term follow-up. A MAG III renal isotope scan may be indicated if there is hydronephrosis or ureteric dilatation to exclude obstruction (pelvi-ureteric junction (PUJ) or vesico-ureteric junction (VUJ) obstruction).

2. *Age 1–5 years.* US and DMSA scans. If scars are detected, or if there are recurrent UTIs proceed to an MCUG (this investigation involves catheterization and is unpleasant for an older child).

3. *Age more than 5 years.* US only. Other investigations are indicated only if US is abnormal.

Prevention of reflux nephropathy

Simple measures which may help prevent UTIs include a good fluid intake, regular voiding of the bladder and correction of constipation.

If VUR is detected, prophylactic low-dose antibiotics should be given to prevent further UTIs, as evidence suggests that reflux of sterile urine does not cause scarring. New scars probably do not develop after the age of 5 years, but some centres continue prophylactic antibiotics to the age of 10 years. Compliance becomes a problem the longer antibiotics are continued. Prophylactic antibiotics may have a place in the treatment of older children with recurrent symptomatic UTIs. A small number of children with severe reflux, recurrent UTIs despite prophylactic antibiotics and evidence of new scars developing, proceed to surgery such as reimplantation of the ureters or silicone injection of the VU junctions.

Antenatally diagnosed renal tract abnormalities

With the introduction of routine US scanning, the antenatal detection of renal tract abnormalities has increased. The commonest abnormality detected is hydronephrosis but dysplastic or cystic kidneys may also be found. Hydronephrosis may be due to obstruction or marked VUR, and if still persistent on postnatal US may be investigated with renal isotope scans and MCUG. Even if hydronephrosis is due to a degree of PUJ obstruction, it may resolve spontaneously, and only a small number will require surgery (pyeloplasty) for worsening function, symptoms or increasing dilatation. The outcome of infants with mild to moderate hydronephrosis is still unclear and requires ongoing audit. It is important to detect the small number of infants who have correctable abnormalities, but we must be careful not to provoke unnecessary parental anxiety in those with minor abnormalities which will have no long-term significance.

Further reading

Guidelines for the management of acute urinary tract infection in childhood. Report of a working party. *Journal of the Royal College of Physicians of London,* 1991; **25** (1): 36–42.

Merrick MV, Notghi A, Chalmers N, Wilkinson AG, Uttley WS. Long term follow up to determine the prognostic value of imaging after urinary tract infections. *Archives of Disease in Childhood,* 1995; **72:** 388–96.

Smellie JM, Rigden SPA, Prescod NP. Urinary tract infection. Comparison of four methods of investigation. *Archives of Disease in Childhood,* 1995; **72:** 247–50.

Related topics of interest

Chronic renal failure (p. 82)
Haematuria (p. 176)

VISION

Normal vision depends on precise motor and sensory optic functions in addition to numerous central interactions which interpret the information received. Abnormalities of vision in childhood may be minor, e.g. mild refractive errors, or major, resulting in severe visual impairment and disability.

Refractive errors

These are the most common visual problem in childhood. Images are not formed precisely on the retina. If the eye is otherwise healthy, errors may be corrected by wearing lenses. Hypermetropia is uncommon. Myopia frequently presents during school years and there is a familial tendency. Astigmatism produces a distorted image because the corneal curvature is non-uniform, but may be corrected by appropriate lenses.

Squints

Squints (strabismus) affect 5% of children. A squint is an abnormal alignment of the eyes which prevents the occurrence of single binocular vision. Pseudosquints may occur if the child has wide epicanthic folds. Squints are usually concomitant in children, i.e. the angle of squint is the same in all directions of gaze. If the squint is incomitant (paralytic), eye movement is impaired due to a defective extraocular muscle and the angle of squint alters with different positions of gaze, or with changes of fixation. Manifest squints are readily apparent at examination and are demonstrated by the cover test. Latent squints are detected at times of tiredness or stress, or by specific clinical examination (alternate cover test). Early detection of squints is important for the diagnosis of treatable causes, e.g. cataracts, and to prevent the development of amblyopia. Squint is more common in children with Down's syndrome, prematurity, cerebral palsy, and other neurological disorders. There is often a family history of strabismus.

Amblyopia

Amblyopia results when the brain has suppressed or failed to develop the ability to perceive a detailed image from one eye and is usually defined as a reduction of at least two lines on the Snellen chart. Loss of acuity may be severe, and prevention by successful detection and treatment of squints is of great importance.

Defects of colour vision

These occur in 8% of boys and 0.5% of girls, and chiefly affect red–green perception. Many types are X-linked recessive. Detection can be important for careers guidance (certain occupations barred) and may be relevant if classroom methods are colour coded.

Serious impairment of vision

Severe visual handicap has an estimated prevalence of 1 in 2500 children. Those registered blind have a visual acuity of 3/60 or less in their better eye. Those registered partially sighted have acuity of 6/24 or 4/60 in their better eye. The aetiology of such serious defects includes cataracts, optic atrophy, retinal disease (retinoblastoma, retinopathy of prematurity, chorioretinitis), congenital eye defects and severe refractive errors. Corneal ulceration is the commonest cause of blindness world-wide. Neoplasia of the optic nerve or tract may cause blindness.

History

A full history should include family history of visual problems, pregnancy and birth history. Predisposing conditions include Down's syndrome, congenital rubella, prematurity and hydrocephalus. Significant post-natal events such as head injury or meningitis must also be noted. Parental concerns about the child's visual performance may be expressed, and the symptoms of nystagmus with roving eye movements, light gazing, photophobia or eye pressing may be reported. Language and motor development may be delayed. Parental concerns are important at any age.

Testing of vision

Early detection of a visual defect is important in order to allow treatment, and optimal development. Squints should be excluded by shining a light source (looking for asymmetrical reflection if there is a squint) and use of the cover and uncover test.

Screening at 6 weeks of age should include testing of pupil reactions, fixing and following, examination of the red reflex with an ophthalmoscope.

Screening for non-disabling visual defects in children under 2 years of age should be confined to history and observation. Children at any age with a suspected visual defect, strong family history or a neurological disorder should have formal visual assessment.

A visual acuity test should be carried out at school entry, covering each eye in turn. Picture tests (Kay, Elliott), single letters (the Stycar test or the Sheridan–Gardner cards) or a Snellen chart may be used.

Tests of colour vision are the Ishihara and Sheridan–Gardiner screening tests, and also the City University test.

Videorefraction is a newer technique. Electroretinography and visually evoked potentials may be useful in the neonate or severely handicapped child.

Management

Refractive errors may be corrected by appropriate lenses. Squints may be treated by exercises, occlusion ('patching'), spectacles or surgery, aiming to restore binocular vision before amblyopia occurs. Other remediable conditions must be treated early, e.g. retinopathy of prematurity by cryotherapy, surgical removal of cataracts. For the severely visually impaired child, management depends on early intervention programmes to maximize the use of the child's other special senses. Special educational provision must be made for their learning needs, and skills in learning Braille may be taught. Genetic counselling is important in some cases of blindness.

Further reading

Hall DMB, ed. *Health for all Children. A Programme for Child Health Surveillance*, 3rd edn. Oxford: Oxford University Press, 1996.

Lawson J, Timms C. Understanding squints: diagnosis and management. *Current Paediatrics,* 1997; **7:** 23–7.

Sonksen PM. Developmental aspects of visual disorders. *Current Paediatrics,* 1997; **7:** 18–22.

Related topics of interest

Developmental assessment (p. 111)
Developmental delay (p. 115)
Fetal medicine (p. 141)
Hearing and speech (p. 185)

VOMITING

Vomiting is a very common symptom in childhood. The causes are numerous but a good history and examination will often give an indication as to the underlying problem. The differential diagnosis will depend on the age of the child and the presence or absence of associated symptoms (e.g. fever, diarrhoea, headache). Posseting is the regurgitation of small amounts of milk in an otherwise well and thriving infant. Effortless regurgitation of larger volumes of milk may occur with gastro-oesophageal reflux. Bile-stained vomiting suggests an obstruction distal to the duodenum, although an older child who has vomited several times may then vomit bile in the absence of an intestinal obstruction. In an older child, vomiting first thing in the morning, particularly if associated with headache, is very worrying and raises the possibility of raised intracranial pressure.

Causes

1. *Neonatal*

- Intestinal obstruction, e.g. atresias, malrotation, meconium ileus, strangulated hernia.
- Infection, e.g. meningitis, UTI.
- Necrotizing enterocolitis.
- Respiratory distress, e.g. surfactant deficiency, meconium aspiration.
- Metabolic/endocrine disorder, e.g. inborn errors of metabolism, congenital adrenal hyperplasia.
- Raised intracranial pressure, e.g. hydrocephalus.

2. *Infancy*

- Any infection – gastroenteritis, UTI, upper respiratory tract infections, meningitis, pneumonia.
- Gastro-oesophageal reflux.
- Pyloric stenosis.
- Intussusception (see related topic Abdominal pain – acute, p. 1).
- Other causes of intestinal obstruction, e.g. malrotation/volvulus, strangulated hernia.
- Respiratory distress (e.g. bronchiolitis, whooping cough).
- Food allergy/intolerance, e.g. cow's milk, eggs.
- Cerebral, e.g. minor head injury, subdural haematoma (accidental/non-accidental), hydrocephalus.
- Metabolic, e.g. inborn errors of metabolism, Reye's syndrome, hypercalcaemia.

3. *Older child*

- Any infection.
- Minor head injury.
- Respiratory disorders, e.g. acute exacerbation of asthma, whooping cough.

- Metabolic/endocrine disorders – diabetic ketoacidosis, Reye's syndrome, uraemia, hypoadrenalism.
- Raised intracranial pressure, e.g. tumour, subdural haematoma.
- Intestinal obstruction, e.g. due to adhesions from previous surgery, strangulated hernia.
- Drugs and toxins, e.g. alcohol, cytotoxics, theophylline, antibiotics (particularly erythromycin).
- Eating disorder – bulimia.
- Cyclical vomiting, motion sickness, excitement or anxiety.

History

The differential diagnosis will depend on the age of the child (see above). The onset, nature (e.g. projectile, effortless), and frequency of vomiting should be established. Enquiry should be made about the presence of bile or blood in the vomit and any associated symptoms (e.g. fever, headache, diarrhoea).

Examination

- Plot height and weight, (and head circumference in infancy) on a centile chart.
- Assess the state of hydration.
- Look particularly for signs of infection, abdominal pathology (e.g. distension, tenderness, or masses), and raised intracranial pressure.

Subsequent investigations and management depend on the likely cause. If the history and examination are unhelpful in establishing this, a period of in-patient observation may be of value.

Gastro-oesophageal reflux (GOR)

Clinical features

GOR is very common in infancy and, although messy and inconvenient for the parents, it is not a major cause for concern as long as the infant continues to gain weight. The condition usually improves with age and resolves with the child assuming a more upright posture. Regurgitation and vomiting of large amounts of feed can occasionally result in failure to thrive and reflux may also be associated with symptoms of oesophagitis (irritability, dysphagia, haematemesis, iron deficiency anaemia and rarely melaena, neurobehavioural symptoms). When vomiting is persistent or associated with failure to thrive or oesophagitis, 24-hour oesophageal pH monitoring is the method of choice for confirming and quantifying reflux. Barium studies may miss the dynamic process of GOR, but are of value in detecting anatomical lesions, e.g. malrotation, hiatus hernia. Reflux is more common in children with neurodevelopmental problems such as cerebral palsy, and may lead to respiratory problems due to recurrent aspiration. 'Silent' reflux is reflux that occurs in the absence of vomiting and this may be responsible for recurrent respiratory symptoms and apparent life-threatening events in otherwise healthy infants.

Management

Simple measures such as stopping regularly during feeds for winding and keeping the baby upright after feeds may decrease the vomiting. Although GOR is reduced when the infant is put to sleep in the prone position, this can no longer be recommended because of the increased risk of sudden infant death syndrome. The left lateral position is therefore preferred. With more significant reflux, thickening of the feeds (e.g. with Carobel) or the addition of gaviscon may be sufficient. H_2-receptor antagonists (e.g. ranitidine), prokinetic agents (e.g. cisapride), and omeprazole may be considered if there is no improvement (see Further reading). Surgery (e.g. Nissen fundoplication) is occasionally indicated for severe reflux not responding to medical treatment particularly in children with cerebral palsy.

Hypertrophic pyloric stenosis

Presentation with projectile vomiting between the ages of 3 and 8 weeks is typical. Hypertrophy of the smooth circular muscle of the pylorus results in obstruction to the passage of feeds. Vomiting may be infrequent initially but gradually increases as the obstruction progresses. Boys are more commonly affected than girls and there is often a family history of the condition. Associated features include prolonged jaundice, constipation and failure to thrive. On examination the infant will feed hungrily and often has a 'worried' expression. There may be signs of dehydration. The diagnosis is confirmed on a test feed by the presence of visible waves of peristalsis moving from left to right across the abdomen and a palpable pyloric mass in the right hypochondrium (sometimes called a 'tumour' but this can cause a great deal of unnecessary parental anxiety). Ultrasound or barium contrast studies are sometimes indicated if the diagnosis is uncertain clinically. Hypochloraemic hypokalaemic alkalosis with hyponatraemia is typical. Correction of electrolyte disturbances and dehydration with i.v. fluids should always precede surgery (Ramstedt's pyloromyotomy).

Further reading

Booth IW. Silent reflux: how much do we miss? *Archives of Disease in Childhood,* 1992; **67:** 1325–7.

Davies AEM, Sandhu BK. Diagnosis and treatment of gastro-oesophageal reflux. *Archives of Disease in Childhood,* 1995; **73:** 82–6 .

Sullivan PB, Brueton MJ. Vomiting in infants and children. *Current Paediatrics*, 1991; **1** (1): 13–6.

Related topics of interest

Abdominal pain – acute (p. 1)
Gastroenteritis (p. 152)

INDEX